PREFIXES • ABBREVIATIONS • PRONUNCIA

ROOTS • COMBINING FORMS • SUFFIXES •

Medical Terminology
A SYSTEMS APPROACH

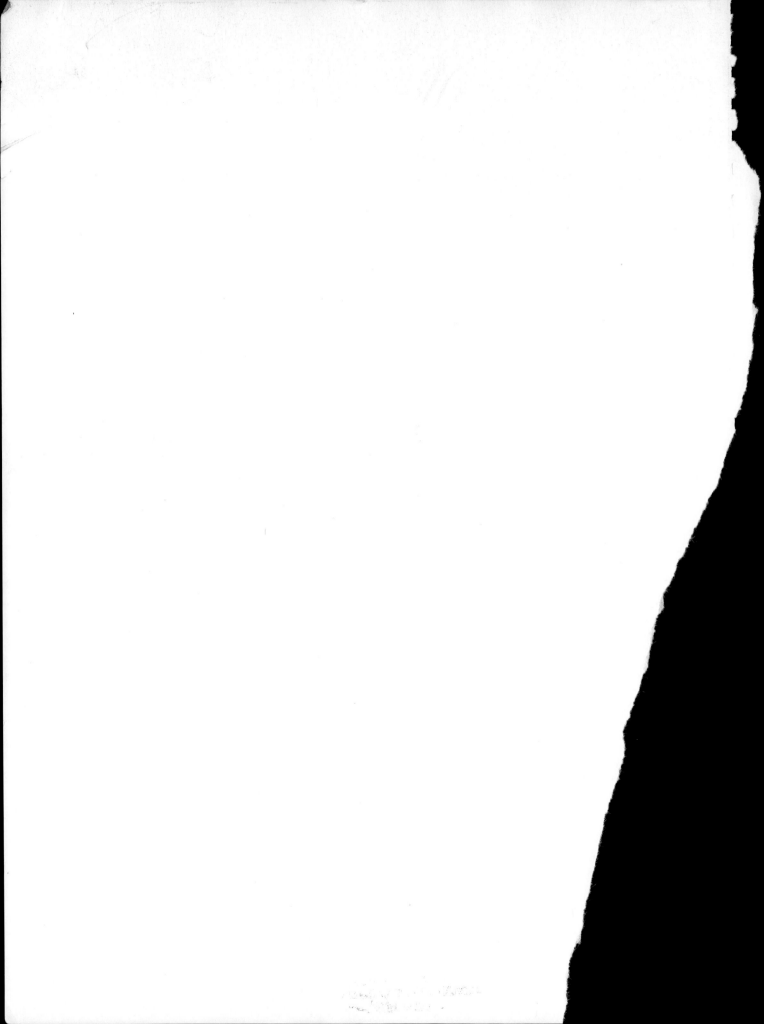

FOURTH EDITION

PREFIXES • ABBREVIATIONS • PRONUNC

ROOTS • COMBINING FORMS • SUFFIXES •

Barbara A. Gylys, MEd, CMA-A

Professor Emerita of Health and Human Services

Medical Assisting Technology

University of Toledo Community and Technical College

Toledo, Ohio

Mary Ellen Wedding, MEd, MT(ASCP), CMA

Professor of Health and Human Services

Director of Medical Assisting Technology

University of Toledo Community and Technical College

Toledo, Ohio

Medical Terminology

A SYSTEMS APPROACH

 F. A. DAVIS COMPANY • Philadelphia

F. A. Davis Company
1915 Arch Street
Philadelphia, PA 19103

Printed in the United States of America

Last digit indicates print number: 10 9 8 7 6 5 4 3 2

Publisher, Health Professions: Jean-François Vilain
Developmental Editor: Marianne Fithian
Production Editor: Stephen D. Johnson
Cover Designer: Louis J. Forgione

As new scientific information becomes available through basic and clinical research, recommended treatments and drug therapies undergo changes. The authors and publisher have done everything possible to make this book accurate, up to date, and in accord with accepted standards at the time of publication. The authors, editors, and publisher are not responsible for errors or omissions or for consequences from application of the book, and make no warranty, expressed or implied, in regard to the contents of the book. Any practice described in this book should be applied by the reader in accordance with professional standards of care used in regard to the unique circumstances that may apply in each situation. The reader is advised always to check product information (package inserts) for changes and new information regarding dose and contraindications before administering any drug. Caution is especially urged when using new or infrequently ordered drugs.

Library of Congress Cataloging-in-Publication Data

Gylys, Barbara A.
    Medical terminology : a systems approach / Barbara A. Gylys,
Mary Ellen Wedding.—4th ed.
    p. cm.
Includes bibliographical references and index.
ISBN 0-8036-0394-0 (alk. paper)
1. Medicine—Terminology.   I. Wedding, Mary Ellen.   II. Title.
R123 -G94   1999
616′ .01′4—dc21

                                                                    98-48638
                                                                        CIP

This book is dedicated with love

■ ■ ■ ■ ■

to my best friend, colleague,
and husband, Julius A. Gylys
and
to my children,
Regina Maria and Julius A., II
and
to Andrew Masters,
Julia Masters,
and Caitlin Masters

B.A.G.

to my little ones,
Andrew Arthur Kurtz,
Katherine Louise Kurtz,
and Daniel Keith Wedding, II

M.E.W.

ACKNOWLEDGMENTS

The authors express special and sincere appreciation for the effort of the following individuals who, through their professionalism and skill, improved the fourth edition of the textbook. The reviewers included:

Joseph R. Bittengle, MEd, RT(R)(ARRT)
Chairman and Assistant Professor
Department of Radiologic Technology
University of Arkansas for Medical Sciences
Little Rock, Arkansas

Sue A. Hunt, MA, RN, CMA
Professor of Medical Assisting
Department of Medical Assisting
Middlesex Community College
Lowell, Massachusetts

Beverly M. Kovanda, PhD, MS, MT(ASCP)
Professor/Coordinator
Multicompetency Health Technology Department
Columbus State Community College
Westerville, Ohio

Anthony Kremnetz, RT(R)
Department of Radiology
Medical College of Ohio
Toledo, Ohio

Carol Masker, BS
Medical Terminology Instructor
Adult Education
Morris County School of Technology
Denville, New Jersey

We also thank the editors and production staff of F. A. Davis Company, especially:

- Jean-François Vilain, Publisher, Health Professions, for his efforts, encouragement, and contributions to this project.

- Marianne Fithian, Developmental Editor, who edited the manuscript and assisted with the review process for the book.
- Stephen D. Johnson, Production Editor, for his thoroughness and diligence in successfully completing the project.
- Samuel A. Rondinelli, Production Manager, for his meticulous review and overseeing the production process.
- Jack Brandt, Illustration Specialist, for his expertise with the art program.
- Robert Butler, Director of Production, whose expertise made the production of this book possible.

Finally, we would like to express our appreciation and acknowledge the following individuals for their contributions with the *Instructor's Guide*.

- Patricia Goshorn, MA, RN, CMA-C, Consumnes River College, Sacramento, California, for developing the medical records.
- Ralph Zickgraf, Managing Editor, Electronic Publishing, for developing the crossword puzzles.
- Michelle Bishop, for providing computer skills in our transition from the third to the fourth edition.
- Barbara Blank, instructor at Toledo University Community and Technical College, for retyping the medical records.

PREFACE

The fourth edition of *Medical Terminology: A Systems Approach* lives up to its well-established track record to provide medical word building principles that are based on the criteria of a competency-based curriculum. The book is designed as a classroom teaching text with the underlying pedagogy of a textbook-workbook format. Its design employs traditional lecture and recitation methods. However, various self-instructional features allow students to develop an extensive medical vocabulary independently and at their own pace.

The principal objectives of the textbook are twofold. First, it provides the basic techniques of medical word building. Once learned, these techniques can readily be applied to acquire an extensive medical vocabulary. Secondly, it presents material at a level that is easily understood by the average student. Thus, no previous knowledge of anatomy, physiology, or pathology is necessary.

Full color has been incorporated as a pedagogic tool in both the text and figures. This feature enables the student to more clearly identify anatomical structures and pathological disorders. It also provides easier recognition of graphics and table content. Many topics in each chapter have been updated and strengthened to be consistent with current technological changes in medicine. To develop a complete state-of-the-art teaching and learning package, suggestions from educators and medical practitioners have been addressed and incorporated. Nevertheless, the popular basic features have been enhanced but do remain the same as in previous editions. Some of the highlights of the fourth edition are enumerated here.

- **Chapter 1** explains the techniques of medical word building using basic word elements.
- **Chapter 2** categorizes major suffixes in the following groups: surgical, diagnostic, symptomatic, and related suffixes. Pronunciations and definitions of suffixes are included as they are presented.
- **Chapter 3** contains suffixes denoting adjective, noun, singular, and plural forms of medical words.
- **Chapter 4** includes major prefixes in the following groups: position, number and measurement, negation, direction, and other prefixes.
- **Chapter 5** introduces anatomical, physiological, and pathological terms. Combining forms denoting anatomical directions, regions of the body, anatomical structures, colors, and other combining forms related to body structure are presented.
- **Chapters 6 to 16** are organized according to body systems and may be taught in any sequence. These chapters include anatomy and physiology; combining forms, suffixes, and prefixes; pathology; diagnostic, symptomatic, and therapeutic terms; diagnostic procedures; surgical and therapeutic procedures; pharmacology terms; abbreviations; a medical record; and worksheets that include medical record analyses. The worksheets provide a means of self-assessment and evaluation of competency for each chapter.

- **Appendix A: Answer Key** contains worksheet answers to validate medical terminology competency and provides immediate feedback for student assessment.
- **Appendix B: Abbreviations** include a comprehensive list of medical abbreviations and their meanings.
- **Appendix C: Index of Medical Word Elements** contains alphabetical lists of medical word elements with corresponding pronunciations and meanings. This appendix employs two methods for word-element indexing—first by medical word element, then by English term.
- **Appendix D: Index of Genetic Disorders** lists the genetic disorders covered in the textbook.
- **Appendix E: Index of Diagnostic Imaging Procedures** lists the radiographic and other diagnostic imaging procedures covered in the textbook.
- **Appendix F: Index of Pharmacology** lists the medications covered in the textbook.
- **Appendix G: Index of Oncological Terms** lists the terms related to oncology covered in the textbook.

TEACHING AIDS

The following teaching aids are available for instructors who adopt the fourth edition of *Medical Terminology: A Systems Approach*.

Audiocassette Tapes are included with the text (at the instructor's option*) or available through the instructor. Use them to strengthen and reinforce spelling and pronunciation of medical words.

Instructor's Guide is a comprehensive text detailing teaching methods for terminology instructors. It includes a test bank of over 800 questions in a variety of formats; medical records with an analysis of each record; and a list of journals, films, and community resources to help instructors develop various teaching activities. Crossword puzzles provide a review of the elements and medical words in the chapters, as well as a challenge and fun for the student.

Interactive CD-ROM is available (at the instructor's option*) with the text. The **Interactive Medical Terminology** software is a competency-based, self-paced multimedia program. It includes graphics, audio, a pull-down dictionary based on *Taber's Cyclopedic Medical Dictionary, edition 18*, and help menus along with numerous interactive learning activities designed at a 90 percent competency level. This program provides immediate feedback regarding student competency. A printout of student's progress is also available.

CyberTest testbank is designed to help instructors create chapter, midterm, and final tests in a short period of time. Users can specify question format and choose (or randomly select) from over 800 questions. It runs in Windows 3.X, Windows 95, Windows 98, and Windows NT and is available for Mac on request.

Taber's Cyclopedic Medical Dictionary, edition 18 is the recommended companion reference because it includes etymologies for nearly all of the main entries presented in the textbook.

B.A.G.
M.E.W.

---

*The instructor may choose to adopt 1) the book with CD-ROM package, 2) the book shrink-wrapped with two audiocassette tapes, 3) the book with CD-ROM and two audiocassettes, or 4) the book by itself. Instructors who adopt the book alone may make copies, for their students, of the two audiocassette masters included in the complimentary instructor's package.

CONTENTS

Chapter 1
BASIC ELEMENTS OF A MEDICAL WORD 1
CHAPTER OUTLINE   1
STUDENT OBJECTIVES   1
WORD ROOTS   2
COMBINING FORMS   2
SUFFIXES   2
PREFIXES   3
BASIC RULES FOR BUILDING AND DEFINING MEDICAL WORDS   3
Building Medical Words   3
Defining Medical Words   4
PRONUNCIATION GUIDELINES   5
WORKSHEETS   7

Chapter 2
SUFFIXES: SURGICAL, DIAGNOSTIC, SYMPTOMATIC, AND RELATED 11
CHAPTER OUTLINE   11
STUDENT OBJECTIVES   11
SUFFIXES   12
SURGICAL SUFFIXES   13
Suffixes Denoting Incisions   13
Suffixes Denoting Reconstructive Surgeries   14
Suffixes Denoting Refracturing, Loosening, or Crushing   14
DIAGNOSTIC, SYMPTOMATIC, AND RELATED SUFFIXES   14
WORKSHEETS   17

Chapter 3
SUFFIXES: ADJECTIVE, NOUN, DIMINUTIVE, SINGULAR, PLURAL 25
CHAPTER OUTLINE   25
STUDENT OBJECTIVES   25
ADJECTIVE SUFFIXES   26
NOUN SUFFIXES   26
DIMINUTIVE SUFFIXES   27
PLURAL SUFFIXES   27
WORKSHEETS   28

Chapter 4
PREFIXES 31
CHAPTER OUTLINE   31
STUDENT OBJECTIVES   31

xi

PREFIXES   32
  Prefixes of Position   32
  Prefixes of Number and Measurement   33
  Prefixes of Negation   34
  Prefixes of Direction   34
  Other Prefixes   35
WORKSHEETS   36

Chapter 5
BODY STRUCTURE 41

CHAPTER OUTLINE   41
STUDENT OBJECTIVES   41
LEVELS OF ORGANIZATION   42
  Cells   42
  Tissues   42
  Organs   42
  Systems   43
  Organism   43
THE DISEASE PROCESS   43
ANATOMICAL POSITION   43
PLANES OF THE BODY   44
BODY CAVITIES   45
ABDOMINOPELVIC REGION   46
DIAGNOSTIC IMAGING   47
THE SPINE   48
DIRECTIONAL TERMS   48
COMBINING FORMS   49
  Combining Forms Denoting Cellular Structure   49
  Combining Forms Denoting Anatomical Directions   49
  Combining Forms Denoting Regions of the Body   50
  Combining Forms Denoting Colors   50
  Other Combining Forms Related to Body Structure   51
SUFFIXES   52
PREFIXES   52
DIAGNOSTIC, SYMPTOMATIC, AND THERAPEUTIC TERMS   53
DIAGNOSTIC PROCEDURES   53
SURGICAL AND THERAPEUTIC PROCEDURES   54
ABBREVIATIONS   54
MEDICAL RECORD   55
  Radiology Report of Cervical and Lumbar Spine   55
WORKSHEETS   56

Chapter 6
INTEGUMENTARY SYSTEM 63

CHAPTER OUTLINE   63
STUDENT OBJECTIVES   63
ANATOMY AND PHYSIOLOGY   64
  Skin   64
  Appendages of the Skin   65
    Hair   65
    Glands   65
    Nails   65
    Breasts   65
COMBINING FORMS   66
SUFFIXES   68
PREFIXES   68
PATHOLOGY   68
  Primary Skin Lesions   68
  Secondary Skin Lesions   68
  Burns   70
  Frostbite   71
  Oncology   71
    Basal Cell Carcinoma   71
    Breast Cancer   72

Squamous Cell Carcinoma   72
Malignant Melanoma   72
DIAGNOSTIC, SYMPTOMATIC, AND THERAPEUTIC TERMS   72
DIAGNOSTIC PROCEDURES   75
Imaging Procedures   75
SURGICAL AND THERAPEUTIC PROCEDURES   75
PHARMACOLOGY   76
ABBREVIATIONS   76
MEDICAL RECORD   77
Pathology Report of Skin Lesion   77
WORKSHEETS   78

Chapter 7
GASTROINTESTINAL SYSTEM... 85
CHAPTER OUTLINE   85
STUDENT OBJECTIVES   85
ANATOMY AND PHYSIOLOGY   86
Mouth (Oral or Buccal Cavity)   86
Stomach   87
Small Intestine (Small Bowel)   89
Large Intestine (Large Bowel)   89
ACCESSORY ORGANS OF DIGESTION   89
Liver   89
Pancreas   90
Gallbladder   90
COMBINING FORMS   91
Mouth   91
Pharynx, Stomach, and Esophagus   91
Small Intestine and Colon (Large Intestine)   92
Accessory Organs of Digestion: Liver, Pancreas, and Biliary System   92
SUFFIXES   93
PREFIXES   93
PATHOLOGY   94
Ulcers   94
Hernias   94
Bowel Obstructions   95
Hemorrhoids   96
Liver Disorders   96
Diverticulosis   96
Oncology   96
DIAGNOSTIC, SYMPTOMATIC, AND THERAPEUTIC TERMS   98
DIAGNOSTIC PROCEDURES   100
Imaging Procedures   100
Endoscopic Procedures   101
Laboratory Procedures   101
SURGICAL AND THERAPEUTIC PROCEDURES   102
PHARMACOLOGY   102
ABBREVIATIONS   103
MEDICAL RECORD   104
GI Evaluation   104
WORKSHEETS   105

Chapter 8
RESPIRATORY SYSTEM... 115
CHAPTER OUTLINE   115
STUDENT OBJECTIVES   115
ANATOMY AND PHYSIOLOGY   116
Internal Respiration   116
External Respiration   116
Respiratory System   116
COMBINING FORMS   118
SUFFIXES   120
PREFIXES   120

PATHOLOGY   120
   Chronic Obstructive Pulmonary Disease   120
   Influenza   121
   Pleural Effusions   121
   Tuberculosis   122
   Bronchopneumonia   122
   Cystic Fibrosis   123
   Respiratory Distress Syndrome   123
   Oncology   123
     Primary Pulmonary Cancer   123
DIAGNOSTIC, SYMPTOMATIC, AND THERAPEUTIC TERMS   125
DIAGNOSTIC PROCEDURES   126
   Imaging Procedures   126
   Endoscopic Procedures   127
   Clinical Procedures   127
   Laboratory Procedures   127
SURGICAL AND THERAPEUTIC PROCEDURES   128
PHARMACOLOGY   128
ABBREVIATIONS   128
MEDICAL RECORD   129
   Respiratory Evaluation   129
WORKSHEETS   130

Chapter 9

CARDIOVASCULAR SYSTEM 137
CHAPTER OUTLINE   137
STUDENT OBJECTIVES   137
ANATOMY AND PHYSIOLOGY   138
   Vascular System   138
     Arteries   138
     Capillaries   138
     Veins   139
   Heart   140
   Conduction System of the Heart   142
   Blood Pressure   142
   Fetal Circulation   144
COMBINING FORMS   145
SUFFIXES   145
PREFIXES   146
PATHOLOGY   146
   Atherosclerosis   146
   Coronary Artery Disease   147
   Infective Endocarditis   148
   Varicose Veins   148
   Oncology   149
DIAGNOSTIC, SYMPTOMATIC, AND THERAPEUTIC TERMS   149
DIAGNOSTIC PROCEDURES   151
   Imaging Procedures   151
   Clinical Procedures   152
   Laboratory Procedures   153
SURGICAL AND THERAPEUTIC PROCEDURES   153
PHARMACOLOGY   154
ABBREVIATIONS   154
MEDICAL RECORD   155
   Acute Myocardial Infarction   155
WORKSHEETS   156

Chapter 10

BLOOD, LYMPH, AND IMMUNE SYSTEMS 163
CHAPTER OUTLINE   163
STUDENT OBJECTIVES   163

ANATOMY AND PHYSIOLOGY   164
  Blood   164
    Red Blood Cells (Erythrocytes)   164
    White Blood Cells (Leukocytes)   166
    Platelets   167
    Plasma   168
  Lymph System   168
  Immune System   170
    Blood Groups   173
COMBINING FORMS   173
SUFFIXES   175
PREFIXES   175
PATHOLOGY   176
  Anemias   176
  Acquired Immunodeficiency Syndrome (AIDS)   176
  Autoimmune Diseases   177
  Edema   177
  Hemophilia   177
  Infectious Mononucleosis   178
  Allergy   179
  Oncology   179
    Leukemia   179
    Hodgkin's Disease   179
    Kaposi's Sarcoma   179
DIAGNOSTIC, SYMPTOMATIC, AND THERAPEUTIC TERMS   180
DIAGNOSTIC PROCEDURES   180
  Imaging Procedures   180
  Laboratory Procedures   180
SURGICAL AND THERAPEUTIC PROCEDURES   181
PHARMACOLOGY   182
ABBREVIATIONS   182
MEDICAL RECORD   183
  Therapeutic Plasmapharesis   183
WORKSHEETS   184

Chapter 11

MUSCULOSKELETAL SYSTEM 189

CHAPTER OUTLINE   189
STUDENT OBJECTIVES   189
ANATOMY AND PHYSIOLOGY   190
  Skeletal System   190
    Functions   190
    Structure and Types of Bones   190
    Divisions of the Skeletal System: Axial and Appendicular Skeleton   192
    Projections and Depressions in Bones   195
    Joints or Articulations   195
  Muscles   195
  Attachments   196
COMBINING FORMS   199
  Skeletal System   199
    Bones of Upper Extremities   199
    Bones of Lower Extremities   199
    Other Combining Forms   200
  Muscular System   201
SUFFIXES   201
PATHOLOGY   202
  Bones   202
    Fractures   202
    Osteoporosis   202
    Spinal Disorders   203
  Joints   204
  Muscles   204
  Oncology   205
DIAGNOSTIC, SYMPTOMATIC, AND THERAPEUTIC TERMS   205

DIAGNOSTIC PROCEDURES   206
  Imaging Procedures   206
SURGICAL AND THERAPEUTIC PROCEDURES   207
PHARMACOLOGY   207
ABBREVIATIONS   208
MEDICAL RECORD   209
  Radiographic Consultation: Injury of Left Wrist and Hand   209
WORKSHEETS   210

Chapter 12
GENITOURINARY SYSTEM... 219

CHAPTER OUTLINE   219
STUDENT OBJECTIVES   219
ANATOMY AND PHYSIOLOGY   220
  Urinary System   220
    Macroscopic Structures   221
    Microscopic Structures   222
  Male Reproductive System   224
COMBINING FORMS   225
SUFFIXES   226
PATHOLOGY   227
  Pyelonephritis   227
  Glomerulonephritis   227
  Nephrolithiasis   227
  Bladder Neck Obstruction   227
  Benign Prostatic Hyperplasia   227
  Cryptorchidism   228
  Acute Tubular Necrosis   228
  Oncology   228
    Carcinoma of the Prostate   228
DIAGNOSTIC, SYMPTOMATIC, AND THERAPEUTIC TERMS   228
  Urinary System   228
  Male Reproductive System   229
DIAGNOSTIC PROCEDURES   230
  Imaging Procedures   230
  Endoscopic Procedures   230
  Laboratory Procedures   231
SURGICAL AND THERAPEUTIC PROCEDURES   231
PHARMACOLOGY   232
ABBREVIATIONS   232
MEDICAL RECORD   233
  Operative Report   233
WORKSHEETS   234

Chapter 13
FEMALE REPRODUCTIVE SYSTEM 243

CHAPTER OUTLINE   243
STUDENT OBJECTIVES   243
ANATOMY AND PHYSIOLOGY   244
  Internal Organs of Reproduction   245
    Ovaries   245
    Fallopian Tubes   245
    Uterus and Vagina   246
  Menstrual Cycle   247
    Menstrual Phase   247
    Follicular Phase   247
    Luteal Phase   247
  Pregnancy   247
  Labor and Childbirth   247
  Menopause   248
COMBINING FORMS   249
SUFFIXES   250

PREFIXES 250
PATHOLOGY 250
  Menstrual Disturbances 250
  Premenstrual Syndrome 251
  Endometriosis 251
  Pelvic Infections 251
  Vaginal Infections 251
  Sexually Transmitted Diseases 251
  Uterine Tumors 253
  Oncology 253
    Cervical Cancer 253
DIAGNOSTIC, SYMPTOMATIC, AND THERAPEUTIC TERMS 254
  Female Reproductive System 254
  Obstetrics 255
DIAGNOSTIC PROCEDURES 256
  Imaging Procedures 256
  Endoscopic Procedures 256
  Laboratory Procedures 256
SURGICAL AND THERAPEUTIC PROCEDURES 257
PHARMACOLOGY 258
ABBREVIATIONS 259
  Maternal-Gynecological and Related Abbreviations 259
  Fetal-Obstetric Abbreviations 260
MEDICAL RECORD 260
  Primary Herpes Infection 260
WORKSHEETS 261

Chapter 14
ENDOCRINE SYSTEM 269
CHAPTER OUTLINE 269
STUDENT OBJECTIVES 269
ANATOMY AND PHYSIOLOGY 270
  Pituitary Gland 270
  Thyroid Gland 271
  Parathyroid Glands 274
  Adrenal Glands 274
    Adrenal Cortex 275
    Adrenal Medulla 275
  Pancreas (Islets of Langerhans) 275
  Pineal Gland 276
COMBINING FORMS 277
SUFFIXES 277
PATHOLOGY 278
  Pituitary Disorders 278
  Thyroid Disorders 278
  Parathyroid Disorders 279
  Disorders of the Adrenal Glands 279
    Adrenal Medulla 279
    Adrenal Cortex 279
  Pancreatic Disorders 280
  Oncology 281
    Pancreatic Cancer 281
    Pituitary Tumors 281
    Thyroid Cancer 281
DIAGNOSTIC, SYMPTOMATIC, AND THERAPEUTIC TERMS 282
DIAGNOSTIC PROCEDURES 283
  Imaging Procedures 283
  Laboratory Procedures 284
SURGICAL AND THERAPEUTIC PROCEDURES 284
PHARMACOLOGY 284
ABBREVIATIONS 285
MEDICAL RECORD 286
  Hyperparathyroidism and Diabetes Mellitus 286
WORKSHEETS 287

Chapter 15
NERVOUS SYSTEM..293

CHAPTER OUTLINE   293
STUDENT OBJECTIVES   293
ANATOMY AND PHYSIOLOGY   294
  Nervous Tissue   294
    Neurons   294
    Neuroglia   296
  Subdivisions of the Nervous System   296
  Brain   299
  Spinal Cord   300
  Meninges   300
COMBINING FORMS   301
SUFFIXES   301
PREFIXES   302
PATHOLOGY   302
  Bell's Palsy   302
  Cerebrovascular Disease   302
  Seizure Disorders   302
  Parkinson's Disease   303
  Multiple Sclerosis   303
  Alzheimer's Disease   303
  Oncology   303
DIAGNOSTIC, SYMPTOMATIC, AND THERAPEUTIC TERMS   304
DIAGNOSTIC PROCEDURES   307
  Imaging Procedures   307
SURGICAL AND THERAPEUTIC PROCEDURES   308
PHARMACOLOGY   308
ABBREVIATIONS   308
MEDICAL RECORD   309
  Subarachnoid Hemorrhage   309
WORKSHEETS   310

Chapter 16
SPECIAL SENSES..317

CHAPTER OUTLINE   317
STUDENT OBJECTIVES   317
ANATOMY AND PHYSIOLOGY   318
  The Eye   318
  The Ear   320
    Hearing   320
    Equilibrium   321
COMBINING FORMS   321
SUFFIXES   322
PREFIXES   322
PATHOLOGY   323
  Errors of Refraction   323
  Cataracts   324
  Glaucoma   324
  Strabismus   324
  Macular Degeneration   325
  Otitis Media   325
  Otosclerosis   325
  Oncology   326
DIAGNOSTIC, SYMPTOMATIC, AND THERAPEUTIC TERMS   326
DIAGNOSTIC PROCEDURES   327
  Endoscopic Procedures   327
  Imaging Procedures   328
  Clinical Procedures   328
SURGICAL AND THERAPEUTIC PROCEDURES   328
PHARMACOLOGY   329
ABBREVIATIONS   329
MEDICAL RECORD   330
  Operative Report   330
WORKSHEETS   331

Appendix A
ANSWER KEY..339

Appendix B
ABBREVIATIONS...351

Appendix C
INDEX OF MEDICAL WORD ELEMENTS....................................361

    Part I: Medical Word Element to English Term   361
    Part II: English Term to Medical Word Element   369

Appendix D
INDEX OF GENETIC DISORDERS...381

Appendix E
INDEX OF DIAGNOSTIC IMAGING PROCEDURES.........................383

Appendix F
INDEX OF PHARMACOLOGY..385

Appendix G
INDEX OF ONCOLOGICAL TERMS...387

Index..389

Chapter 1

BASIC ELEMENTS OF A MEDICAL WORD

Chapter Outline

Student Objectives
Word Roots
Combining Forms
Suffixes
Prefixes

Basic Rules for Building and Defining Medical Words
Building Medical Words
Defining Medical Words
Pronunciation Guidelines
Worksheets

Student Objectives

Upon completion of this chapter, you will be able to do the following:

1. Define and provide several examples of word roots, combining forms, suffixes, and prefixes.

2. Divide medical words into their component parts.

3. Describe how medical words are formed.

4. Explain the two basic rules for building medical words.

5. Explain the three basic guidelines for defining medical words.

6. Demonstrate your knowledge of the chapter by completing the worksheets.

Medical word building follows simple rules. Once these rules are learned, numerous words can be formed and defined. As in all languages, some words are exceptions to such rules. Fortunately, in medical terminology few words are subject to irregularities.

To analyze medical words, the student needs to identify the four elements that may be used to form words: word roots, combining forms, suffixes, and prefixes.

WORD ROOTS

The main part or stem of a word is called a **word root (WR)**. A WR is usually derived from the Greek or Latin language and frequently indicates a body part. Most medical words have one or more roots.

Examples of Word Roots

Greek Word	Word Root
kardia (heart)	cardi
gaster (stomach)	gastr
hepar (liver)	hepat
nephros (kidney)	nephr
osteon (bone)	oste

COMBINING FORMS

The **combining form (CF)** is a WR plus a vowel, usually an "o." Like the WR, the CF usually indicates a body part. In this text, a CF will be listed as word root/vowel (e.g., cardi/o), as illustrated in the following chart.

Examples of Combining Forms

Word Root	+	Combining Vowel	=	Combining Form	Meaning
cardi/	+	o	=	cardi/o	heart
gastr/	+	o	=	gastr/o	stomach
hepat/	+	o	=	hepat/o	liver
nephr/	+	o	=	nephr/o	kidney
oste/	+	o	=	oste/o	bone

Try to learn the CF rather than the WR because the CF makes many words easier to pronounce. For example, in the previous list, the WRs gastr and nephr are difficult to pronounce, whereas their CFs gastr/o and nephr/o are easy to pronounce.

SUFFIXES

A **suffix** is a word ending. In the words tonsill/*itis*, and tonsill/*ectomy*, the suffixes are -*itis* (inflammation) and -*ectomy* (excision, removal). Changing the suffix gives medical words a new meaning. In medical terminology, a suffix usually indicates a procedure, condition, disease, or part of speech. Many suffixes are derived from Greek or Latin words.

Examples of Suffixes

Combining Form	+ Suffix	= Medical Word	Meaning
arthr/o (joint)	-centesis (puncture)	arthrocentesis	puncture of a joint
thorac/o (chest)	-tomy (incision)	thoracotomy	incision of the chest
gastr/o (stomach)	-megaly (enlargement)	gastromegaly	enlargement of the stomach

PREFIXES

A **prefix** is a word element located at the beginning of a word. Prefixes are frequently found in general language as well as in medical and scientific terminology. When a medical word contains a prefix, the meaning of the word is altered. The prefix usually indicates a number, time, position, direction, color, or sense of negation.

Examples of Prefixes

Prefix	+ Word Root	+ Suffix	= Medical Word	Meaning
a- (without)	mast (breast)	-ia (condition)	amastia	without a breast
hyper- (excessive)	therm (heat)	-ia (condition)	hyperthermia	condition of excessive heat
intra- (in, within)	muscul (muscle)	-ar (relating to)	intramuscular	relating to within the muscles
macro- (large)	gloss (tongue)	-ia (condition)	macroglossia	condition of a large tongue
micro- (small)	card (heart)	-ia (condition)	microcardia	condition of a small heart

BASIC RULES FOR BUILDING AND DEFINING MEDICAL WORDS

Building Medical Words

There are two basic rules for building medical words.

Rule 1   A WR is used before a suffix that begins with a vowel.

Word Root	Suffix	Medical Word	Meaning
scler/ (hardening)	+ osis (abnormal condition)	= sclerosis	abnormal condition of hardening

Rule 2   A combining vowel is used to link a WR to a suffix that begins with a consonant and to link a WR to another WR to form a compound word.

- Here is an example of a combining vowel linking a WR to a suffix that begins with a consonant.

Word Root and Combining Vowel	Suffix	Medical Word	Meaning
colon/o (colon)	+ scope (instrument to view)	= colonoscope	instrument to view the colon

- Here are two examples of a combining vowel linking one WR to another WR to form a compound word.

Word Root	Combining Vowel	Word Root	Suffix	Medical Word	Meaning
oste/ (bone)	o/	chondr/ (cartilage)	+ itis (inflammation)	= osteochondritis	inflammation of bone and cartilage

Word Root	Combining Vowel	Word Root	Suffix	Medical Word	Meaning
oste/ (bone)	o/	arthr/ (joint)	+ itis (inflammation)	= osteoarthritis	inflammation of bone and joint

In most instances, the combining vowel is retained between two roots even if the second root begins with a vowel, as illustrated in the preceding example, oste/o/arthr/itis.

Defining Medical Words

There are three basic steps for defining medical words.
- First, define the **suffix**, or last part of the word.
- Second, define the **prefix**, or first part of the word.
- Last, define the **middle** of the word.

Here is an example.

gastr/o stomach (2)	enter/ intestine (3)	itis inflammation (1)

Read as follows:
1. Inflammation (of) [suffix]
2. Stomach (and) [first part of the word]
3. Intestine [middle]

The definition of gastr/o/enter/itis is "inflammation (of) stomach and intestine."

PRONUNCIATION GUIDELINES

Although medical words usually follow the rules that govern the pronunciation of English words, they may be difficult to pronounce when you first encounter them. Here are some general rules you will find helpful:

- For **ae** and **oe**, only the second vowel is pronounced.

  EXAMPLES
  burs**ae**, pleur**ae**, r**oe**ntgen

- **c** and **g** are given the soft sound of s and j, respectively, before e, i, and y in words of both Greek and Latin origins.

  EXAMPLES
  cerebrum, **c**ircumcision, **c**ycle, **g**el, **g**ingivitis, **g**iant, **g**yrate

- **c** and **g** have a hard sound before other letters.

  EXAMPLES
  cardiac, **c**ast, **g**astric, **g**onad

- **e** and **es**, when forming the final letter or letters of a word, are often pronounced as separate syllables.

  EXAMPLES
  syncop**e**, systol**e**, nar**es**

- **ch** is sometimes pronounced like k.

  EXAMPLES
  cholesterol, **ch**olera, **ch**olemia

- **i** at the end of a word (to form a plural) is pronounced "eye."

  EXAMPLES
  bronch**i**, fung**i**, nucle**i**

- **pn** at the beginning of a word is pronounced with only the n sound.

  EXAMPLES
  pneumonia, **pn**eumotoxin

- **pn** in the middle of a word is pronounced with a hard p and a hard n.

  EXAMPLES
  ortho**pn**ea, hyper**pn**ea

- **ps** is pronounced like s.

  EXAMPLES
  psychology, **ps**ychosis

- All other vowels and consonants have ordinary English sounds.

Most medical words in this textbook are spelled phonetically in order to teach their correct pronunciation. Diacritical marks, the macron (ˉ) and breve (˘), are used for long and short vowel pronunciations, respectively.

The macron (ˉ) indicates the long sound of vowels, as in the following:

ā in rate
ē in rebirth
ī in isle
ō in over
ū in unite

The breve (˘) indicates the short sound of vowels, as in the following:

ă in apple
ĕ in ever
ĭ in it
ŏ in not
ŭ in cut

Capitalization is used to indicate emphasis on certain syllables, as in LĔT-ter.

WORKSHEET 1

1. List the four elements used to form words: _____

2. A root is the main part or foundation of a word. In the words *teacher*, *teaches*, and *teaching*, the root

   is _____.

Answer the following statements either true or false.

3. _____ A combining vowel is usually an "e."

4. _____ A combining vowel is not used before a suffix that begins with a vowel.

5. _____ A combining vowel is used to link one root to another root.

6. _____ A combining vowel is not used before a suffix that begins with a consonant.

7. _____ To define a medical word, first define the prefix.

Check your answers in Appendix A. Review any material that you did not answer correctly.

WORKSHEET 2

Underline the WR in each of following CFs.

1. rhin/o (nose)

2. splen/o (spleen)

3. hyster/o (uterus)

4. enter/o (intestine)

5. neur/o (nerve)

6. ot/o (ear)

7. dermat/o (skin)

8. hydr/o (water)

9. hepat/o (liver)

10. toxic/o (poison)

WORKSHEET 3

Underline the WR in the following words. Recall that in most instances the root designates a body part.

Word	Meaning
1. nephritis	inflammation of the kidneys
2. arthrodesis	surgical fixation of a joint
3. phlebotomy	incision of a vein
4. dentist	specialist in teeth
5. gastrectomy	excision of the stomach
6. lumpectomy	excision of a lump
7. hepatoma	tumor of the liver
8. cardiologist	specialist in the heart
9. gastria	condition of the stomach
10. thermometer	instrument for measuring heat

WORKSHEET 4

Underline the elements that are CFs.

1. hepat   6. nephr/o

2. pancreat   7. cyt

3. cardi/o   8. arthr

4. oste/o   9. erythr/o

5. gastr/o   10. dent/o

WORKSHEET 5

■ ■ ■ ■ ■ ■ ■ ■ ■ ■ ■ ■ ■ ■

In the space provided, change the roots to CFs.

Root	*Combining Form*
1. mast (breast)	*mast/o*
2. hepat (liver)	_____
3. arthr (joint)	_____
4. cyst (bladder)	_____
5. phleb (vein)	_____
6. thorac (chest)	_____
7. abdomin (abdomen)	_____
8. trache (trachea)	_____
9. leuk (white)	_____
10. gastr (stomach)	_____

SUFFIXES: SURGICAL, DIAGNOSTIC, SYMPTOMATIC, AND RELATED

Chapter Outline

Student Objectives

Suffixes
Surgical Suffixes

Diagnostic, Symptomatic, and Related Suffixes

Worksheets

Student Objectives

Upon completion of this chapter, you will be able to do the following:

1. Define and provide examples of operative, diagnostic, and symptomatic suffixes.
2. Determine the use of a combining form and word root when linking these elements to a suffix.
3. Demonstrate your knowledge of the chapter by completing the worksheets.

SUFFIXES

In medical words a *suffix* is added to the end of a root or combining form to change its meaning. For example, the combining form **gastr/o** means stomach. The suffix **-megaly** means enlargement, and **-itis** means inflammation. Gastr/o/megaly is an enlargement of the stomach, and gastr/itis is an inflammation of the stomach. Whenever you change the suffix, the word takes on a new meaning. Suffixes are also used to denote singular and plural forms of a word as well as a part of speech (see Chap. 3 for more in-depth discussion).

Following are additional examples applying rule 1 of medical word building.

A Word Root Is Used before a Suffix That Begins with a Vowel

Word Root	+	Suffix	=	Medical Word	Pronunciation
gastr (stomach)	+	itis (inflammation)	=	gastritis inflammation of the stomach	găs-TRĪ-tĭs
cephal (head)	+	algia (pain)	=	cephalalgia pain in the head, headache	sĕf-ă-LĂL-jē-ă
mast (breast)	+	ectomy (excision)	=	mastectomy excision of a breast	măs-TĔK-tō-mē

Following are additional examples applying rule 2 of medical word building.

A Combining Vowel Is Used before a Suffix That Begins with a Consonant

Combining Form (WR + o)	+	Suffix	=	Medical Word	Pronunciation
phleb + o (vein)	+	tomy (incision)	=	phlebotomy incision of a vein	flĕ-BŎT-ō-mē
colon + o (colon)	+	scopy (visual examination)	=	colonoscopy visual examination of colon	kō-lŏn-ŎS-kō-pē
arthr + o (joint)	+	centesis (puncture)	=	arthrocentesis puncture of a joint	ăr-thrō-sĕn-TĒ-sĭs
thorac + o (chest)	+	tomy (incision)	=	thoracotomy incision of the chest	thō-răk-ŎT-ō-mē

A Combining Vowel Is Used to Link a Word Root to Another Word Root to Form a Compound Word

Combining Form (WR + o)	+ WR	+ Suffix	Medical Word	Pronunciation
gastr + o (stomach)	+ enter (intestine)	+ itis (inflammation)	gastroenteritis inflammation of stomach and intestine	găs-trō-ĕn-tĕr-Ī-tĭs
oste + o (bone)	+ arthr (joint)	+ itis (inflammation)	osteoarthritis inflammation of bone and joint	ŏs-tē-ō-ăr-THRĪ-tĭs
encephal + o (brain)	+ mening (meninges)	+ itis (inflammation)	encephalomeningitis inflammation of brain and meninges	ĕn-sĕf-ă-lō-mĕn-ĭn-JĪ-tĭs

An effective strategy in mastering medical terminology is learning the major suffixes first. To become proficient in medical terminology, review the examples in each section and say each word by referring to its phonetic pronunciation. Define medical words by following the three basic steps outlined in Chapter 1: First, *define the suffix*, or end of the word; second, *define the prefix*, or first part of the word. *Last, define the middle* of the word. For example, gastr/o/enter/itis is defined as inflammation of the stomach and intestine; append/ectomy is defined as excision of the appendix.

Surgical Suffixes

Suffixes Denoting Incisions

Suffix	Meaning	Example	Pronunciation
-centesis	puncture	arthr/o/centesis joint	ăr-thrō-sĕn-TĒ-sĭs
-ectomy	excision, removal	append/ectomy appendix	ăp-ĕn-DĔK-tŏ-mē
-stomy	forming an opening (mouth)	col/o/stomy colon	kŏ-LŎS-tō-mē
-tome	instrument to cut	oste/o/tome bone	ŎS-tē-ō-tōm
-tomy	incision, cut into	phleb/o/tomy vein	flĕ-BŎT-ō-mē

Suffixes Denoting Reconstructive Surgeries

Suffix	Meaning	Example	Pronunciation
-desis	binding, fixation (of a bone or joint)	arthr/o/desis joint	ăr-thrō-DĒ-sĭs
-pexy	suspension, fixation (of an organ)	mast/o/pexy breast	MĂS-tō-pěks-ē
-rrhaphy	suture	my/o/rrhaphy muscle	mī-OR-ă-fē
-plasty	surgical repair	rhin/o/plasty nose	RĪ-nō-plăs-tē

Suffixes Denoting Refracturing, Loosening, or Crushing

Suffix	Meaning	Example	Pronunciation
-clasis	break, fracture	oste/o/clasis bone	ŏs-tē-ŎK-lă-sĭs
-lysis	separation, destruction, loosening	enter/o/lysis intestine	ěn-těr-ŎL-ĭ-sĭs
-tripsy	crushing	lith/o/tripsy stone, calculus	LĬTH-ō-trĭp-sē

Diagnostic, Symptomatic, and Related Suffixes

Suffix	Meaning	Example	Pronunciation
-algia	pain	cephal/algia head	sěf-ă-LĂL-jē-ă
-dynia		gastr/o/dynia stomach	găs-trō-DĬN-ē-ă
-cele	hernia, swelling	hepat/o/cele liver	HĔP-ă-tō-sēl
-ectasis	dilation, expansion	bronchi/ectasis bronchus	brŏng-kē-ĔK-tă-sĭs
-emesis	vomiting	hyper/emesis excessive	hī-pěr-ĔM-ě-sĭs
-emia	blood condition	leuk/emia white	loo-KĒ-mē-ă
-gen	forming, producing, origin	carcin/o/gen cancer	kăr-SĬN-ō-jěn
-genesis		oste/o/genesis bone	ŏs-tē-ō-JĔN-ě-sĭs
-gram	record, a writing	cardi/o/gram heart	KĂR-dē-ō-grăm

Diagnostic, Symptomatic, and Related Suffixes *(Continued)*

Suffix	Meaning	Example	Pronunciation
-graph	instrument for recording	cardi/o/graph heart	KĂR-dē-ō-grăf
-graphy	process of recording	cardi/o/graphy heart	kăr-dē-ŎG-ră-fē
-iasis	abnormal condition (produced by something specified)*	chole/lith/iasis gall stone	kō-lē-lĭ-THĪ-ă-sĭs
-itis	inflammation	gastr/itis stomach	găs-TRĪ-tĭs
-lith	stone, calculus	chol/e/lith gall	KŌ-lē-lĭth
-logist	specialist in the study of	dermat/o/logist skin	dĕr-mă-TŎL-ō-jĭst
-logy	study of	psych/o/logy mind	sī-KŎL-ō-jē
-malacia	softening	oste/o/malacia bone	ŏs-tē-ō-mă-LĀ-shē-ă
-megaly	enlargement	hepat/o/megaly liver	hĕp-ă-tō-MĔG-ă-lē
-meter	instrument for measuring	therm/o/meter heat	thĕr-MŎM-ĕ-tĕr
-metry	act of measuring	pelv/i/metry pelvis	pĕl-VĬM-ĕt-rē
-oid	resembling	lip/oid fat	LĬP-oyd
-oma	tumor	aden/oma gland	ăd-ĕ-NŌ-mă
-osis	abnormal condition, increase (used primarily with blood cells)	dermat/osis skin erythr/o/cyt/osis red cell	dĕr-mă-TŌ-sĭs ĕ-rĭth-rō-sī-TŌ-sĭs
-para†	to bear (offspring)	multi/para many, much	mŭl-TĬP-ă-ră
-paresis	partial paralysis	hemi/paresis half	hĕm-ē-PĂR-ĕ-sĭs
-pathy	disease	neur/o/pathy nerve	nū-RŎP-ă-thē
-penia	decrease, deficiency	leuk/o/penia white (cell)	loo-kō-PĒ-nē-ă
-phagia	eating, swallowing	dys/phagia difficult, painful	dĭs-FĀ-jē-ă

*There are few exceptions to this rule.
†-para may also be used as a prefix, at which time it means near, beside, beyond.

Diagnostic, Symptomatic, and Related Suffixes *(Continued)*

Suffix	Meaning	Example	Pronunciation
-phasia	speech	a/phasia without	ăh-FĀ-zē-ă
-philia	attraction to	hem/o/philia blood	hē-mō-FĬL-ē-ă
-phobia	fear	claustr/o/phobia confined place	klaws-trō-FŌ-bē-ă
-plasia	formation, growth	hyper/plasia excessive	hī-pĕr-PLĀ-zē-ă
-plegia	paralysis, stroke	hemi/plegia half	hĕm-ĕ-PLĒ-jē-ă
-poiesis	formation, production	hem/o/poiesis blood	hē-mō-poy-Ē-sĭs
-ptosis	prolapse, downward displacement	hyster/o/ptosis uterus	hĭs-tĕr-ŏp-TŌ-sĭs
-rrhage	bursting forth	hem/o/rrhage blood	HĔM-ĕ-rĭj
-rrhagia		men/o/rrhagia menses	mĕn-ō-RĀ-jē-ă
-rrhea	discharge, flow	dia/rrhea through	dī-ă-RĒ-ă
-rrhexis	rupture	angi/o/rrhexis vessel	ăn-jĭ-ō-RĔK-sĭs
-scope	instrument to view or examine	gastr/o/scope stomach	GĂS-trō-skōp
-scopy	visual examination	proct/o/scopy anus, rectum	prŏk-TŎS-kō-pē
-spasm	involuntary contraction, twitching	blephar/o/spasm eyelid	BLĔF-ă-rō-spăzm
-stasis	standing still	hem/o/stasis blood	hē-mō-STĀ-sĭs
-stenosis	narrowing, stricture	arteri/o/stenosis artery	ăr-tē-rē-ō-stĕ-NŌ-sĭs
-toxic	poison	thyr/o/toxic thyroid	thī-rō-TŎKS-ĭk
-trophy	development, nourishment	a/trophy without	ĂT-rō-fē

WORKSHEET 1

■ ■ ■ ■ ■ ■ ■ ■ ■ ■ ■ ■ ■ ■ ■

SURGICAL SUFFIXES DENOTING INCISIONS*

Use the meaning column to complete the words on the left.

Incomplete Word   **Meaning**

1. episi/o/ _t o m y_   incision of the perineum

2. col _ _ _ _ _ _ _   excision (of all or part) of the colon

3. arthr/o/ _ _ _ _ _ _ _ _ _   puncture of a joint (to remove fluid)

4. splen _ _ _ _ _ _ _   excision of the spleen

5. col/o/ _ _ _ _ _ _   forming a permanent opening into the colon

6. derma _ _ _ _ _   instrument to cut skin

7. tympan/o/ _ _ _ _ _   incision of the tympanic membrane

8. trache/o/ _ _ _ _ _ _   forming an opening into the trachea

9. mast _ _ _ _ _ _ _   excision of a breast

10. lith/o/ _ _ _ _ _   incision to remove a stone or calculus

11. hemorrhoid _ _ _ _ _ _ _   excision of hemorrhoids

Cover the meaning column in the previous section. Use the word list to build words meaning:

12. forming an opening into the colon *colostomy* _____

13. excision of the colon _____

14. instrument to cut skin _____

15. puncture of a joint _____

16. incision to remove a stone _____

17. excision of a breast _____

18. incision of the tympanic membrane _____

19. forming an opening into the trachea _____

20. excision of the spleen _____

_____

*In Worksheets 1 and 2 the word roots are underlined.

WORKSHEET 2

. . . .

SURGICAL SUFFIXES DENOTING RECONSTRUCTIVE SURGERIES*

Use the meaning column to complete the words on the left.

Incomplete Word	*Meaning*
1. arthr/o/ _ _ _ _ _ _	fixation or binding of a joint
2. rhin/ _ / _ _ _ _ _ _ _	surgical repair of the nose
3. ten/o/ _ _ _ _ _ _ _	surgical repair of tendons
4. my/o/ _ _ _ _ _ _ _	suture of muscle
5. mast/ _ / _ _ _ _ _	fixation of a (pendulous) breast
6. cyst/ _ / _ _ _ _ _ _ _	suture of the bladder

SURGICAL SUFFIXES DENOTING REFRACTURING, LOOSENING, OR CRUSHING

7. oste/o/ _ _ _ _ _ _ _	to break or fracture a bone
8. lith/ _ / _ _ _ _ _ _ _	crushing a stone
9. enter/ _ / _ _ _ _ _ _	separating intestinal (adhesions)
10. neur/ _ / _ _ _ _ _ _ _	crushing a nerve

Cover the meaning column in the previous section. Use the word list to build medical words meaning:

11. surgical repair of the nose ⎯⎯⎯⎯⎯⎯⎯⎯⎯⎯⎯⎯⎯⎯⎯⎯⎯⎯⎯⎯⎯⎯⎯

12. fixation of a joint ⎯⎯⎯⎯⎯⎯⎯⎯⎯⎯⎯⎯⎯⎯⎯⎯⎯⎯⎯⎯⎯⎯⎯⎯⎯⎯⎯⎯

13. suture of (a torn) muscle ⎯⎯⎯⎯⎯⎯⎯⎯⎯⎯⎯⎯⎯⎯⎯⎯⎯⎯⎯⎯⎯⎯⎯

14. fixation of a (pendulous) breast ⎯⎯⎯⎯⎯⎯⎯⎯⎯⎯⎯⎯⎯⎯⎯⎯⎯⎯⎯

15. suture of the bladder ⎯⎯⎯⎯⎯⎯⎯⎯⎯⎯⎯⎯⎯⎯⎯⎯⎯⎯⎯⎯⎯⎯⎯⎯⎯⎯

16. repair of tendons ⎯⎯⎯⎯⎯⎯⎯⎯⎯⎯⎯⎯⎯⎯⎯⎯⎯⎯⎯⎯⎯⎯⎯⎯⎯⎯⎯⎯⎯

17. refracturing a bone ⎯⎯⎯⎯⎯⎯⎯⎯⎯⎯⎯⎯⎯⎯⎯⎯⎯⎯⎯⎯⎯⎯⎯⎯⎯⎯⎯

18. crushing stones ⎯⎯⎯⎯⎯⎯⎯⎯⎯⎯⎯⎯⎯⎯⎯⎯⎯⎯⎯⎯⎯⎯⎯⎯⎯⎯⎯⎯⎯⎯

19. freeing intestinal (adhesions) ⎯⎯⎯⎯⎯⎯⎯⎯⎯⎯⎯⎯⎯⎯⎯⎯⎯⎯⎯⎯⎯

20. crushing a nerve ⎯⎯⎯⎯⎯⎯⎯⎯⎯⎯⎯⎯⎯⎯⎯⎯⎯⎯⎯⎯⎯⎯⎯⎯⎯⎯⎯⎯⎯

⎯⎯⎯⎯⎯⎯⎯⎯⎯⎯⎯⎯

*In Worksheets 1 and 2 the word roots are underlined.

WORKSHEET 3

▪ ▪ ▪ ▪ ▪ ▪ ▪ ▪ ▪ ▪ ▪ ▪ ▪ ▪ ▪ ▪ ▪

DIAGNOSTIC, SYMPTOMATIC, AND RELATED SUFFIXES

Fill in the blanks to complete each medical word.

Incomplete Word   *Meaning*

1. bronchi_ _ _ _ _ _ _ _   dilation of a bronchus

2. gastr/o/_ _ _ _ _ _   pain in the stomach

3. nephr_ _ _ _ _   abnormal condition of the kidneys

4. chole_ _ _ _ _   gallstone

5. carcin/o/_ _ _   forming or producing cancer

6. psych/o/_ _ _ _ _   study of the mind

7. oste/_ _/_ _ _ _ _ _ _ _ _   softening of bone

8. hepat/_ _/_ _ _ _ _ _ _   enlargement of the liver

9. cholelith_ _ _ _ _ _   abnormal condition of gallstones

10. therm/_ _/_ _ _ _ _ _ _   instrument for measuring heat

11. hepat/_ _/_ _ _ _ _   herniation of the liver

12. lip_ _ _ _   resembling fat

13. neur/o/_ _ _ _ _ _   disease of the nerves

14. dermat_ _ _ _ _   abnormal condition of the skin

15. hemi_ _ _ _ _ _ _ _   paralysis of one half of the body

16. proct/o/_ _ _ _ _ _   visual examination of the colon

17. dys_ _ _ _ _ _ _ _   difficult swallowing

18. a_ _ _ _ _ _ _   without speech or absence of speech

19. cephal_ _ _ _ _ _   pain in the head; headache

20. blephar/_ _/_ _ _ _ _ _ _   twitching of the eyelid

21. angi/_ _/_ _ _ _ _ _ _ _ _   rupture of a blood vessel

22. hem/_ _/_ _ _ _ _ _ _ _ _   development or formation of blood

Incomplete Word	*Meaning*
23. hyster/o/ _ _ _ _ _ _	prolapse of the uterus
24. hemi _ _ _ _ _ _ _	paralysis of one half (of the body)
25. hyper _ _ _ _ _ _	excessive formation (of an organ or tissue)

WORKSHEET 4

■ ■ ■ ■ ■ ■ ■ ■ ■ ■ ■ ■ ■ ■ ■ ■

SURGICAL SUFFIXES REVIEW

-centesis	-lysis	-stomy
-clasis	-pexy	-tome
-desis	-plasty	-tomy
-ectomy	-rrhaphy	-tripsy

Use the suffixes in the list above to form surgical terms meaning:

1. crushing a stone   lith/o/ _____

2. puncture of a joint (to remove fluid)   arthr/o/ _____

3. excision of the spleen   splen/ _____

4. forming an opening into the colon   col/o/ _____

5. instrument to cut skin   derma/ _____

6. forming an opening into the trachea   trache/o/ _____

7. incision to remove a stone or calculus   lith/ __ / _____

8. excision of a breast   mast/ _____

9. excision of hemorrhoids   hemorrhoid/ _____

10. incision of the trachea   trache/ __ / _____

11. fixation of a (pendulous) breast   mast/ __ / _____

12. excision (of part or all) of the colon   col/ _____

13. suture of the stomach (wall)   gastr/ __ / _____

14. fixation of the uterus   hyster/ __ / _____

15. surgical repair of the nose   rhin/ __ / _____

16. fixation or binding of a joint   arthr/ __ / _____

17. to break or fracture a bone   oste/ __ / _____

18. loosening of nerve (tissue)   neur/ __ / _____

19. suture of muscle   my/o/ _____

20. incision of the tympanic membrane   tympan/ __ / _____

WORKSHEET 5

▪ ▪ ▪ ▪ ▪ ▪ ▪ ▪ ▪ ▪ ▪ ▪

DIAGNOSTIC, SYMPTOMATIC, AND RELATED SUFFIXES REVIEW

-algia	-malacia	-phasia
-cele	-megaly	-plegia
-dynia	-metry	-poiesis
-ectasis	-oid	-rrhage
-emia	-oma	-rrhea
-genesis	-osis	-rrhexis
-graph	-pathy	-spasm
-iasis	-penia	-stenosis
-itis	-phagia	

Use the suffixes in the list above to form diagnostic and symptomatic terms meaning:

1. dilation of a bronchus   bronchi/ _____

2. pain (along the course) of a nerve   neur/ _____

3. inflammation of the stomach   gastr/ _____

4. headache; pain in the head   cephal/o/ _____

5. tumor of the liver   hepat/ _____

6. producing or forming cancer   carcin/o/ _____

7. abnormal condition of the skin   dermat/ _____

8. resembling fat   lip/ _____

9. enlarged kidney   nephr/o/ _____

10. narrowing or stricture of the pylorus   pylor/__/ _____

11. discharge or flow from the ear   ot/__/ _____

12. production or formation of blood   hem/o/ _____

13. rupture of the uterus   hyster/__/ _____

14. spasm or twitching of the eyelid   blephar/__/ _____

15. herniation of the bladder   cyst/__/ _____

16. bursting forth (of) blood   hem/o/ _____

17. abnormal condition of a stone or calculus   lith/ _____

18. paralysis affecting one side (of the body)   hemi/ _____

19. diseases of muscle (tissue)   my/＿/ _____

20. difficult or painful eating   dys/ _____

21. softening of the bones   oste/＿/ _____

22. without, or absence of, speech   a/ _____

23. white blood   leuk/ _____

24. deficiency in number of red blood cells   erythr/＿/ _____

25. measuring the pelvis   pelv/i/ _____

Chapter 3

SUFFIXES: ADJECTIVE, NOUN, DIMINUTIVE, SINGULAR, PLURAL

Chapter Outline
Student Objectives
Adjective Suffixes
Noun Suffixes

Diminutive Suffixes
Plural Suffixes
Worksheets

Student Objectives

Upon completion of this chapter, you will be able to do the following:

1. List and define diminutive suffixes.
2. List and define adjective suffixes, and apply this knowledge by completing Worksheet 1.
3. List and define noun suffixes, and apply this knowledge by completing Worksheet 2.
4. Define the rules for changing singular words to plural words, and apply this knowledge by completing Worksheet 3.

The suffixes discussed in this chapter are added to word roots to indicate either a part of speech or a singular or plural form of a medical word.

ADJECTIVE SUFFIXES

Adjectives are words used to modify nouns. The adjective suffixes that mean "pertaining to" or "relating to," or both, are summarized here.

Adjective Suffix	Example	Adjective Suffix	Example
-ac*	cardi/ac heart	-ic	hypo/ derm/ic under skin
-al	neur/al nerve	-ical†	med/ical medicine
-ar	muscul/ar muscle	-ory	audit/ory hearing
-ary	saliv/ary saliva	-ous	cutane/ous skin
-eal	mening/eal meninges	-tic	acous/tic sound

* -ac ending is rarely used.
† -ical is a combination of -ic and -al.

NOUN SUFFIXES

Nouns are names of persons, places, things, conditions, or states of being. The noun suffixes added to word roots to indicate a noun are summarized here.

Noun Suffix	Meaning	Example
-ia		pneumon/ia lung
-ism	condition	alcohol/ism alcohol
-y		path/y disease
-iatrics, -iatry	treatment, medicine	ped/iatrics child pod/iatry foot
-ist	specialist	ur/o/log/ist urine study (of)

DIMINUTIVE SUFFIXES

A diminutive suffix forms a word designating a smaller version of the object indicated by the word root. They are summarized here.

Dimunitive Suffix	Meaning	Example
-icle		part/icle piece
-ole		arteri/ole artery
-ula	small, minute, little	mac/ula spot
-ule		ven/ule vein

PLURAL SUFFIXES

The rules for forming plural words from singular words are summarized in the following chart.

Form Singular	Form Plural	Rule	Example Singular	Example Plural
a	ae	Retain the a and add e.	pleura	pleurae
ax	aces	Drop the x and add ces.	thorax	thoraces
en	ina	Drop the en and add ina.	lumen	lumina
is	es	Drop the is and add es.	diagnosis	diagnoses
ix ex	ices	Drop the ix or ex and add ices.	appendix apex	appendices apices
on	a	Drop the on and add a.	ganglion	ganglia
um	a	Drop the um and add a.	bacterium	bacteria
us	i	Drop the us and add i.	bronchus	bronchi
y	ies	Drop the y and add ies.	deformity	deformities
ma	mata	Retain the ma and add ta.	carcinoma	carcinomata

WORKSHEET 1

Use the following adjective suffixes to complete a medical term. When in doubt about the validity of a medical term, refer to a medical dictionary.

-ac	-eal	-tic
-al	-ic	-tix
-ary	-ous	

Element	Medical Term	Meaning
1. thorac/	*thoracic*	pertaining to the chest
2. gastr/		pertaining to the stomach
3. bacteri/		pertaining to bacteria
4. aqua/		pertaining to water
5. axill/		pertaining to the armpit
6. cardi/		pertaining to the heart
7. spin/		pertaining to the spine
8. membran/		pertaining to a membrane

WORKSHEET 2

■ ■ ■ ■ ■ ■ ■ ■ ■ ■ ■ ■ ■ ■ ■

Use the following noun suffixes to form a medical term. When in doubt about the validity of a medical term, refer to a medical dictionary.

-er	-is	-ist
-ia	-ism	-y

Element	Medical Term	Meaning
1. intern/	*internist*	specialist in internal medicine
2. leuk/em/		condition of "white" blood
3. sigmoid/o/scop/		visual examination of the sigmoid colon
4. alcohol/		condition of (excessive) alcohol
5. allerg/		specialist in allergies
6. senil/		condition associated with aging
7. man/		condition of madness
8. orth/o/ped/		specialist in orthopedics

WORSHEET 3

Write the plural form for each word and briefly state the pertinent rule. Use the dictionary as a reference.

Singular	Plural	Rule
1. diagno<u>sis</u>	*diagnoses*	*Drop the is and add es.*
2. forn<u>ix</u>		
3. burs<u>a</u>		
4. vertebr<u>a</u>		
5. kerato<u>sis</u>		
6. bronch<u>us</u>		
7. spermatozo<u>on</u>		
8. sept<u>um</u>		
9. coc<u>cus</u>		
10. ap<u>ex</u>		
11. gang<u>lion</u>		
12. progno<u>sis</u>		
13. thromb<u>us</u>		
14. append<u>ix</u>		
15. bacteri<u>um</u>		
16. rad<u>ius</u>		
17. test<u>is</u>		
18. nev<u>us</u>		

Chapter 4

PREFIXES • ABBREVIATIONS • PRONUNCIATION

ROOTS • COMBINING FORMS • SUFFIXES

PREFIXES

Chapter Outline

Student Objectives

Prefixes
Prefixes of Position
Prefixes of Number
    and Measurement

Prefixes of Negation
Prefixes of Direction
Other Prefixes

Worksheets

Student Objectives

Upon completion of this chapter, you will be able to do the following:

1. Explain the use of prefixes in medical terminology.
2. Explain how a prefix changes the meaning of a medical word.
3. Identify prefixes of position, number and measurement, negation, and direction.
4. Demonstrate your knowledge of this chapter by completing the worksheets.

This chapter emphasizes major prefixes used in building a medical vocabulary. It completes the information necessary to develop a basic foundation for learning medical words. Once you understand the basic components, medical terms will be much easier to define.

PREFIXES

A prefix is a word element located at the beginning of a word. Substituting one prefix for another alters the meaning of a medical word. Many medical words contain a prefix.

Consider the terms eu/pnea and dys/pnea. **Eupnea** means breathing that is normal; **dyspnea** means breathing that is painful or difficult.

The prefix **eu-** means good, normal; the prefix **dys-** means bad, painful, difficult; the suffix **-pnea** means breathing. Carefully study the components of both words and see how substituting **dys-** for **eu-** changes the meaning of the word.

Review the following examples to see how prefixes change the meaning of a word.

Prefix	Word Root	Suffix	Medical Word	Meaning
pre (before)	+ nat (birth)	+ al (pertaining to)	= prenatal	pertaining to (the period) before birth

Prefix	Word Root	Suffix	Medical Word	Meaning
peri (around)	+ nat (birth)	+ al (pertaining to)	= perinatal	pertaining to (the period) around birth

Prefix	Word Root	Suffix	Medical Word	Meaning
post (after)	+ nat (birth)	+ al (pertaining to)	= postnatal	pertaining to (the period) after birth

Prefixes of Position

Prefix	Meaning	Example	Pronunciation
ante-		ante/cubit/ al elbow pertaining to	ăn-tē-KŪ-bǐ-tăl
pre-	before, in front	pre/operative operation	prē-ŎP-ĕr-ă-tǐv
pro-		pro/ot/ ic ear pertaining to	prō-ŎT-ǐk
epi-	above, upon	epi/derm/is skin noun ending	ĕp-ǐ-DĔR-mǐs
hypo-		hypo/derm/ic skin relating to	hī-pō-DĔR-mǐk
infra-	under, below	infra/pub/ ic pubis relating to	ǐn-fră-PŪ-bǐk
sub-		sub/nas/ al nose pertaining to	sŭb-NĀ-zăl

Prefixes of Position (Continued)

Prefix	Meaning	Example	Pronunciation
inter-	between	inter/cost/al ribs pertaining to	ĭn-tĕr-KŌS-tăl
medi-	middle	medi/al pertaining to	MĒ-dē-ăl
meso-		meso/derm skin	MĔS-ō-dĕrm
post-	after, behind	post/nat/ al birth pertaining to	pōst-NĀ-tăl
retro-	backward, behind	retro/peritone/ al peritoneum pertaining to	rĕt-rō-pĕr-ĭ-tō-NĒ-ăl

Prefixes of Number and Measurement

Prefix	Meaning	Example	Pronunciation
bi-	two	bi/later/al side relating to	bī-LĂT-er-ăl
dipl-	double, twofold	dipl/opia vision	dĭp-LŌ-pē-ă
diplo-		diplo/cocci spherical bacteria	dĭp-lō-KŎK-sī
hemi-	half	hemi/plegia paralysis	hĕm-ē-PLĒ-jē-ă
semi-		semi/circul/ar circle pertaining to	sĕm-ē-SŬR-kū-lăr
hyper-	excessive, above normal	hyper/glyc/ emia glucose, sugar blood	hī-pĕr-glī-SĒ-mē-ă
macro-	large	macro/cephal/y head noun ending	măk-rō-SĔF-ă-lē
micro-	small	micro/scope instrument to view	MĪ-krō-skōp
mono-	one	mono/nucle/ ar nucleus pertaining to	mŏn-ō-NŪ-klē-ăr
uni-		uni/para to bear (offspring)	ū-NĬP-ă-ră
multi-	many, much	multi/para to bear (offspring)	mŭl-TĬP-ă-ră
poly-		poly/phobia fear(s)	pŏl-ē-FŌ-bē-ă
primi-	first	primi/gravida pregnancy	prī-mĭ-GRĂV-ĭ-dă
quadri-	four	quadri/plegia paralysis	kwŏd-rĭ-PLĒ-jē-ă
tri-	three	tri/ceps heads	TRĪ-sĕps

Prefixes of Negation

Prefix	Meaning	Example	Pronunciation
a-*	without, not	a/mast/ ia breast condition	ă-MĂS-tē-ă
an-†		an/esthes/ ia sensation condition	ăn-ĕs-THĒ-zē-ă
im-	in, not	im/potency potent	ĬM-pō-tĕn-sĭ
in-		in/sane sound	ĭn-SĀN

*Usually used before a consonant.
† Usually used before a vowel.

Prefixes of Direction

Prefix	Meaning	Example	Pronunciation
ab-	from, away from	ab/norm/ al regular, pertaining to usual	ăb-NOR-măl
ad-	toward	ad/stern/ al sternum, relating to breastbone	ăd-STĔR-năl
circum-	around	circum/or/ al mouth pertaining to	sĕr-kŭm-Ō-răl
peri-		peri/oste/ itis bone inflammation	pĕr-ē-ŏs-tē-Ĭ-tĭs
ec-	out, out from	ec/top/ ia place condition	ĕk-TŌ-pē-ă
ex-		ex/cise to cut	ĕk-SĪZ
dia-	through, across	dia/rrhea flow	dī-ă-RĒ-ă
trans-		trans/fusion a pouring	trăns-FŪ-zhŭn
ecto-	outside, outward	ecto/derm skin	ĔK-tō-dĕrm
exo-		exo/trop/ ia turning condition	ĕks-ō-TRŌ-pē-ă
extra-		extra/ocul/ar eye pertaining to	ĕks-tră-ŎK-ū-lăr
endo-	in, within	endo/cardi/ um heart noun ending	ĕn-dō-KĂR-dē-ŭm
intra-		intra/muscul/ar muscle relating to	ĭn-tră-MŬS-kū-lăr
para-*	near, beside, beyond	para/nas/ al nose pertaining to	păr-ă-NĂ-săl
super-	above, excessive	super/sensitive sensation	soo-pĕr-SĔNS-ĭ-tĭv
supra-		supra/ren/ al kidney pertaining to	soo-pră-RĒ-năl

*para- may also be used as a suffix, at which time it means to bear (offspring).

Other Prefixes

Prefix	Meaning	Example	Pronunciation
anti-	against	anti/bacteria/al bacteria pertaining to	ăn-tī-băk-TĒ-rē-ăl
contra-		contra/ception conceiving	kŏn-tră-SĔP-shŭn
brady-	slow	brady/card/ ia heart noun ending, condition	brăd-ē-KĂR-dē-ă
dys-	bad, painful, difficult	dys/pep/sia digestion	dĭs-PĔP-sē-ă
eu-	good, normal	eu/pnea breathing	ūp-NĒ-ă
hetero-	different	hetero/sex/ual sex pertaining to	hĕt-ĕr-ō-SĔK-shū-ăl
homo-	same	homo/sex/ual sex pertaining to	hō-mō-SĔK-shū-ăl
mal-	bad	mal/nutrition food substances	măl-nū-TRĬSH-ŭn
pan-	all	pan/hyster/ ectomy uterus excision	păn-hĭs-tĕr-ĔK-tō-mē
pseudo-	false	pseudo/plegia paralysis	soo-dō-PLĒ-jē-ă
syn-*	union, together, joined	syn/arthr/osis joint abnormal condition	sĭn-ăr-THRŌ-sĭs
tachy-	rapid	tachy/pnea breathing	tăk-ĭp-NĒ-ă

*Appears as sym- before b, p, ph, or m.

WORSHEET 1

Place a slash after each prefix, and then define the prefix.

Word	Definition of Prefix
1. inter/dental	between
2. hypodermic	
3. epigastrium	
4. retroactive	
5. subnasal	
6. medial	
7. infrapatellar	
8. postnatal	
9. quadriplegia	
10. hyperlipidemia	
11. primipara	
12. microcephaly	
13. triceps	
14. polydipsia	
15. impotent	
16. anaerobic	
17. macrocephaly	
18. intramuscular	
19. suprarenal	
20. diarrhea	
21. circumrenal	
22. adhesion	
23. perirenal	
24. bradycardia	
25. tachypnea	

26. dyspnea   _____

27. eupnea   _____

28. heterograft   _____

29. malfunction   _____

30. periosteum   _____

WORKSHEET 2

. . . .

Match the medical words that follow with the definitions in the numbered list.

diarrhea   macrocephaly   preoperative
ectoderm   medial   primigravida
epidermis   microscope   quadriplegia
hemiplegia   monocyte   retroperitoneal
hypodermic   periosteum   subnasal
impotent   polyphobia   suprarenal
intercostal   postoperative

PREFIXES OF POSITION AND DIRECTION

1. _____ pertaining to behind the peritoneum

2. _____ pertaining to under the skin

3. _____ before surgery

4. _____ pertaining to under the nose

5. _____ after surgery

6. _____ pertaining to between the ribs

7. _____ pertaining to the middle

8. _____ around the bone

9. _____ flow through (watery bowel movement)

10. _____ outside the skin

11. _____ above the kidney

PREFIXES OF NUMBER AND MEASUREMENT

12. _____ paralysis of one half of the body

13. _____ paralysis of four limbs

14. _____ abnormally large head

15. _____ instrument to view minute objects

16. _____ many fears

17. _____ first pregnancy

WORKSHEET 3

Prefixes of Negation and Other Prefixes

Match the following medical words with the definitions in the numbered list.

amastia	dyspepsia	malnutrition
anesthesia	dysphagia	pseudomembranous
antibacterial	eupnea	synarthosis
bradycardia	heterosexual	tachycardia
contraception	homosexual	

1. _____ difficult digestion

2. _____ pertaining to the opposite sex

3. _____ pertaining to a false membrane

4. _____ against bacteria

5. _____ slow heartbeat

6. _____ poor or bad nutrition

7. _____ without a breast

8. _____ without sensation

9. _____ good or normal breathing

10. _____ abnormal condition of a united joint

11. _____ rapid heartbeat

12. _____ against conception

13. _____ pertaining to the same sex

BODY STRUCTURE

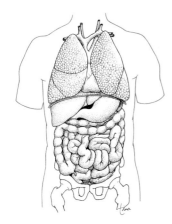

Chapter Outline

Student Objectives

Levels of Organization
Cells
Tissues
Organs
Systems
Organism

The Disease Process

Anatomical Position

Planes of the Body

Body Cavities

Abdominopelvic Region

Diagnostic Imaging

The Spine

Directional Terms

Combining Forms
Combining Forms Denoting Cellular
Structures

Combining Forms Denoting
Anatomical Directions
Combining Forms Denoting Regions
of the Body
Combining Forms Denoting Colors
Other Combining Forms Related
to Body Structure

Suffixes

Prefixes

**Diagnostic, Symptomatic,
and Therapeutic Terms**

Diagnostic Procedures
Imaging Procedures

Surgical and Therapeutic Procedures

Abbreviations

Medical Record
Radiology Report of Cervical
and Lumbar Spine

Worksheets

Student Objectives

Upon completion of this chapter, you will be able to do the following:

1. List and briefly define the levels of organization in the human body.

2. Demonstrate an understanding of the disease process by defining medical terms associated with pathology.

3. List and identify four body planes.

4. List two dorsal cavities and two ventral cavities, and identify at least one organ within each cavity.

5. List and locate nine sections of the abdominopelvic region and the four quadrants of the same area.

6. Demonstrate an understanding of body imaging by defining terms associated with radiology, computed tomography, magnetic resonance imaging, and ultrasonography.

Student Objectives (Continued)

7. Define directional terms and be able to use them correctly.
8. Identify combining forms, suffixes, and prefixes related to body structure.
9. Identify diagnostic, symptomatic, and therapeutic terms related to the body structure.
10. Identify diagnostic procedures related to body structure.
11. Identify surgical and therapeutic procedures related to the body structure.
12. Define the abbreviations related to body structure.
13. Demonstrate your knowledge of the chapter by completing the worksheets.

This chapter is an overview of body structure and presents terms related to the body as a whole, rather than to any specific body system. Review the material carefully because it provides a foundation for the remaining chapters of the book.

LEVELS OF ORGANIZATION

The body is composed of different levels of structure and function. Each of these levels incorporates the structures and functions of the previous level, contributing to the entire organism. The levels of organization are as follows:

Cellular level → Tissue level → Organ level → System level → Organismic level

Cells

The **cell** is the structural and functional unit of life. Although it is small in size, it is composed of many intricate organelles that are responsible for a variety of specialized functions. Individual cells perform all activities that we associate with living (eating, eliminating waste, breathing, reproducing). The way different cells undertake these activities may vary considerably, but the end result is the same. The study of the body at the cellular level is called **cytology**. An understanding of cytology is important because the disease process originates at the cellular level.

Tissues

Groups of cells that perform a specialized activity are called **tissues**. The study of tissues is called **histology**. The four major tissues of the body are:

- **Epithelial tissue**, composed of cells arranged in a continuous sheet consisting of one or several layers; forms the epidermis of the skin, covers surfaces of organs, lines cavities and canals, forms tubes, ducts, and secreting portions of glands
- **Connective tissue**, supports and connects other tissues and organs
- **Muscle tissue**, contractile tissue of the body
- **Nervous tissue**, tissue capable of transmitting electrical impulses

Organs

Organs are body structures composed of at least two different tissue types that perform specialized functions. For example, the stomach is composed of muscle tissue and epithelial tissue. The muscle tissue moves food through the stomach, and epithelial tissue secretes enzymes and gastric products for digestion.

Systems

The next level of organization is a **system**. A body system is composed of at least one organ and accessory structures that have similar or interrelated functions. For example, the organs and accessory structures of the gastrointestinal system include the esophagus, stomach, and small intestine. The purpose of this system is to digest food, extract nutrients from it, and eliminate waste products. Some of the other body systems are the reproductive, respiratory, and cardiovascular systems.

Organism

The highest level of organization is the **organism**. This is a complete living entity capable of independent existence. All complex organisms, including humans, are composed of several body systems that work together to sustain life.

THE DISEASE PROCESS

Although most people understand the concept of **disease**, a clinical definition is quite complex. From the clinical point of view, disease is a **pathological** or **morbid condition** of the body that presents a group of **signs, symptoms,** and **clinical findings**. Signs are objective indicators that are observable by others. A palpable mass and tissue redness are examples of signs. In contrast, a symptom is subjective and is experienced only by the patient. Dizziness, pain, and malaise are examples of symptoms. Clinical findings are results of laboratory examinations and other tests performed on the patient.

All body cells require oxygen and nutrients for survival. They also need a stable internal environment that provides a narrow range of temperature, water, acidity, and salt concentration. This stable internal environment is called **homeostasis**. When homeostasis is significantly interrupted and cells, tissues, organs, or systems are unable to meet the challenges of everyday life, the condition is called **pathology**. As each phase of pathology progresses, signs, symptoms, and clinical findings change. The study of the progression of a disease is called **pathogenesis**. Pathogenesis varies from disease to disease.

Etiology is the study of all factors involved in the development of a disease. The following list identifies several types of diseases and gives an example.

- Metabolic (diabetes)
- Infectious (measles, mumps)
- Congenital (cleft lip)
- Hereditary (hemophilia)
- Environmental (burns, trauma)
- Neoplastic (cancer)

Establishing the cause and nature of a disease is referred to as **diagnosis**. Determining a diagnosis helps the physician to select a method of treatment. A **prognosis** is the prediction of the course of a disease and its probable outcome. Any disease whose cause is unknown is said to be **idiopathic**.

ANATOMICAL POSITION

The **anatomical position** is placement of the body in a stance that is accepted by anatomists throughout the world. In this position, the body is erect and the eyes are looking forward. The

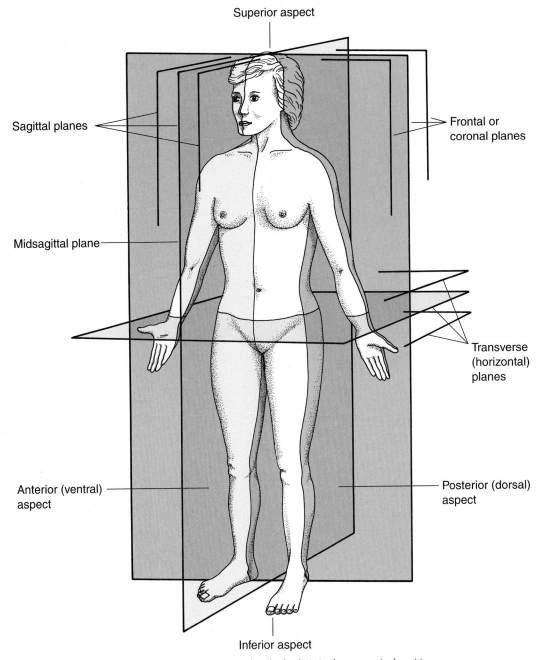

Figure 5–1   Body planes. Note that the body is in the anatomical position.

upper limbs hang to the sides, with the palms facing to the front; the lower limbs are parallel, with the toes pointing forward. Regardless of whether the body actually lies facing upward or downward, or how the limbs are actually placed, the positions and relationships of a structure are always described as if the body were in the anatomical position (Fig. 5–1).

PLANES OF THE BODY

An **anatomical plane** of the body is an imaginary flat surface that passes through the body at different places in order to divide it for anatomical purposes. Several commonly used anatomical planes are illustrated in Figure 5–1. Table 5–1 lists body planes and describes their anatomical divisions.

Table 5–1   PLANES OF THE BODY

Body Plane	Anatomical Division
Midsagittal or median	Right and left halves
Sagittal	Unequal right and left sides
Coronal or frontal	Front side (anterior or ventral aspect) and back side (posterior or dorsal aspect)
Transverse or horizontal	Upper portion (superior aspect) and lower portion (inferior aspect)

BODY CAVITIES

The body has two major cavities: the **dorsal cavity** (posterior) and the **ventral cavity** (anterior). Each of these cavities has further subdivisions that are shown in Figure 5–2. Table 5–2 lists the body cavities and some of the major organs found within them. The thoracic cavity is separated from the abdominopelvic cavity by a muscular wall, the **diaphragm**.

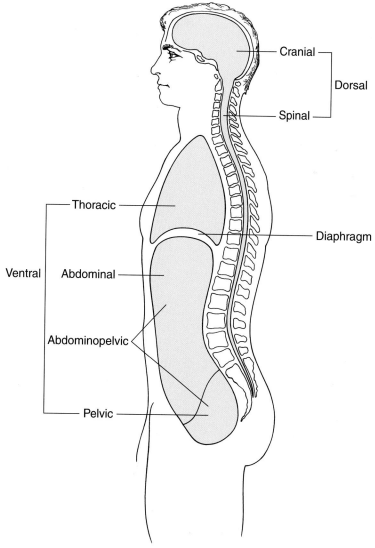

Figure 5–2   Body cavities.

Table 5–2 BODY CAVITIES

Cavity	Major Organ(s) Found in the Cavity
Dorsal	
Cranial	Brain
Spinal	Spinal cord
Ventral	
Thoracic	Heart, lungs, and associated structures
Abdominopelvic	Digestive, excretory, and reproductive systems and associated structures

ABDOMINOPELVIC REGION

The abdominopelvic region may be divided into nine major sections by constructing an imaginary "tic-tac-toe" over this region. This provides divisions to locate the placement of internal or **visceral** organs. Operative reports frequently refer to these divisions as a point of reference to designate

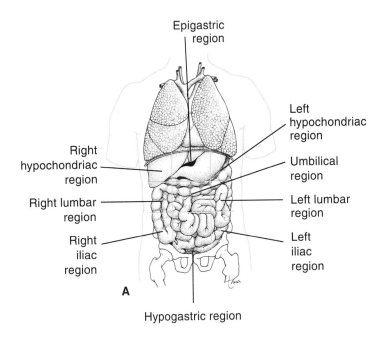

Epigastric region

Left hypochondriac region

Right hypochondriac region

Umbilical region

Right lumbar region

Left lumbar region

Right iliac region

Left iliac region

A

Hypogastric region

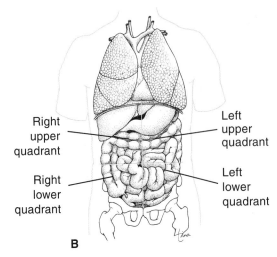

Right upper quadrant

Left upper quadrant

Right lower quadrant

Left lower quadrant

B

Figure 5–3 Areas of the abdomen. (A) Nine regions. (B) Four quadrants. (Adapted from Scanlon, VC and Sanders, T: Understanding Human Structure and Function. F.A. Davis, Philadelphia, 1997, p 15, with permission.)

exact locations of tumors, ulcers, and body structures. The nine regions of the body (Fig. 5–3A) from left to right and top to bottom are as follows:

Region	Location
Epigastric	Region of the stomach
Right hypochondriac	Upper right region beneath the ribs
Left hypochondriac	Upper left region beneath the ribs
Right lumbar	Right middle lateral region
Umbilical	Region of the navel
Left lumbar	Left middle lateral region
Right iliac	Right lower lateral region
Hypogastric	Lower middle region beneath the navel
Left iliac	Left lower lateral region

For purposes of clinical evaluation, the abdominopelvic region may be divided into four quadrants (sections) by an imaginary cross (Fig. 5–3B).

Right upper quadrant (RUQ)	Left upper quadrant (LUQ)
Right lower quadrant (RLQ)	Left lower quadrant (LLQ)

DIAGNOSTIC IMAGING

Recent advances in body imaging procedures have greatly reduced the need for exploratory surgery. Current techniques for examining underlying structures include radiography, computed tomography (CT) scan, magnetic resonance imaging (MRI), and ultrasonography (echography, sonography).

The oldest and most widely used of these methods is **radiography (roentgenography)**, more commonly called **x-ray examination**. In this technique, an energy beam in the x band of the radiation spectrum passes through the area of the body to be examined. Although some x-rays are absorbed by the structures through which the beam passes, the remainder of the x-rays falls on the radiographic film placed behind the area to be examined. Denser tissue absorbs more of the beam than does tissue of a lesser density. Because of the difference in densities of various tissues, an image, called a radiograph or x-ray film, is produced. It is a negative image similar to a photographic negative produced by a camera.

In its early applications, radiography was used almost exclusively to visualize bones because bones are very dense and abnormalities are easily seen. With the advent of **radiopaque materials** (substances that absorb x-rays), the use of radiography expanded to include visualization of many soft tissues of the body.

Computed tomography (CT) scan is a variation of the radiographic technique just described. CT scan, however, is more sensitive than conventional radiographic examination and is particularly valuable in detecting soft body tissue diseases. In this procedure, the x-ray beam circles around a central axis of the body or an organ. The data obtained are computerized and then reconstructed to generate an image. This image appears as a "slice" of an organ or body part. The term *tomography* literally means "a recording or record of a slice."

Magnetic resonance imaging (MRI) is another type of scanning technique. However, a magnetic field rather than an x-ray beam is used to produce the image. A magnetic field induces tissue to produce **radiofrequency (RF)** waves. These waves are sensed by a receiving device called an **RF detector coil**, which sends them to a computer. The computer then generates an image of the tissue and provides three views from different angles: axial, sagittal, and coronal. Different tissues can be distinguished because each emits a different radio signal. MRI often produces sharper images of soft tissue than those obtained using CT scans. MRI also has the advantage over CT scans in that it does not employ the potentially harmful radiation associated with x-rays.

Ultrasonography is a technique that reflects high-frequency sound (ultrasonic) waves off internal tissues. A detector called a transducer converts ultrasonic waves to electrical impulses and then displays them on a video monitor. The resultant images are not as clear as those produced with x-rays or RF waves, but ultrasonography is easy to use and inexpensive and causes little or no risk to the patient. Ultrasonography is used extensively in maternofetal diagnostics.

THE SPINE

The spine is divided into sections corresponding to the vertebrae, which are located in the spinal column. (For a more complete discussion, refer to Chapter 11, Musculoskeletal System.) These divisions are as follows:

- Cervical (neck)
- Thoracic (chest)
- Lumbar (loin)
- Sacral (lower back)
- Coccyx (tailbone)

DIRECTIONAL TERMS

Directional terms are used to indicate the position of a structure in relation to another structure. For example, the kidneys are superior to (above) the urinary bladder. The directional term "superior to" denotes "above" the structure, which, in this example, is the urinary bladder. In the following list, opposing terms are presented consecutively to aid in memorization.

Superficial	Toward the surface of the body
Deep	Away from the surface of the body (internal)
Abduction	Movement away from the median plane of the body or one of its parts
Adduction	Movement toward the median plane of the body
Medial	Pertaining to the midline of the body or structure
Lateral	Pertaining to a side
Superior (Cephalad)	Toward the head or upper portion of a structure
Inferior (Caudal)	Away from the head, or toward the tail or lower part of a structure
Proximal	Near the attachment of an extremity to the trunk or a structure
Distal	Farther from the attachment of an extremity to the trunk or a structure
Anterior (Ventral)	Near the front of the body
Posterior (Dorsal)	Near the back of the body
Parietal	Pertaining to the outer wall of the body cavity
Visceral	Pertaining to an organ
Prone	Lying horizontal with the face downward, or denoting the hand with palms turned downward

Supine	Lying on the back with the face upward, or denoting the position of the hand or foot with the palm or foot facing upward
Inversion	Turning inward or inside out
Eversion	Turning outward
Palmar	Pertaining to the palm of the hand
Plantar	Pertaining to the sole of the foot

COMBINING FORMS

Combining Forms Denoting Cellular Structure

Combining Form	Meaning	Example	Pronunciation
cyt/o	cell	cyt/o/logist one who studies	sī-TŎL-ō-jĭst
hist/o	tissue	hist/o/logy study of	hĭs-TŎL-ō-jē
nucle/o	nucleus	nucle/o/toxin poison	NŪ-klē-ō-tŏk-sĭn

Combining Forms Denoting Anatomical Directions

Combining Form	Meaning	Example	Pronunciation
anter/o	anterior, front	anter/o/posterior behind	ăn-tĕr-ō-pŏs-TĒ-rē-ŏr
caud/o	tail	caud/al pertaining to	KAW-dăl
dist/o	far, farthest	dist/al pertaining to	DĬS-tăl
dors/o	back (of body)	dors/al pertaining to	DOR-săl
infer/o	lower, below	infer/ior pertaining to	ĭn-FĒ-rē-or
later/o	side, to one side	later/o/abdomin/al abdomen pertaining to	lăt-ĕr-ō-ăb-DŎM-ĭ-năl
medi/o	middle	medi/o/later/al side pertaining to	mē-dē-ō-LĂT-ĕr-ăl
poster/o	back (of body), behind, posterior	poster/o/later/al side pertaining to	pŏs-tĕr-ō-LĂT-ĕr-ăl
proxim/o	near, nearest	proxim/al pertaining to	PRŎK-sĭm-ăl
ventr/o	belly, belly-side	ventr/al pertaining to	VĔN-trăl

Combining Forms Denoting Regions of the Body

Combining Form	Meaning	Example	Pronunciation
abdomin/o	abdomen	abdomin/o/pelv/ ic pelvis pertaining to	ăb-DŎM-ĭ-nō-PĔL-vĭk
acr/o	extremity	acr/o/megaly enlargement	ăk-RŌ-mĕg-ă-lē
inguin/o	groin	inguin/al pertaining to	ĬNG-gwĭ-năl
lumb/o	loin	lumb/o/dynia pain	lŭm-bō-DĬN-ē-ă
omphal/o	navel (umbilicus)	omphal/o/cele herniation	ŏm-FĂL-ō-sēl
pelv/i	pelvis	pelv/i/metry measuring	pĕl-VĬM-ĕ-trē
pelv/o		pelv/o/scopy visual examination	pĕl-VŎS-kō-pē

Combining Forms Denoting Colors

Combining Form	Meaning	Example	Pronunciation
albin/o	white	albin/ism condition	ĂL-bĭn-ĭzm
leuc/o		leuc/o/cyte cell	LOO-kō-sīt
leuk/o		leuk/o/derma skin	loo-kō-DĔR-mă
anthrac/o	black, coal	anthrac/osis abnormal condition	ăn-thră-KŌ-sĭs
chlor/o	green	chlor/o/cyte cell	KLŌ-rō-sīt
cirrh/o	yellow	cirrh/osis abnormal condition	sĭr-RŌ-sĭs
jaund/o		jaund/ice noun ending	JAWN-dĭs
xanth/o		xanth/emia blood	zăn-THĒ-mē-ă
cyan/o	blue	cyan/o/derma skin	sī-ă-nō-DĔR-mă

Combining Forms Denoting Colors (Continued)

Combining Form	Meaning	Example	Pronunciation
erythem/o		erythem/a noun ending	ĕr-ĭ-THĒ-mă
erythr/o	red	erythr/o/cyte cell	ĕ-RĬTH-rō-sīt
rube/o		rube/osis abnormal condition	roo-bē-Ō-sĭs
melan/o	black	melan/oma tumor	mĕl-ă-NŌ-mă
poli/o	gray	poli/o/myel/ itis spinal cord inflammation	pōl-ē-ō-mī-ĕl-Ī-tĭs

Note: In some instances, combining forms of color are also used as prefixes.

Other Combining Forms Related to Body Structure

Combining Form	Meaning	Example	Pronunciation
fasci/o	band	fasci/itis inflammation	făs-ē-Ī-tĭs
home/o	same, alike	home/o/stasis standing still	hō-mē-ō-STĀ-sĭs
idi/o	unknown, peculiar	idi/o/path/ ic disease pertaining to	ĭd-ē-ō-PĂTH-ĭk
path/o	disease	path/o/gen to produce	PĂTH-ō-jĕn
radi/o	radiation, x-ray	radi/o/graphy process of recording	rā-dē-ŎG-ră-fē
somat/o	body	somat/o/path/ ic disease pertaining to	sō-mă-tō-PĂTH-ĭk
viscer/o	internal organs, viscera	viscer/o/megaly enlargement	vĭs-ĕr-ō-MĔG-ă-lē
xen/o	foreign, strange	xen/o/graft tissue transplant	ZĔN-ō-grăft
xer/o	dry	xer/osis abnormal condition	zē-RŌ-sĭs

SUFFIXES

Suffix	Meaning	Example	Pronunciation
-genesis	forming, producing, origin	path/o/genesis disease	păth-ō-JĔN-ĕ-sĭs
-gnosis	knowing	pro/gnosis before	prŏg-NŌ-sĭs
-gram	record, a writing	son/o/gram sound	SŌ-nō-grăm
-graph	instrument for recording	son/o/graph sound	SŌ-nō-grăf
-graphy	process of recording	myel/o/graphy spinal cord	mī-ĕ-LŎG-ră-fē
-pathy	disease	cyt/o/pathy cell	sī-TŎP-ĭ-thē

PREFIXES

Prefix	Meaning	Example	Pronunciation
ab-	from, away from	ab/axi/ al axis pertaining to	ăb-ĂK-sē-ăl
ad-	toward	ad/duction movement	ă-DŬK-shŭn
allo-	other, differing from the usual	allo/plasty surgical repair	ĂL-ō-plăs-tē
infra-	below, under	infra/cost/al rib pertaining to	ĭn-fră-KŎS-tăl
peri-	around	peri/cardi/ um heart noun ending	pĕr-ĭ-KĂR-dē-ŭm
super-	upper, above	super/ior pertaining to	soo-PĒ-rē-or
trans-	across, through	trans/ocul/ar eye pertaining to	trăns-ŎK-ū-lăr
ultra-	excess, beyond	ultra/sound sound	ŬL-tră-sound

DIAGNOSTIC, SYMPTOMATIC, AND THERAPEUTIC TERMS

Term	Meaning
ablation ăb-LĀ-shŭn	removal of a part, pathway, or function by surgery, chemical destruction, electrocautery, or radiofrequency (RF)
adhesion ăd-HĒ-zhŭn	a uniting or holding together of two surfaces or parts, as in wound healing
dehiscence dē-HĬS-ĕns	the bursting open of a wound, especially a surgical abdominal wound
nuclear medicine NŪ-klē-ăr	the branch of medicine involved with the use of radioactive substances for diagnosis, therapy, and research
polyp PŎL-ĭp	a tumor with a pedicle, commonly found in vascular organs such as the nose, uterus, and rectum
radiopharmaceutical rā-dē-ō-fărm-ă-SŪ-tĭ-kăl	radioactive chemicals used in testing the location, size, outline, or function of tissues, organs, vessels, or body fluids
sepsis SĔP-sĭs	pathological state, usually febrile, resulting from the presence of microorganisms or their products in the bloodstream
suppurative SŬP-ū-rā-tĭv	producing or associated with generation of pus

DIAGNOSTIC PROCEDURES

Imaging Procedure	Description
digital radiography (computerized radiography) DĬJ-ĕt-ăl rā-dē-ŎG-ră-fē	radiographic imaging procedure using a computer screen instead of conventional x-ray film
fluoroscopy floo-or-ŎS-kō-pē	a technique that uses an x-ray to project an image onto a television monitor; this provides live images and allows the observer to study the function of the organ as well as its structures
magnetic resonance angiography măg-NĔT-ĭc RĔZ-ĕn-ăns ăn-jē-ŎG-ră-fē	an imaging technique that uses a magnetic filed to visualize vascular structures
magnetic resonance imaging (MRI) măg-NĔT-ĭc RĔZ-ĕn-ăns ĬM-ĭj-ĭng	a noninvasive imaging technique that uses a magnetic field rather than an x-ray beam to produce an image, especially of the brain, spine, joints, and internal organs, which are usually poorly seen on conventional radiographs and CT scans
positron emission tomography (PET) scan PŎZ-ĭ-trŏn ē-MĬSH-ŭn tō-MŎG-ră-fē	a cross-sectional transverse plane that identifies metabolic and physiological function in tissues
sonography sō-NŎG-ră-fē	a technique that uses high-frequency sound waves to produce an image; used to display various body parts, including breast, major veins and arteries (Doppler), kidney, spleen, and eye, and is a valuable diagnostic tool for prenatal evaluation of the fetus
stereoradiography stĕr-ē-ō-rā-dē-Ŏg-ră-fē	the process of taking x-rays from two slightly different angles so that when they are viewed through a stereoscope the structure has the appearance of solidity and relief as though seen in three dimensions

SURGICAL AND THERAPEUTIC PROCEDURES

Procedure	Description
anastomosis ă-năs-tō-MŌ-sĭs	the joining together of two ducts or blood vessels to allow flow from one to the other; bypass
biopsy BĪ-ŏp-sē	the obtaining of a representative tissue sample for microscopic examination, usually to establish a diagnosis
needle	the removal of tissue by use of a needle, usually attached to a syringe
punch	removal of a small bit of tissue by use of a hollow punch
cauterize KAW-tĕr-īz	to destroy tissue by electricity, freezing, heat, or corrosive chemicals
curettage kū-rĕ-TĂZH	scraping of a body cavity with a spoon-shaped instrument called a curette (curet)
frozen section	microscopic examination of slides prepared with fresh tissue; used for rapid diagnosis of malignancy, while patient awaits surgery, to determine conservative or radical approach
incision and drainage (I&D) ĭn-SĬZH-ŭn DRĀN-ĭj	a incision made to allow the free flow or withdrawal of fluids from a wound or cavity
laser surgery LĀ-zĕr SŬR-jĕr-ē	a surgical procedure that employs a device that emits intense heat and power at close range. The device converts various frequencies of light into one small and extremely intense unified beam of one-wavelength radiation
ligation lī-GĀ-shŭn	the process of binding or tying using a band, bandage, thread, or wire
resection rē-SĔK-shŭn	partial excision of a bone, organ, or other structure
radical dissection RĂD-ĭ-kăl dī-SĔK-shŭn	the surgical removal of tissue in an extensive area surrounding the surgical site, in an attempt to excise all tissue that may possibly be malignant to decrease the chance of recurrence (e.g., radical mastectomy)

ABBREVIATIONS

Abbreviations	Meaning
AP	anteroposterior
CNS	central nervous system
CT scan, CAT scan	computed tomography scan, computed axial tomography scan
CV	cardiovascular
Dx	diagnosis
GI	gastrointestinal

ABBREVIATIONS (Continued)

Abbreviations	Meaning
GU	genitourinary
I&D	incision and drainage
LAT, lat	lateral
LLQ	left lower quadrant
LUQ	left upper quadrant
MRI	magnetic resonance imaging
MS	musculoskeletal
PA	posteroanterior
RLQ	right lower quadrant
ROM	range of motion
RUQ	right upper quadrant
sono	sonogram, sonography
U&L, U/L	upper and lower

MEDICAL RECORD

Radiology Report of Cervical and Lumbar Spine

AP, lateral, and odontoid views of the cervical spine demonstrate some reversal of normal cervical curvature, as seen on lateral projection. There is some right lateral scoliosis of the cervical spine. The vertebral bodies, however, appear to be well maintained in height; the intervertebral spaces are well maintained. The odontoid is visualized and appears to be intact. The atlantoaxial joint appears symmetrical.

Impression   Films of the cervical spine demonstrate some reversal of normal cervical curvature and a minimal scoliosis, possibly secondary to muscle spasm, without evidence of recent bony disease or injury.

AP and lateral films of the lumbar spine, with spots of the lumbosacral junction, demonstrate an apparent minimal spina bifida occulta of the first sacral segment. The vertebral bodies, however, are well maintained in height; the intervertebral spaces appear well maintained.

Pathological Diagnosis   Right lateral scoliosis with some reversal of normal cervical curvature.

Worksheet 5 provides a dictionary and reading application and an analysis of this medical record.

WORSHEET 1

Match the following elements with the definitions in the numbered list.

hist/o   ventr/o   infra-
home/o   -cyte   mono-
later/o   -gram   peri-
nucle/o   -graphy   ultra-

1. _____ tissue

2. _____ record, a writing

3. _____ excess, beyond

4. _____ belly side

5. _____ same

6. _____ cell

7. _____ below, under

8. _____ process of recording

9. _____ around

10. _____ to one side

WORKSHEET 2

■ ■ ■ ■ ■ ■ ■ ■ ■ ■ ■ ■ ■ ■

Match the following directional terms with the definitions in the numbered list.

abduction   inferior   proximal
adduction   inversion   superior
anterior   lateral   supine
digital   medial   umbilical
distal   posterior
eversion   prone

1. _____ pertaining to the side

2. _____ pertaining to the midline of the body or structure

3. _____ farther from the attachment of an extremity to the trunk or structure

4. _____ near the attachment of an extremity to the trunk or a structure

5. _____ lying on the back with the face upward

6. _____ lying horizontal with the face downward

7. _____ movement toward the median plane

8. _____ movement away from the median plane

9. _____ toward the head or upper portion of the body or structure

10. _____ away from the head or toward the tail or lower part of a structure

11. _____ near the front of the body (ventral)

12. _____ near the back of the body (dorsal)

13. _____ turning inward or inside out

14. _____ turning outward

WORSHEET 3

■ ■ ■ ■ ■ ■ ■ ■ ■ ■ ■ ■

Match the following medical words with the definitions in the numbered list.

diagnosis   pathologist   symptom
etiology   prognosis   tomography
homeostasis   radiography   ultrasonography
MRI   radiologist   x-ray
morbid   radiopaque material
pathogenesis   sign

1. _____ study of the cause of disease

2. _____ specialist in the study of radiography

3. _____ specialist in study of disease

4. _____ diseased or pathological

5. _____ origin or development of a disease

6. _____ objective indicator of a disease

7. _____ a subjective experience such as pain or dizziness

8. _____ the probable outcome of a disease

9. _____ the determination of the cause and nature of a disease

10. _____ a stable internal environment

11. _____ substance that absorbs x-rays, used to visualize soft tissue

12. _____ literally means a "record of a slice"

13. _____ uses a magnetic field rather than an x-ray beam to produce an image

14. _____ a technique that reflects high-frequency sound waves off internal tissues to produce an image

15. _____ the beam of radiation used to produce a radiographic image

WORKSHEET 4

Match the following medical words with the definitions in the numbered list.

ablation   dissection   radiopharmaceutical
adhesion   I&D   resection
anastomosis   laser surgery   sepsis
curettage   ligation   suppurative
cauterize   nuclear medicine   ultrasonography
dehiscence   radical surgery

1. _____ pathological state, resulting from the presence of microorganisms or their products in the blood

2. _____ a uniting or holding together of two surfaces or parts

3. _____ removal of a part, pathway, or function by surgery, chemical destruction, electrocautery, or radiofrequency

4. _____ pus forming, associated with the production of pus

5. _____ radioactive chemicals used in testing the location, size, outline, or function of tissues, organs, vessels, or body fluids

6. _____ the branch of medicine involved with the use of radioactive substances for diagnosis, therapy, and research

7. _____ a bursting open of a wound, especially a surgical abdominal wound

8. _____ scraping of a body cavity with a spoon-shaped instrument

9. _____ surgical procedure that employs intense heat and power at close range

10. _____ an incision made to allow the free flow or withdrawal of fluids from a wound or cavity

11. _____ partial excision of a bone, organ, or other structure

12. _____ the removal of tissue in an extensive area surrounding the surgical site

13. _____ the process of binding or typing using a band, bandage, thread, or wire

14. _____ the joining together of two ducts or vessels to allow the flow from one to the other; bypass

15. _____ to destroy tissue by electricity, freezing, heat, or corrosive chemicals

WORSHEET 5

■ ■ ■ ■ ■ ■ ■ ■ ■ ■ ■ ■ ■

MEDICAL RECORD: RADIOLOGY REPORT OF CERVICAL AND LUMBAR SPINE

Underline the following terms in the medical record (see p. 55). Use a medical dictionary and other resources to define the terms and to determine their pronunciation; then practice reading the medical record aloud.

AP _____

atlantoaxial joint _____

cervical _____

intervertebral spaces _____

lateral _____

lumbar spine _____

lumbosacral _____

odontoid _____

scoliosis _____

spasm _____

spina bifida occulta _____

vertebral _____

MEDICAL RECORD EVALUATION: RADIOLOGY REPORT OF CERVICAL AND LUMBAR SPINE

1. *Why was an x-ray film taken of the cervical spine?*

2. *Did the patient appear to have experienced any type of recent injury to the spine?*

3. *What cervical vertebrae form the atlantoaxial joint?*

4. *Was the odontoid process fractured?*

5. *What did the radiologist believe was the possible cause of the minimal scoliosis?*

WORKSHEET 6

. . . .

Label the abdominopelvic regions on Figure A and label the body quadrants on Figure B.
Compare your answers with Figure 5–3A and B, page 46.

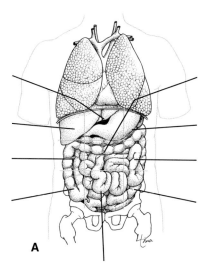

A

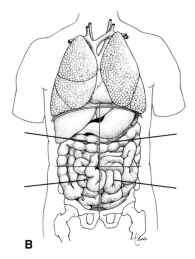

B

Epigastric region
Hypogastric region
Left hypochondriac region
Left iliac region
Left lower quadrant
Left lumbar region
Left upper quadrant
Right hypochondriac region
Right iliac region
Right lower quadrant
Right lumbar region
Right upper quadrant
Umbilical region

Chapter 6

INTEGUMENTARY SYSTEM

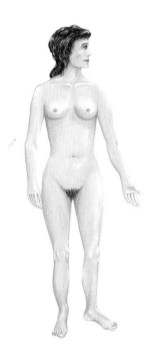

Chapter Outline

Student Objectives

Anatomy and Physiology
Skin
Appendages of the Skin
  Hair
  Glands
  Nails
  Breasts

Combining Forms

Suffixes

Prefixes

Pathology
Primary Skin Lesions
Secondary Skin Lesions
Burns
Frostbite

Oncology
  Basal Cell Carcinoma
  Breast Cancer
  Squamous Cell Carcinoma
  Malignant Melanoma

**Diagnostic, Symptomatic,
  and Therapeutic Terms**

Diagnostic Procedures
Imaging Procedures

Surgical and Therapeutic Procedures

Pharmacology

Abbreviations

Medical Record
Pathology Report of Skin Lesion

Worksheets

Student Objectives

Upon completion of this chapter, you will be able to do the following:

1. Define the main functions of the integumentary system and its appendages.
2. List the appendages of the integumentary system.
3. Identify combining forms, suffixes, and prefixes related to the integumentary system.
4. Identify several primary and secondary skin lesions.
5. Explain and identify major skin problems caused by exposure.
6. Identify diagnostic, symptomatic, and therapeutic terms related to the integumentary system.
7. Identify the diagnostic procedures related to the integumentary system.
8. Identify surgical and therapeutic procedures related to the integumentary system.
9. Define the abbreviations related to the integumentary system.
10. Explain pharmacology related to the treatment of integumentary disorders.
11. Demonstrate your knowledge by completing the worksheets.

ANATOMY AND PHYSIOLOGY

The largest organ in the body is the skin (**integument**). Together with the hair, nails, glands, and breasts, the skin constitutes the **integumentary system**.

Skin

The skin covers all outer surfaces of the body and performs many important functions. It protects against injuries and bacterial invasion, aids in regulation of body temperature, and prevents dehydration. The skin also acts as a reservoir for food and water, works as a sensory receptor, and is responsible for the synthesis of vitamin D when exposed to sunlight. The skin is composed of two layers, the epidermis and the dermis, as shown in Figure 6–1.

The (1) **epidermis**, a layer of tissue with no blood or nerve supply, is the outermost layer of skin. It is made up of cells in several **strata** or sublayers called **stratified squamous epithelium**. The most important of these four or five sublayers are the (2) **stratum corneum** and the (3) **stratum germinativum**.

The stratum germinativum includes a basal layer where new cells are formed. As the cells move toward the outermost layer of the epidermis, the stratum corneum, they die and become filled with a hard protein material called **keratin**. The relatively waterproof characteristic of keratin

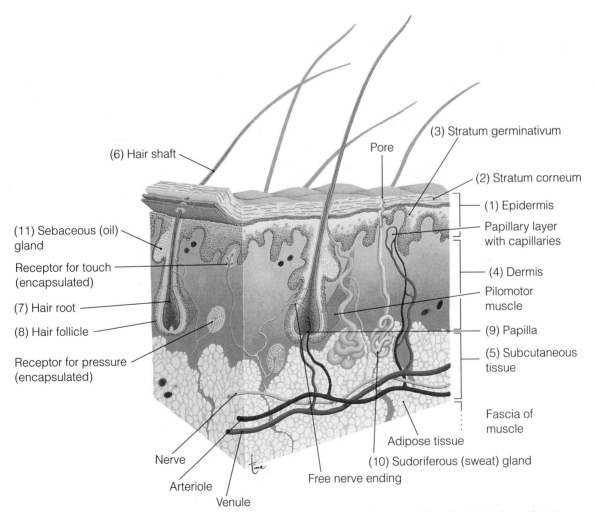

Figure 6–1   Structure of the skin and subcutaneous tissue. (Adapted from Scanlon, VC and Sanders, T: Understanding Human Structure and Function. F.A. Davis, Philadelphia, 1997, p 75, with permission.)

prevents body fluids from evaporating and atmospheric moisture from entering the body. Eventually, the keratinized cells are worn off and replaced by underlying cells that, in turn, become keratinized and die. The entire process by which a cell forms in the basal layers, rises to the surface, becomes keratinized, and sloughs off takes about 1 month.

The (4) **dermis**, or **corium**, is the layer of skin lying immediately under the epidermis. It is composed of living tissue that consists of numerous capillaries, lymphatics, and nerve endings. Hair follicles, sebaceous (oil) glands, and sweat glands are also located in the dermis. The (5) **subcutaneous tissue**, or **hypodermis**, is an underlying connective tissue layer that contains fat or adipose tissue and connects the skin to underlying organs.

Appendages of the Skin

Hair

The visible part of the hair is referred to as the (6) **hair shaft**, whereas the part that is embedded in the dermis is called the (7) **hair root**. The root, together with its coverings, forms the (8) **hair follicle**. At the bottom of the follicle is a loop of capillaries enclosed in a covering called the (9) **papilla**. The cluster of epithelial cells lying over the papilla reproduces and is responsible for the eventual formation of the hair shaft. As long as these cells remain alive, hair will regenerate even if it is cut, plucked, or otherwise removed. Baldness (**alopecia**) occurs when the hairs of the scalp are not replaced because of death of these cells.

Glands

Two important glands in the skin that produce secretions are the (10) **sudoriferous (sweat) glands** and the (11) **sebaceous (oil) glands**.

The sudoriferous glands are small structures that open as **pores** on the surface of the skin. They are found on the palms, soles, forehead, and armpits (axillae). The main functions of the sudoriferous glands are to cool the body by evaporation, to excrete waste products through the pores of the skin, and to moisten surface cells.

The sebaceous glands are the oil-secreting glands of the skin. These glands are filled with cells, the centers of which are saturated with fatty droplets. As these cells disintegrate, they yield an oily secretion called **sebum**. The acidic nature of sebum helps to destroy harmful organisms on the skin's surface and thus to prevent infection. Sebaceous glands are present over the entire body, except on the soles of the feet and the palms of the hands. They are especially prevalent on the scalp and face; around openings such as the nose, mouth, external ear, and anus; and on the upper back and scrotum.

Nails

The nails protect the tips of the fingers and toes from bruises and other kinds of injuries. The nailbed covers the dorsal surface of the last bone of each finger and toe. Most of the nail body appears pink because of the underlying vascular tissue. The crescent-shaped white area near the root of the nailbed is the **lunula**. It has a whitish appearance because the vascular tissue underneath does not show through. The lunula is the area in which new growth occurs.

Breasts

The breasts (Fig. 6–2), or mammary glands, are located in the upper anterior aspect of the chest. During puberty, the woman's breasts develop as a result of periodic stimulation of ovarian hormones estrogen and progesterone. Estrogen is responsible for (1) **adipose tissue** and increased size of the breasts as they reach full maturity. The size of the breast is basically determined by the amount of fat around the glandular tissue, but breast size is not indicative of functional ability. The other ovarian hormone, progesterone, forms the lobules that are present in the breast. Each breast has approximately 20 lobes of (2) **glandular tissue**. Milk in these lobes is drained by a

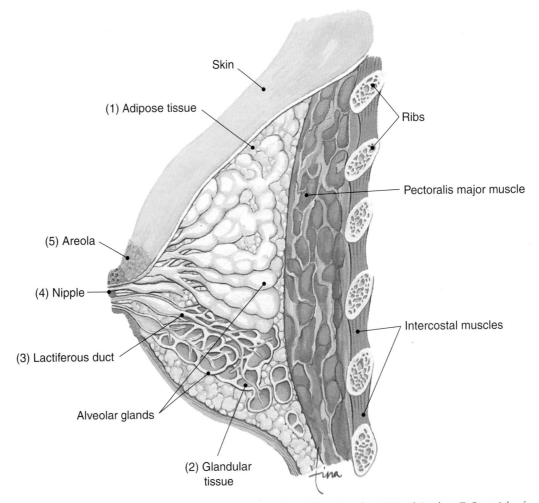

Skin

(1) Adipose tissue

Ribs

Pectoralis major muscle

(5) Areola

(4) Nipple

Intercostal muscles

(3) Lactiferous duct

Alveolar glands

(2) Glandular tissue

Figure 6–2 Mammary gland shown in midsagittal section. (Adapted from Scanlon, VC and Sanders, T: Essentials of Anatomy and Physiology, ed 2. F.A. Davis, Philadelphia, 1995, p 468, with permission.)

(3) **lactiferous duct** that opens on the tip of the raised (4) **nipple**. Circling the nipple is a border of slightly darker skin called the (5) **areola**.

The main purpose of the breasts is to secrete milk for the nourishment of newborn infants. Thus, pregnancy causes the breasts to enlarge for this function. In women, breasts fully develop by age 16. At menopause, breast tissue begins to atrophy.

COMBINING FORMS

Combining Form	Meaning	Example	Pronunciation
aden/o	gland	aden/o/pathy disease	ăd-ĕ-NŎP-ă-thē
adip/o		adip/oma tumor	ă-dĭ-PŌ-mă
lip/o	fat	lip/oid resembling	LĬP-oyd
steat/o		steat/oma tumor	stē-ă-TŌ-mă
crypt/o	hidden	onych/o/crypt/osis nail abnormal condition	ŏn-ĭ-kō-krĭp-TŌ-sĭs
cutane/o		sub/cutane/ous under pertaining to	sŭb-kū-TĀ-nē-ŭs
dermat/o	skin	dermat/itis inflammation	dĕr-mă-TĪ-tĭs
derm/o		derm/is noun ending	DĔR-mĭs
hidr/o	sweat	hidr/aden/ oma gland tumor	hī-drăd-ĕ-NŌ-mă
ichthy/o	dry, scaly	ichthy/osis abnormal condition	ĭk-thē-Ō-sĭs
kerat/o	horny tissue, hard, cornea	kerat/osis abnormal condition	kĕr-ă-TŌ-sĭs
lact/o	milk	lact/ic pertaining to	LĂK-tĭk
mamm/o		mamm/o/plasty surgical repair	MĂM-ō-plăs-tē
mast/o	breast	mast/ectomy excision	măs-TĔK-tŏ-mē
myc/o	fungus	dermat/o/myc/osis skin abnormal condition	dĕr-mă-tō-mī-KŌ-sĭs
onych/o		onych/o/malacia softening	ŏn-ĭ-kō-mă-LĀ-sē-ă
ungu/o	nail	ungu/al pertaining to	ŬNG-gwăl
pil/o		pil/o/nid/ al nest pertaining to	pī-lō-NĪ-dăl
trich/o	hair	trich/o/pathy disease	trĭk-ŎP-ă-thē
scler/o	hardening	scler/osis abnormal condition	sklĕ-RŌ-sĭs
squam/o	scaly	squam/ous pertaining to	SKWĀ-mŭs
thel/o	nipple	thel/itis inflammation	thē-LĪ-tĭs
xer/o	dry	xer/o/derma skin	zē-rō-DĔR-mă

SUFFIXES

Suffix	Meaning	Example	Pronunciation
-cyte	cell	lip/o/cyte fat	LĬP-ō-sīt
-derma	skin	scler/o/derma hardening	sklĕr-ă-DĔR-mă
-gram	record	mamm/o/gram breast	MĂM-ō-grăm
-graph	instrument for recording	mamm/o/graph breast	MĂM-ō-grăf
-graphy	process of recording	mamm/o/graphy breast	măm-ŎG-ră-fē
-logist	specialist in the study of	dermat/o/logist skin	dĕr-mă-TŎL-ō-jĭst
-logy	study of	dermat/o/logy skin	dĕr-mă-TŎL-ō-jē
-therapy	treatment	dermat/o/therapy skin	dĕr-mă-tō-THĔR-ă-pē

PREFIXES

Prefix	Meaning	Example	Pronunciation
epi-	above, upon	epi/derm/ is skin noun ending	ĕp-ĭ-DĔR-mĭs
hyper-	excessive, above normal	hyper/hidr/ osis sweat abnormal condition	hī-pĕr-hī-DRŌ-sĭs
hypo-	under, below	hypo/derm/ic skin pertaining to	hī-pō-DĔR-mĭk
sub-	under, below	sub/cutane/ous skin pertaining to	sŭb-kū-TĀ-nē-ŭs

PATHOLOGY

Primary Skin Lesions

Areas of pathologically altered tissue are called **lesions**. Figure 6–3 illustrates and Table 6–1 describes several primary skin lesions.

Secondary Skin Lesions

Secondary skin lesions are pathological skin alterations that are a result of a primary skin lesion. During the healing process, scabs **(crustations)** form over sores and wounds. The crusts are composed of dry pus, lymph, or blood and may vary in color and thickness.

When trauma, chemicals, or burns cause a superficial loss of tissue, the resulting skin lesion is called an **excoriation**. Excoriation is often caused by a scraping or rubbing away **(abrasion)** of

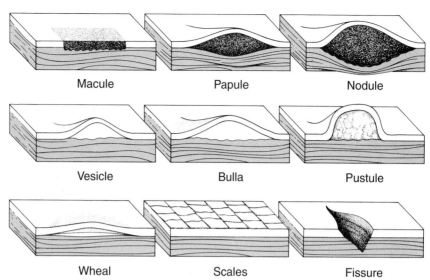

Figure 6–3 Skin lesions. (From Gylys, BA and Masters, RM: Medical Terminology Simplified, ed 2. F.A. Davis, Philadelphia, 1998, p 163, with permission.)

epidermal tissue. When tissue injury exists without skin breakage, it is called a bruise (**contusion**). A more serious injury results when a wound is produced by the tearing of body tissue (**laceration**), as distinguished from a cut or incision. A laceration may be small or large and may be caused in many ways. Some common causes are a blow from a blunt instrument, a fall against a rough surface, and an accident with machinery.

Table 6–1   SKIN LESIONS

Type	Characteristics	Example
Flat Lesion		
Macule	Flat, discolored, circumscribed lesion of any size	Freckle, flat mole, hyperpigmentation
Elevated Lesion		
Papule	Solid elevated lesion, <1 cm in diameter	Nevus, warts, pimples
Nodule	Palpable circumscribed lesion, larger than a papule, 1–2 cm in diameter	Benign or malignant tumor
Wheal	Dome-shaped or flat-topped elevated lesion, slightly reddened and often changing in size and shape, usually accompanied by intense itching	Hives
Vesicle and bulla	Elevated lesion that contains fluid; a bulla is a vesicle >0.5 cm	Blister, herpes zoster, second-degree burn
Pustule	Elevated lesion containing pus that may be sterile or contaminated with bacteria; small abscess on the skin	Acne, pustular psoriasis
Scale	Excessive dry exfoliation shed from upper layers of the skin	Psoriasis, ichtryosis
Cyst	Elevated, encapsulated mass of dermis or subcutaneous layers, solid or fluid-filled	Sebaceous cyst
Tumor	Swelling; well-demarcated, elevated lesion >2 cm in diameter	Fibroma, lipoma, steatoma, melanoma, hemangioma
Depressed Lesion		
Fissure	Small cracklike sore or break exposing the dermis; usually red	Athlete's foot, cheilosis
Ulcer	Loss of epidermis and dermis within a distinct border	Pressure sore, basal cell carcinoma

Ulcers are open wounds. As they heal, a scar (**cicatrix**) often develops. Excessive scarring may produce an enlarged thickened scar (**keloid**) that may grow for a prolonged period of time. A predisposition to keloid formation is thought to be hereditary and occurs more often in dark-skinned people. Although this complication can have serious cosmetic implications, it is not life-threatening.

Burns

Burns are thermal injuries to the outer surfaces of the body. They can be classified according to three major categories, depending on the degree of severity (Fig. 6–4).

First-degree burns are superficial burns. The skin damage is limited to the top layers of the epidermis. These burns are distinguished by redness of the skin (**erythema**) and extreme sensitivity (**hyperesthesia**) to sensory stimuli, especially touch.

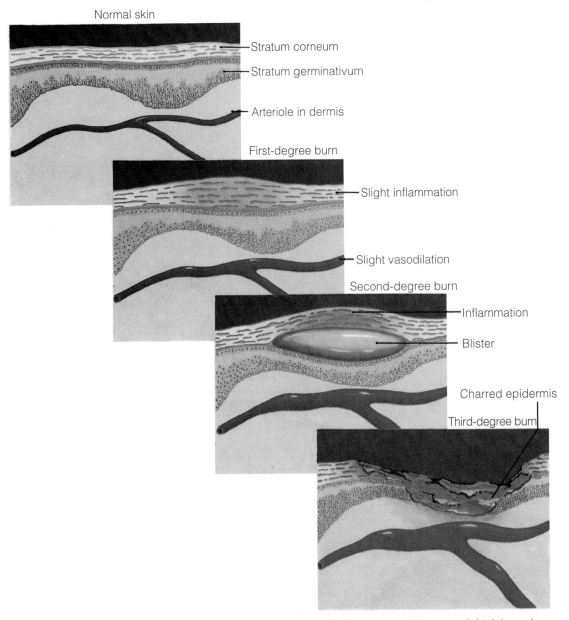

Figure 6–4 Normal skin section and representative sections showing first-degree, second degree, and third degree burns. (From Scanlon, VC and Sanders, T: Essentials of Anatomy and Physiology, ed 2. F.A. Davis, Philadelphia, 1995, p 90, with permission.)

Second-degree burns are characterized by the formation of fluid-filled blisters (**vesicles** or **bullae**), caused by deeper penetration of heat. In most instances, a second-degree burn will not result in the formation of scar tissue.

Third-degree burns, which penetrate both the epidermis and the dermis, cause complete destruction of skin tissue and represent the most serious type of burn. This type of burn usually results in scar formation, which can be altered only by the process of skin grafting (**dermatoplasty**). When more than two-thirds of the body's skin is destroyed, death usually results because of excessive loss of body fluids. Without the proper amount of body fluids, the brain, heart, and other organs cannot perform their normal functions.

Frostbite

Frostbite causes a local destruction of the skin as a result of freezing. Like burns, frostbite is classified according to its degree of severity: first-, second-, and third-degree.

Oncology

New autonomous growths (**neoplasms**) must be **microscopically** examined to determine if they are **malignant** or **benign**. Tumors are considered malignant when they invade normal tissue and eventually establish additional malignancies in other parts of the body (**metastasize**). Malignant neoplasms constitute the disease known as cancer. The location (**site**) and type of malignancy influence the spread of cancer through the body. Pathologists **grade** and **stage** tumors to help in diagnosis and treatment of the disease. Tumor grading (Table 6–2) is an evaluation of the degree of malignancy in a tumor. The TNM system of staging (Table 6–3) determines the extent to which a tumor has spread through the body. **T** refers to size and extent of the primary **tumor**. **N** indicates number of area lymph **nodes** involved. **M** refers to any **metastases** of the primary tumor.

The treatment of cancer includes chemotherapy and radiation, both of which can cause hair loss (**alopecia**). These treatments cause alopecia by damaging stem cells and hair follicles. The hair becomes brittle and may fall out or break off at the surface of the scalp. Loss of other body hair is less common. Hair loss is a minor problem compared with the potentially life-threatening consequences of malignancy.

Basal Cell Carcinoma

Basal cell carcinoma, the most common type of skin cancer, which is often caused by overexposure to sunlight, is a malignancy of the basal cell layer of the epidermis, the stratum germinativum (see Fig. 6–1). These tumors grow slowly, but as they increase in size they often ulcerate and develop crusting that is firm to the touch. Although metastases occur infrequently with this type of cancer, the disease can invade the tissue sufficiently to destroy an ear, nose, or eyelid.

Table 6–2 TUMOR GRADING

Grading	Characteristics of Tumor
Grade I: Tumor cells well differentiated	Closely resembles normal parent tissue; thus retains some specialized functions
Grade II: Tumor cells moderately differentiated	Less resemblance to tissue of origin; more variation in size and shape of tumor cells; increased mitoses
Grade III: Tumor cells poorly to very poorly differentiated	Does not closely resemble tissue of origin; much variation in shape and size of tumor cells; greatly increased mitoses
Grade IV: Tumor cells very poorly differentiated	No resemblance to tissue of origin; great variation in size and shape of tumor cells

Table 6–3   TNM SYSTEM OF STAGING

T_0	No evidence of primary tumor
T_{IS}	Carcinoma in situ
T_1, T_2, T_3, T_4	Progressive increase in tumor size and involvement
T_X	Tumor cannot be assessed
N_0	Regional lymph nodes not demonstrably abnormal
N_1, N_2, N_3, N_4	Increasing degrees of demonstrable abnormality and increasingly distant location of spread
N_X	Regional lymph nodes cannot be assessed
M_0	No evidence of distant metastasis
M_1, M_2, M_3	Ascending degrees of distant metastasis

Source: Adapted from Classification and Staging of Cancer by Site: A Preliminary Handbook. American Joint Committee for Cancer Staging and End Results Reporting, 1976.

Breast Cancer

Breast cancer, also called **carcinoma of the breast**, is the most common malignancy of women in the United States. This disease seems to be associated with ovarian hormonal function. In addition, a diet high in fats appears to increase the incidence of breast cancer. Other contributing factors include a family history of the disease and possibly the use of estrogen replacement therapy. Women who have not borne children (**nulliparous**) or those who have had an early onset of menstruation (**menarche**) or late onset of menopause are also more likely to develop breast cancer. Because this type of malignancy is highly responsive to treatment when detected early, women are urged to practice breast self-examination monthly and to receive mammography after age 40. Many breast malignancies are detected by the patient.

Squamous Cell Carcinoma

Squamous cell carcinoma is a tumor of the epidermis. There are two types: **in situ** (in position) and **invasive**. Because of its ability to invade and spread, this type of malignancy must be treated.

Malignant Melanoma

Malignant melanoma is a cancerous tumor of the skin originating from pigment cells (**melanocytes**) in the epidermis and dermis. The incidence of melanoma is doubling every 10 to 20 years. There is strong evidence that sunlight exposure is an important contributing factor for this disease. Avoiding the sun and using sunscreen have proved effective in preventing the disease.

Melanoma is diagnosed by biopsy. The primary mode of treatment at this time is excision. The extent of surgery is determined by staging the disease (see Table 6–3).

DIAGNOSTIC, SYMPTOMATIC, AND THERAPEUTIC TERMS

Term	Meaning
abscess ĂB-sĕs	a localized collection of pus in any body part that results from invasion of a pyogenic (pus-forming) bacterium
acne ĂK-nē	papular and pustular eruption of the skin
carbuncle KĂR-bŭng-kĕl	pyogenic infection of the skin
cellulitis sĕl-ū-LĪ-tĭs	inflammation of cellular or connective tissue

DIAGNOSTIC, SYMPTOMATIC, AND THERAPEUTIC TERMS
(Continued)

Term	Meaning
chloasma klō-ĂZ-mă	hyperpigmentation of the skin characterized by yellowish-brown patches or spots
comedo KŎM-ē-dō	blackhead; discolored dried sebum plugging an excretory duct of the skin
decubitus ulcer dē-KŪ-bĭ-tŭs ŬL-sĕr	lesion due to impaired circulation in a portion of the body surface caused by prolonged pressure especially from a bed or chair; most frequently found in skin overlying a bony projection such as the hip, ankle, heel, shoulder, or elbow; also known as a bedsore
dermatomycosis dĕr-mă-tō-mī-KŌ-sĭs	fungal infection of the skin
desquamation dĕs-kwă-MĀ-shŭn	shedding of the epidermis
ecchymosis ĕk-ĭ-MŌ-sĭs	skin discoloration consisting of large, irregularly formed hemorrhagic area, with color changing from blue-black to greenish-brown or yellow (Fig. 6–5)
eczema ĔK-zĕ-mă	inflammatory skin disease with erythema, papules, vesicles, pustules, scales, crusts, and scabs, either alone or in combination
erythema ĕr-ĭ-THĒ-mă	inflammatory redness of the skin
eschar ĔS-kăr	damaged tissue following a severe burn
hirsutism HĔR-soot-ĭzm	condition characterized by the excessive growth of hair or presence of hair in unusual places, especially in women
impetigo ĭm-pĕ-TĪ-gō	inflammatory skin disease characterized by isolated pustules that become crusted and rupture
keratosis kĕr-ă-TŌ-sĭs	thickened area of the epidermis; any horny growth on the skin (i.e., a callus or wart)
lentigo lĕn-TĪ-gō	small brown macules or yellow-brown pigmented areas of skin, sometimes caused by exposure to the sun and weather
pallor PĂL-ŏr	unnatural paleness or absence of color in the skin
pediculosis pē-dĭk-ū-LŌ-sĭs	infestation with lice, transmitted by personal contact or common use of brushes, combs, or headgear

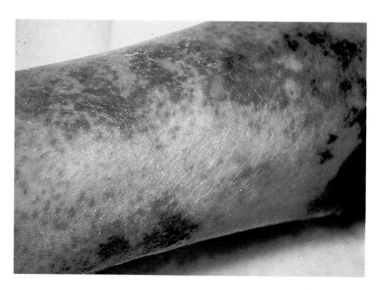

Figure 6–5 Ecchymosis on the skin of a leg. (From Harmening, DM: Clinical Hematology and Fundamentals of Hemostasis, ed 3. F.A. Davis, Philadelphia, 1997, p 527, with permission.)

DIAGNOSTIC, SYMPTOMATIC, AND THERAPEUTIC TERMS (Continued)

Term	Meaning
pemphigus PĔM-fĭ-gŭs	acute or chronic adult disease characterized by the occurrence of successive crops of vesicles (bullae) that appear suddenly on apparently normal skin and then disappear, leaving pigmented spots
petechia, petechiae (pl) pē-TĔ-kē-ă, pē-TĔ-kē-ē	minute or small hemorrhagic spot on the skin (petechia is a smaller version of ecchymosis)
pruritus proo-RĪ-tŭs	an itching
psoriasis sō-RĪ-ă-sĭs	chronic skin disease characterized by itching, red macules, papules, or plaques covered with silvery scales
purpura PŬR-pū-ră	any of several bleeding disorders characterized by hemorrhage into the tissues, particularly beneath the skin or mucous membranes, producing ecchymoses or petechiae
scabies SKĀ-bēz	contagious skin disease transmitted by the itch mite
tinea TĬN-ē-ăh	any fungal skin disease, frequently caused by ringworm, whose name often indicates the body part affected (e.g., tinea barbae [beard], tinea corporis [body], tinea pedis [athlete's foot], tinea versicolor [skin])

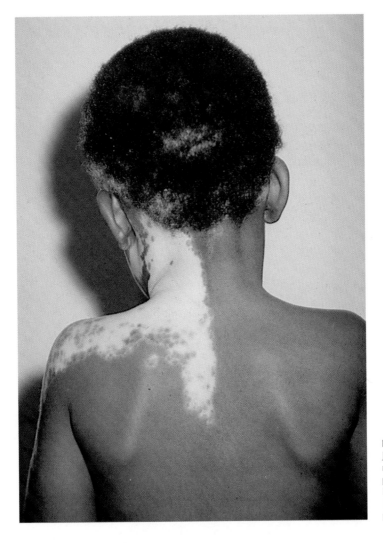

Figure 6–6 Vitiligo. (From Reeves, JRT and Maibach, HI: Clinical Dermatology Illustrated: A Regional Approach, ed 3. MacLennan and Petty Ptd Ltd, Rosebery, Australia, 1998, [distributed by F.A. Davis, Philadelphia], p 265, with permission.)

DIAGNOSTIC, SYMPTOMATIC, AND THERAPEUTIC TERMS
(Continued)

Term	Meaning
urticaria ŭr-tĭ-KĀ-rē-ă	allergic reaction of the skin characterized by the eruption of pale red elevated patches called wheals (hives)
vitiligo vĭt-ĭl-Ī-gō	localized loss of skin pigmentation characterized by milk-white patches (Fig. 6–6)
verruca (wart), verrucae (pl) vĕr-ROO-kă, vĕr-ROO-kē	epidermal growth caused by a virus, which includes plantar warts, juvenile warts, and venereal warts; removable by cryosurgery, electrocautery, or acids; able to regrow if virus remains in the skin

DIAGNOSTIC PROCEDURES

Imaging Procedure	Description
mammography, mammogram măm-ŎG-ră-fē, MĂM-ō-grăm	radiographic examination of the breast to detect abnormalities of breast tissue
xeromammography, xeromammogram, xeroradiography zē-rō-măm-MŎG-ră-fē, zē-rō-MĂM-mō-grăm, zē-rō-rā-dē-ŎG-ră-fē	process to produce x-ray images on paper rather than on x-ray film; especially beneficial in diagnosis of breast tumors and minute breast calcifications

SURGICAL AND THERAPEUTIC PROCEDURES

Procedure	Description
allograft ĂL-ō-grăft	transplant tissue obtained from the same species
biopsy BĪ-ŏp-sē	excision of a small piece of tissue by use of a syringe and needle or through a surgical procedure for microscopic examination; usually performed to establish a diagnosis
debridement dā-brēd-MŎN	removal of foreign material and dead or damaged tissue, especially in a wound
dermabrasion DĔRM-ă-brā-zhŭn	removal of acne scars, nevi, tattoos, or fine wrinkles on the skin through the use of sandpaper, wire brushes, or other abrasive materials on the anesthetized epidermis
fulguration fŭl-gū-RĀ-shŭn	tissue destruction by means of high-frequency electric sparks
lumpectomy lŭm-PĔK-tō-mē	excision of a small primary breast tumor, leaving the remainder of the breast intact
mammoplasty, mastoplasty MĂM-ă-plăs-tē, MĂS-tō-plăs-tē	surgical reconstruction of the breast(s), sometimes augmented by substances such as fat tissue or silicone to alter the size and shape
mastectomy	excision of the breast
radical	removing the breast and any involved skin, pectoral muscles, axillary lymph nodes, and subcutaneous fat
skin graft	using the skin from another part of the body, or from a donor, to repair a defect or trauma of the skin
xenograft	transplant tissue obtained from a different species

PHARMACOLOGY

Medication	Action
anti-infectives, antibacterials, antifungals	agents that eliminate epidermal infections, which can be administered either topically or systemically. Topical medications create a skin environment that is lethal to microbes. Generally, a specific fungicide must be prescribed for a given fungus strain, whereas one antibiotic effectively eliminates several types of bacteria
anti-inflammatory drugs, topical corticosteroids	these topically applied drugs relieve three common symptoms of skin disorders: pruritus (itching), vasodilation, and inflammation
antipruritics	agents that prevent or relieve itching
antiseptics	topically applied agents that destroy bacteria, thus preventing the development of infections in cuts, scratches, and surgical incisions
keratolytics	agents that destroy and soften the outer layer of skin so that it is sloughed off or shed. The strong keratolytics are effective for removing warts and corns and aid in penetration of antifungal drugs. Milder preparations are used to promote shedding of scales and crusts in eczema, psoriasis, seborrheic dermatitis, and other dry, scaly conditions. Very weak keratolytics irritate inflamed skin, acting as tonics to speed up healing
parasiticides	used to destroy insect parasites that infest the skin. Scabicides kill mites and their eggs. Pediculicides destroy lice and their eggs
protectives	function by covering, cooling, drying, or soothing inflamed skin. Protectives do not penetrate the skin or soften it, but form a long-lasting film, which protects the skin from air, water, and clothing during the natural healing process
topical anesthetics	prescribed for pain on skin surfaces or mucous membranes caused by wounds, hemorrhoids, or sunburn. They relieve pain and itching by numbing the skin layers and mucous membranes and are applied directly by means of sprays, creams, gargles, suppositories, and other preparations

ABBREVIATIONS

Abbreviation	Meaning
Bx	biopsy
decub.	decubitus
derm.	dermatology
FS	frozen section
I&D	incision and drainage
ID	intradermal
SC, sc, subcu, subq	subcutaneous
ung	ointment

MEDICAL RECORD

Pathology Report of Skin Lesion

Specimen   Skin on (a) dorsum left wrist and (b) left forearm, ulnar, near elbow.

Clinical Diagnosis   Bowen's disease versus basal cell carcinoma versus dermatitis.

Microscopic Description   (a) There is mild hyperkeratosis and moderate epidermal hyperplasia with full-thickness atypia of squamous-keratinocytes. Squamatization of the basal cell layer exists. A lymphocytic inflammatory infiltrate is present in the papillary dermis. Solar elastosis is present. (b) Nests, strands, and columns of atypical neoplastic basaloid keratinocytes grow down from the epidermis into the underlying dermis. Fibroplasia is present. Solar elastosis is noted.

Pathological Diagnosis   (a) Bowen's disease of left wrist; (b) nodular and infiltrating basal cell carcinoma of left forearm, near elbow.

Worksheet 5 provides a dictionary and reading application and an analysis of this medical record.

WORKSHEET 1

■ ■ ■ ■ ■ ■ ■ ■ ■ ■ ■ ■ ■

Use **mast/o** *(breast) to build medical words meaning:*

1. pain in the breast _____

2. inflammation of a breast _____

3. any disease of the breast _____

4. without or lack of a breast (development) _____

Use **mamm/o** *(breast) to build medical words meaning:*

5. record (x-ray film) of the breast _____

6. pertaining to the breast _____

Use **adip/o** *or* **lip/o** *(fat) to build medical words meaning:*

7. tumor consisting of fat _____

8. hernia containing fat _____

9. resembling fat _____

10. fat cell _____

Use **dermat/o** *(skin) to build medical words meaning:*

11. inflammation of the skin _____

12. specialist in skin (diseases) _____

Use **onych/o** *(nail, nailbed) to build medical words meaning:*

13. inflammation of the nailbed _____

14. tumor of the nailbed _____

15. disease of the nails _____

16. abnormal condition of the nails caused by a fungus _____

17. softening of the nails _____

18. abnormal condition of a hidden (ingrown) nail _____

Use **trich/o** *(hair) to build medical words meaning:*

19. disease of the hair _____

20. abnormal condition of hair caused by a fungus _____

WORSHEET 2

Build a surgical term meaning:

1. excision of a breast _____

2. surgical repair or reconstruction of a breast _____

3. excision of fat (adipose tissue) _____

4. removal of the nail _____

5. incision of a nail _____

6. surgical repair (plastic surgery) of the skin _____

WORKSHEET 3

Match the following medical words with the definitions in the numbered list.

alopecia   pediculosis   tinea
chloasma   pedicterus   urticaria
ecchymosis   petechiae   verruca (wart)
impetigo   scabies   vitiligo

1. _____ infestation with lice

2. _____ depigmentation in areas of the skin characterized by milk-white patches

3. _____ any fungal skin disease, especially ringworm

4. _____ a contagious skin disease transmitted by the itch mite

5. _____ a skin infection characterized by vesicles that become pustular and crusted and then rupture

6. _____ severe itching of the skin, also known as hives

7. _____ hyperpigmentation of the skin, characterized by yellowish-brown patches or spots

8. _____ hemorrhagic spot or bruise on the skin

9. _____ minute or small hemorrhagic spots on the skin

10. _____ loss or absence of hair

WORSHEET 4

Match the following words with the definitions in the numbered list.

antibacterials   desquamation   parasiticides
antipruritics   electrodesiccation   patch test
antiseptics   fulguration   protectives
astringents   keratolytics   pruritus
dermabrasion   mammography

1. _____ agents that prevent or relieve itching

2. _____ topically applied agents that destroy bacteria

3. _____ agents used to shrink the blood vessels locally, dry up seeping lesions and
   secretions, and lessen skin sensitivity

4. _____ use of sandpaper, wire brushes, or other abrasive materials to remove acne
   scars, nevi, tattoos, or fine wrinkles

5. _____ agents that kill parasitic skin infestations

6. _____ agents that soften the outer layer of skin so that it sloughs off

7. _____ shedding of the epidermis

8. _____ substance to be tested is applied topically, usually on forearm

9. _____ agents that cool, dry, and soothe inflamed skin

10. _____ an itching

WORSHEET 5

MEDICAL RECORD: PATHOLOGY REPORT OF SKIN LESION

Underline the following terms in the medical record (see p. 77). Use a medical dictionary and other resources to define the terms and to determine their pronunciation; then practice reading the medical record aloud.

atypia _____

basal cell carcinoma _____

Bowen's disease _____

dermatitis _____

dermis _____

dorsum _____

epidermal hyperplasia _____

fibroplasia _____

hyperkeratosis _____

keratinocytes _____

neoplastic _____

papillary _____

pathology _____

solar elastosis _____

squamous _____

ulnar _____

MEDICAL RECORD EVALUATION: PATHOLOGY REPORT OF SKIN LESION

1. What is the basal cell layer in Figure 6–4 referred to as?

2. What was the inflammatory infiltrate?

3. What was the pathologist's diagnosis for the left forearm?

4. What was the pathologist's diagnosis for the left wrist?

WORSHEET 6

Identify the skin lesions depicted here. To check your answers, refer to Figure 6–3.

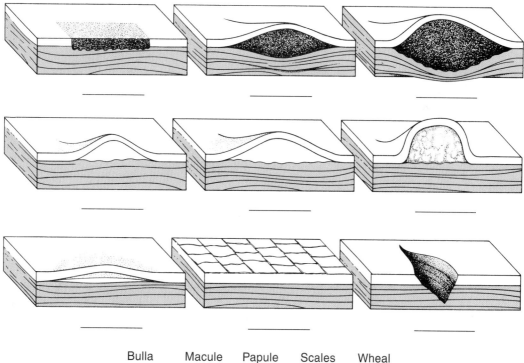

Bulla   Macule   Papule   Scales   Wheal
Fissure   Nodule   Pustule   Vesicle

WORSHEET 7

Label the following illustration. Check your answers by referring to Figure 6–1.

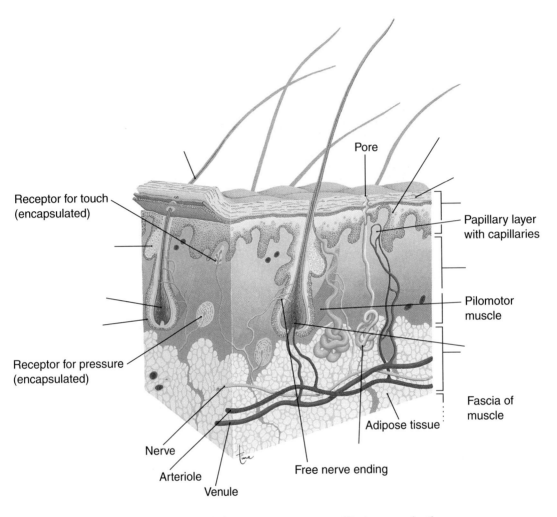

Dermis   Hair shaft   Stratum germinativum
Epidermis   Papilla   Subcutaneous tissue
Hair follicle   Sebaceous (oil) gland   Sudoriferous (sweat) gland
Hair root   Stratum corneum

GASTROINTESTINAL SYSTEM

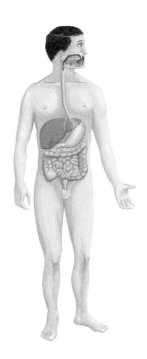

Chapter Outline

Student Objectives

Anatomy and Physiology
Mouth (Oral or Buccal Cavity)
Stomach
Small Intestine (Small Bowel)
Large Intestine (Large Bowel)

Accessory Organs of Digestion
Liver
Pancreas
Gallbladder

Combining Forms
Mouth
Pharynx, Stomach, and Esophagus
Small Intestine and Colon
   (Large Intestine)
Accessory Organs of Digestion: Liver,
   Pancreas, and Biliary System

Suffixes

Prefixes

Pathology
Ulcers
Hernias
Bowel Obstructions
Hemorrhoids
Liver Disorders
Diverticulosis
Oncology

**Diagnostic, Symptomatic,
   and Therapeutic Terms**

Diagnostic Procedures
Imaging Procedures
Endoscopic Procedures
Laboratory Procedures

Surgical and Therapeutic Procedures

Pharmacology

Abbreviations

Medical Record
GI Evaluation

Worksheets

Student Objectives

Upon completion of this chapter, you will be able to do the following:

1. Explain the main functions of the gastrointestinal system.
2. Identify the organs of the alimentary canal.
3. Identify accessory organs of digestion.
4. Explain the role of the liver and gallbladder in digestion.
5. Identify combining forms, suffixes, and prefixes related to the gastrointestinal system.
6. Identify and discuss pathology related to the gastrointestinal system.
7. Identify diagnostic, symptomatic, and therapeutic terms related to the gastrointestinal system.

Student Objectives (Continued)

8. Identify diagnostic procedures related to the gastrointestinal system.
9. Define the abbreviations related to the gastrointestinal system.
10. Explain pharmacology related to treatment of gastrointestinal disorders.
11. Demonstrate your knowledge of the chapter by completing the worksheets.

ANATOMY AND PHYSIOLOGY

The purpose of the gastrointestinal (GI) system is to break down food, prepare it for absorption, and eliminate waste. This system consists of the GI tract, a tube extending from the mouth to the anus. The accessory digestive organs include the teeth, tongue, salivary glands, liver, gallbladder, and pancreas. As you read the following material, refer to Figure 7–1.

Mouth (Oral or Buccal Cavity)

The GI tract begins at the mouth or (1) **oral cavity**. The structures within the oral cavity are the cheeks, or **bucca**, and the (2) **tongue**. The main functions of the tongue are food manipulation during the chewing process, deglutition (swallowing), speech production, and taste. On the upper

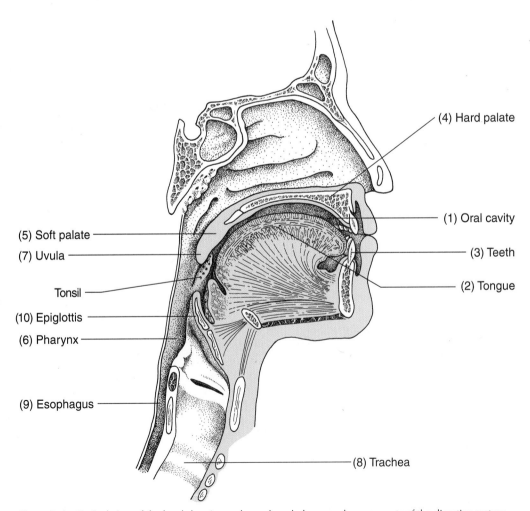

Figure 7–1   Sagittal view of the head showing oral, nasal, and pharyngeal components of the digestive system.

surface of the tongue are small elevations called **papillae**. These sense organs are capable of perceiving four distinct stimuli found in foods: bitterness, sweetness, saltiness, and sourness.

The (3) **teeth**, also found in the oral cavity, play an important role in initial stages of digestion. The chewing process of the teeth, known as **mastication**, mechanically breaks down food into smaller pieces and mixes it with saliva. Teeth are covered by a hard enamel, giving them a white and smooth appearance. Beneath the enamel is the main structure of the tooth, the **dentin**. In the innermost part of the tooth is the **pulp**, which contains nerves and blood vessels. The teeth are imbedded in pink fleshy tissue known as gums, or **gingiva**.

The two structures forming the roof of the mouth are the (4) **hard palate** (the anterior portion) and the (5) **soft palate** (the posterior portion). The soft palate, which forms a partition between the mouth and the nasopharynx, is continuous with the hard palate. The entire oral cavity, like the rest of the digestive tract, is lined with mucous membranes.

After food is chewed, it is formed into a round, sticky mass called a **bolus**, which is pushed by the tongue from the mouth into the (6) **pharynx**, or throat. Its downward movement is guided into the pharynx by the soft, fleshy, V-shaped tissue called the (7) **uvula**.

The pharynx serves as a passageway for air and food. It provides a resonating chamber for speech sounds and has both respiratory and digestive functions.

The funnel-shaped pharynx connects the oral and nasal cavities to the esophagus and trachea. The lowest portion of the pharynx further divides into two tubes: one that leads to the lungs, called the (8) **trachea**, and one that leads to the stomach, called the (9) **esophagus**.

A small flap of tissue, the (10) **epiglottis**, covers the trachea. The main function of the epiglottis is to prevent food from entering the trachea, by channeling it to the stomach through the esophagus.

Stomach

The **stomach** (Fig. 7–2) is a saclike structure located in the left upper quadrant (LUQ) of the abdominal cavity. It extends from the (1) **esophagus** to the first part of the small intestine, the (2) **duodenum**.

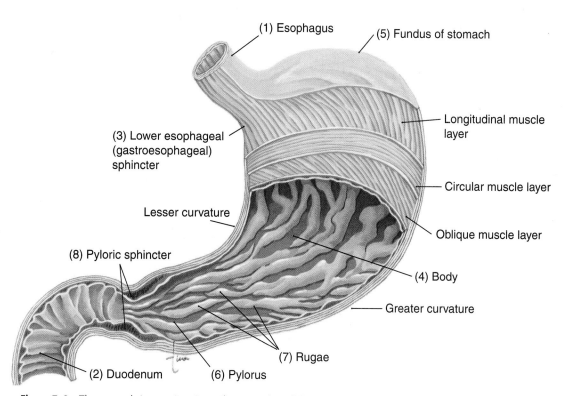

Figure 7–2　The stomach in anterior view. The stomach wall has been sectioned to show the muscle layers and the rugae of the mucosa. (Adapted from Scanlon, VC and Sanders, T: Understanding Human Structure and Function. F.A. Davis, Philadelphia, 1997, p 291, with permission.)

Mechanical and chemical digestion of food takes place in the stomach; food enters the small intestine as a pasty material called **chyme**. The terminal portion of the esophagus is referred to as the (3) **lower esophageal (gastroesophageal) sphincter**, or cardiac sphincter. The muscle fibers of this region constrict after food passes into the stomach, to prevent the stomach contents from being regurgitated into the esophagus. The (4) **body** of the stomach, the large central portion, together with the (5) **fundus**, the upper portion, are mainly storage areas. Most digestion takes place in the funnel-shaped terminal portion, the (6) **pylorus**. The interior lining of the stomach is composed of mucous membranes (mucosa). They are shaped into numerous macroscopic longitudinal folds, called (7) **rugae**, which permit stomach distension. The rugae gradually smooth out as the stomach fills. Located within the rugae are digestive glands, producing hydrochloric acid (HCl) and enzymes. The pylorus narrows to form the duodenal portion of the small intestine

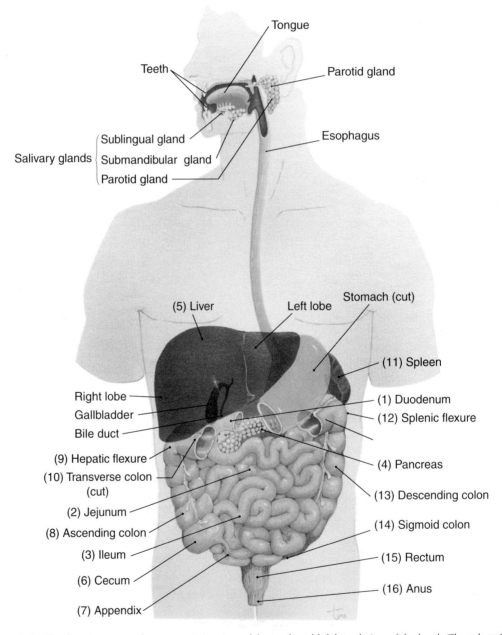

Figure 7–3   The digestive organs shown in anterior view of the trunk and left lateral view of the head. (The spleen is not a digestive organ but is included to show its location relative to the stomach, pancreas, and colon.) (Adapted from Scanlon, VC and Sanders, T: Understanding Human Structure and Function. F.A. Davis, Philadelphia, 1997, p 285, with permission.)

at the (8) **pyloric sphincter**. This junction regulates the movement of chyme into the small intestine and prohibits backflow.

Small Intestine (Small Bowel)

The small intestine, a continuation of the GI tract, is about 21 feet long (Fig. 7–3). Digestion is completed in the small intestine, and the end products of digestion are absorbed into the blood and lymph. The small intestine consists of three parts:

- The (1) **duodenum**, the uppermost division, which is about 10 inches long
- The (2) **jejunum**, which is approximately 8 feet long
- The (3) **ileum**, which is about 12 feet long

Most of the absorption of food takes place in the ileum through tiny, fingerlike projections called **villi**. Inside the villi is a network of fine capillaries, veins, and arterioles that allows food to be absorbed into the bloodstream. Other organs, such as the (4) **pancreas** and (5) **liver**, also produce digestive secretions that combine with chyme in the duodenum.

Large Intestine (Large Bowel)

The large intestine, which is about 5 feet long, extends from the ileum to the anus. It is divided into four major regions: cecum, colon, rectum, and anus (see Fig. 7–3).

The (6) **cecum** is the first 2 or 3 inches of the large intestine. A wormlike projection, the (7) **appendix**, hangs from the cecum. Its function in the digestive system is unknown, but problems arise if it becomes infected or inflamed.

The cecum merges with the colon. The colon is divided into ascending, transverse, descending, and sigmoid portions.

- The (8) **ascending colon** extends from the cecum to the lower border of the liver and turns abruptly to form the (9) **hepatic flexure**.
- The colon continues across the abdomen to the left side as the (10) **transverse colon**, curving beneath the lower end of the (11) **spleen** to form the (12) **splenic flexure**.
- The transverse colon turns downward as the (13) **descending colon** and continues until it forms the (14) **sigmoid colon** and the (15) **rectum**. The rectum, which is the last part of the GI tract, terminates at the (16) **anus**.

The main functions of the colon are to absorb water and minerals and eliminate undigestible material. No digestion takes place in the large intestine. The only secretion of the colonic mucosa is mucus, which lubricates fecal material so it can pass from the body.

ACCESSORY ORGANS OF DIGESTION

Even though food does not pass through the liver, pancreas, and gallbladder, these organs play a vital role in the proper digestion and absorption of nutrients. Refer to Figure 7–4 as you read the following material.

Liver

The (1) **liver**, the largest glandular organ in the body, weighs approximately 3 to 4 lb. It is located beneath the diaphragm in the right upper quadrant (RUQ) of the abdominal cavity. The liver performs many vital activities, and death occurs once its function is lost.

- Production of bile, used in the small intestine to emulsify and absorb fats
- Removal of **glucose** (sugar) from blood, which it synthesizes and stores as **glycogen** (starch)

- Storage of vitamins, such as B_{12}, A, D, E, and K
- Destruction or transformation of some toxic products into less harmful compounds
- Maintenance of normal glucose levels in the blood
- Destruction of old erythrocytes and release of bilirubin
- Production of various blood proteins such as prothrombin and fibrinogen, which aid in the clotting of blood

Pancreas

The (2) **pancreas** is an elongated, somewhat flattened organ that lies posterior and slightly inferior to the stomach. In the digestive system, it provides digestive juice that passes through the (3) **pancreatic duct**. The pancreatic duct extends along the pancreas and, together with the bile duct from the liver, enters the (4) **duodenum**.

Gallbladder

The (5) **gallbladder** serves as a storage area for bile. When bile is needed for digestion, the gallbladder releases it into the duodenum through the (6) **common bile duct**. Bile is also drained from the liver through the (7) **hepatic duct**. The hepatic duct unites with the (8) **cystic duct** and pancreatic duct to form the common bile duct, which transports various digestive juices to the duodenum.

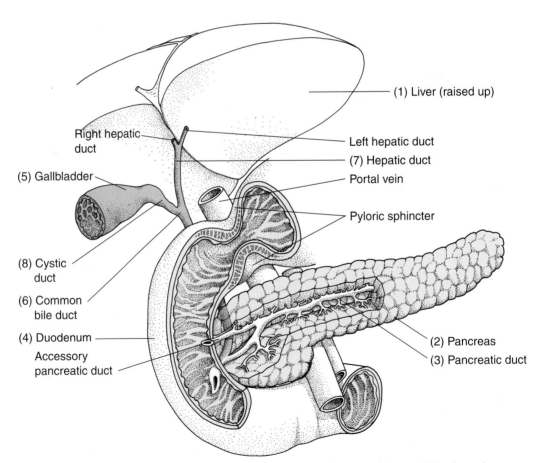

Figure 7–4   The liver, gallbladder, pancreas, and duodenum with associated ducts and blood vessels.

COMBINING FORMS

Mouth

Combining Form	Meaning	Example	Pronunciation
or/o	mouth	or/al pertaining to	OR-ăl
stomat/o		stomat/itis inflammation	stō-mă-TĪ-tĭs
gloss/o	tongue	gloss/ectomy excision	glŏs-ĔK-tō-mē
lingu/o		lingu/al pertaining to	LĬNG-gwăl
bucc/o	cheek	bucc/al pertaining to	BŬK-ăl
cheil/o	lip	cheil/o/plasty surgical repair	KĪ-lō-plăs-tē
labi/o		labi/al pertaining to	LĂ-bē-ăl
dent/o	teeth	dent/ist specialist	DĔN-tĭst
odont/o		orth/odont/ist straight specialist	or-thō-DŎN-tĭst
gingiv/o	gum(s)	gingiv/itis inflammation	jĭn-jĭ-VĪ-tĭs

Pharynx, Stomach, and Esophagus

Combining Form	Meaning	Example	Pronunciation
esophag/o	esophagus	esophag/o/scope instrument to examine	ē-SŎF-ă-gō-skōp
gastr/o	stomach	gastr/o/scopy visual examination	găs-TRŎS-kō-pē
pharyng/o	pharynx (throat)	pharyng/itis inflammation	făr-ĭn-JĪ-tĭs
pylor/o	pylorus	pylor/o/tomy incision, cut into	pī-lor-ŎT-ō-mē

Small Intestine and Colon (Large Intestine)

Combining Form	Meaning	Example	Pronunciation
an/o	anus	an/al 　　pertaining to	Ā-năl
append/o		append/ectomy 　　excision	ăp-ĕn-DĔK-tō-mē
appendic/o	appendix	appendic/itis 　　inflammation	ă-pĕn-dĭ-SĪ-tĭs
col/o		col/o/centesis 　　puncture	kō-lō-sĕn-TĒ-sĭs
colon/o	colon	colon/o/scope 　　instrument to examine	kō-LŎN-ō-skōp
duoden/o	duodenum	duoden/o/stomy 　　forming an opening (mouth)	dū-ŏd-ĕ-NŎS-tō-mē
enter/o	intestine (usually small intestine)	enter/o/pathy 　　disease	ĕn-tĕr-ŎP-ă-thē
ile/o	ileum	ile/o/stomy 　　forming an opening (mouth)	ĭl-ē-ŎS-tō-mē
jejun/o	jejunum	jejun/o/rrhaphy 　　suture	jĕ-joo-NOR-ă-fē
proct/o	anus, rectum	proct/o/plasty 　　surgical repair	PRŎK-tō-plăs-tē
rect/o	rectum	rect/o/cele 　　hernia, swelling	RĔK-tō-sēl
sigmoid/o	sigmoid colon	sigmoid/o/scopy 　　visual examination	sĭg-moy-DŎS-kō-pē

Accessory Organs of Digestion: Liver, Pancreas, and Biliary System

Combining Form	Meaning	Example	Pronunciation
cholangi/o	bile vessel	cholangi/ole 　　small	kō-LĂN-jē-ōl
cholecyst/o	gallbladder	cholecyst/o/gram 　　record	kō-lē-SĬS-tō-grăm
chol/e	bile, gall	chol/emia 　　blood	kō-LĒ-mē-ă
choledoch/o	bile duct	choledoch/o/plasty 　　surgical repair	kō-LĔD-ō-kō-plăs-tē
hepat/o	liver	hepat/oma 　　tumor	hĕp-ă-TŌ-mă

Accessory Organs of Digestion: Liver, Pancreas, and Biliary System (Continued)

Combining Form	Meaning	Example	Pronunciation
pancreat/o	pancreas	pancreat/itis inflammation	păn-krē-ă-TĪ-tĭs
sial/o	saliva, salivary gland	sial/o/lith stone, calculus	sī-ĂL-ō-lĭth

SUFFIXES

Suffix	Meaning	Example	Pronunciation
-emesis	vomiting	hemat/emesis blood	hĕm-ăt-ĔM-ĕ-sĭs
-iasis	abnormal condition (produced by something specified)	chol/e/lith/iasis gall, stone bile	kō-lē-lĭ-THĪ-ă-sĭs
-lith	stone, calculus	chol/e/lith gall, bile	KŌ-lē-lĭth
-megaly	enlargement	hepat/o/megaly liver	hĕp-ă-tō-MĔG-ă-lē
-orexia	appetite	an/orexia without	ăn-ō-RĔK-sē-ă
-pepsia	digestion	dys/pepsia difficult, painful	dĭs-PĔP-sē-ă
-phagia	swallowing, eating	dys/phagia difficult, painful	dĭs-FĀ-jē-ă
-plasty	surgical repair	stomat/o/plasty mouth	STŌ-mă-tō-plăs-tē
-prandial	meal	post/prandial after	pōst-PRĂN-dē-ăl

PREFIXES

Prefix	Meaning	Example	Pronunciation
dia-	through	dia/rrhea flow	dī-ă-RĒ-ă
dys-	bad, painful, difficult	dys/trophy nourishment, development	DĬS-trō-fē
hyper-	excessive	hyper/emesis vomiting	hī-pĕr-ĔM-ĕ-sĭs
peri-	around	peri/an/ al anus pertaining to	pĕr-ē-Ā-năl
sub-	under, below	sub/ling/ ual tongue pertaining to	sŭb-LĬNG-gwăl

PATHOLOGY

Ulcers

An **ulcer** is an open sore (**lesion**) of the skin or mucous membrane. Most ulcers of the alimentary canal occur in the stomach or duodenum. It is not uncommon for ulcers to be accompanied by formation of pus (**pyogenesis**). Current research shows strong support that gastric ulcers (Fig. 7–5) are caused by bacterial infection. Other causes include excess acid and pepsin in gastric juice, which breaks down mucous membranes, causing underlying tissue destruction.

If left untreated, the tissue destruction eventually leads to a hole (**perforation**). When this occurs, food and enzymes enter the abdominal cavity through the **perforated ulcer**, causing contamination of surrounding structures (peritonitis). Antibiotics are used to treat bacterial ulcers; antacids are used to neutralize the effects of acid and pepsin in the stomach or intestine.

Peptic ulcers (named for the enzyme pepsin) are erosions of the mucous membranes of the stomach (see Fig. 7–5) or duodenum. Ulcers develop most commonly in the duodenum, next most frequently in the stomach, and rarely in the lower portion of the esophagus. They may be of long duration (**chronic**) or arise suddenly (**acute**).

Agents that weaken the mucosal lining of the stomach, such as alcohol, smoking, aspirin, and abnormally high secretions of HCl, increase the likelihood of developing peptic ulcers. Many people between the ages of 20 and 45 tend to develop duodenal ulcers rather than other types of ulcers.

Inflammation of the colon with formation of ulcers in the lining of the intestine (**ulcerative colitis**) can occur at any age but is most common in young adults. Anxiety and nervous tension may be the cause (**etiology**) of the disease. The chief symptom of ulcerative colitis is frequent passage of watery bowel movements (**diarrhea**). Patients may feel very weak, lose weight, and sometimes experience anemia. They may also suffer from pain in the joints (**arthralgia**). In severe cases, it may be necessary to create an opening (**stoma**) surgically for bowel evacuation to a bag worn on the abdomen.

Hernias

A **hernia** is a protrusion of an organ, tissue, or structure through the wall of the cavity in which it is naturally contained (Fig. 7–6). This definition may apply to any part of the body (e.g., the

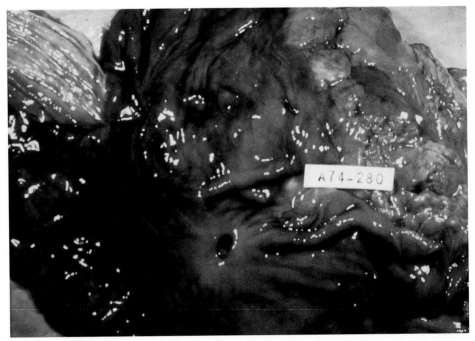

Figure 7–5   Gastric ulcer. (From WRS Group, with permission.)

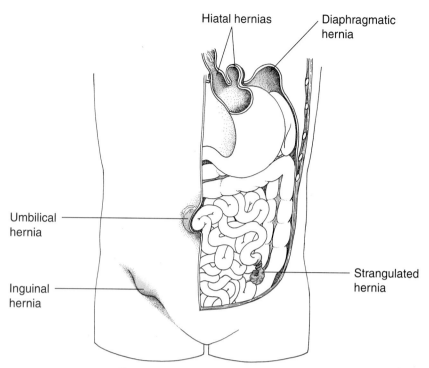

Figure 7–6 Types of abdominal hernias.

protrusion of the brain through a cranial fissure [**encephalocele**]). In general, though, the term is applied to the protrusion of an abdominal organ (**viscus**) through an opening in the abdominal wall.

Hernias are found most commonly in the abdominal region, but they may develop in the diaphragm (**diaphragmatic hernia**) or in the opening where the esophagus passes through the diaphragm (**hiatal hernia**). With this condition, the lower end of the esophagus and the adjacent part of the stomach herniate into the thorax (**gastroesophageal hernia**). This results in gastroesophageal reflux disease (GERD), a condition in which stomach acid backs up into the esophagus.

The **inguinal hernia** develops in the groin where the abdominal folds of flesh meet the thighs. In initial stages, it may hardly be noticeable and appears as a soft lump under the skin, no larger than a marble. In early stages, an inguinal hernia is usually reducible; that is, it can be pushed gently back into its normal place. With this type of hernia, pain may be minimal. As time passes, pressure of the abdomen against the weak abdominal wall may increase the size of the opening as well as the size of the hernia lump. If the blood supply to the hernia is cut off because of pressure (**strangulation**), gangrene (**necrosis**) may develop.

The protrusion of part of the intestine at the navel (**umbilical hernia**) occurs more frequently in obese women and among those who had several pregnancies.

Hernias also occur in newborn infants (**congenital**) or during early childhood. If the defect has not corrected itself by 2 years of age, the deformity can be surgically corrected. Treatment consists of surgical repair of the hernia (**hernioplasty**), with suture of the abdominal wall (**herniorrhaphy**).

Bowel Obstructions

A life-threatening obstruction in which the bowel twists on itself (**volvulus**) with occlusion of the blood supply occurs most frequently in middle-aged and elderly men. The accumulation of gas and fluid coupled with loss of blood supply (**ischemia**) in the trapped bowel eventually leads to tissue death (**necrosis**), perforation, and an inflammation of the peritoneum (**peritonitis**). Surgery is required to untwist the bowel.

Telescoping of the intestine within itself (**intussusception**) occurs when one part of the intestine slips into another part located below it, much as a telescope is shortened by pushing one section into the next. This is a rare type of intestinal obstruction more common in infants 10 to 15 months of age than in adults. Surgery is usually necessary to correct this obstruction.

Hemorrhoids

Enlargement of the veins in the mucous membrane of the anal canal causes hemorrhoids, which may occur inside (**internal**) or outside (**external**) the rectal area.

Hemorrhoids are usually caused by straining to evacuate a fecal concretion or stone (**fecalith**). They sometimes develop during pregnancy because of pressure on the veins from the enlarged uterus. They may also result from pressure on the veins caused by a disorder of the liver or the heart, or may be symptomatic of a tumor that exerts pressure against the veins.

Temporary relief from hemorrhoids can usually be obtained by cold compresses, sitz baths, stool softeners, or an analgesic ointment. Treatment of an advanced hemorrhoidal condition is by surgical removal (**hemorrhoidectomy**).

Liver Disorders

One of the symptoms of many liver disorders is a yellowing of the skin (**jaundice**). This condition, also known as **icterus**, may result when the bile duct is blocked, causing bile to enter the bloodstream. Jaundice is noted in patients who suffer from cirrhosis of the liver and often is related to poor nutrition and excessive alcohol consumption. Icterus may also be exhibited in patients who suffer from **hepatitis**.

A growing public health concern is the increasing incidence of **viral hepatitis**. Even though its mortality rate is low, the disease is easily transmitted and can cause significant morbidity and prolonged loss of time from school or employment. Viral hepatitis includes several forms, the two most common being hepatitis A, also called infectious hepatitis, and hepatitis B, also called serum hepatitis. The most common causes of hepatitis A are ingestion of contaminated food, water, or milk. Hepatitis B is usually transmitted by routes other than the mouth (**parenteral**) (e.g., blood transfusions, semen, and so forth). Because of patient exposure, health care personnel are at increased risk of contracting hepatitis B, but a vaccine that provides immunity to this type is available.

Diverticulosis

Diverticulosis is a condition in which small, blisterlike pockets develop in the walls of the large intestine and may balloon out from the large intestine. These pouchlike areas (**diverticula**; singular, diverticulum) (Fig. 7–7) usually do not cause any problem unless they become inflamed (**diverticulitis**). Pain, usually in the left lower quadrant (LLQ) of the abdomen, extreme constipation (**obstipation**) or diarrhea, fever, abdominal swelling, and occasional blood in the bowel movement are some of the symptoms of diverticulitis. The usual treatment for diverticulitis consists of bedrest, antibiotics, and a soft diet. In severe cases, however, excision of the diverticulum (**diverticulectomy**) may be advised.

Oncology

Although **stomach cancer** is rare in the United States, it is common in many parts of the world where food preservation is questionable. It is significant because of its high mortality rate. Men are more susceptible to stomach cancer than women. The neoplasm nearly always develops from the epithelial or mucosal lining of the stomach in the form of a cancerous glandular tumor (**gastric adenocarcinoma**). Persistent indigestion is one of the important warning signs of stomach cancer. Other types of GI carcinomas include **esophageal carcinomas**, **hepatocellular carcinomas**, and **pancreatic carcinomas**.

Cancer of the colon and rectum (Fig. 7–8) arises from the epithelium lining of the intestine. The effects depend largely on the location of the cancer. Signs and symptoms are changes in bowel

MULTIPLE DIVERTICULA OF THE COLON

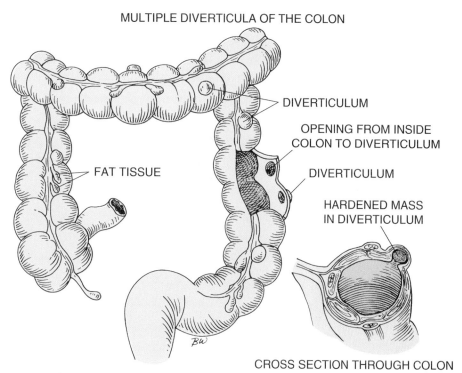

Figure 7–7 Diverticula of the colon. (From Taber's Cyclopedic Medical Dictionary, ed 18. F.A. Davis, Philadelphia, 1997, p 565, with permission.)

habits, the passage of blood in the stools, mucus, rectal or abdominal pain, anemia, weight loss, obstruction, and perforation. A suddenly developing obstruction may be the first symptom of cancer involving the colon anywhere between the cecum and the sigmoid, for in this region, where bowel contents are liquid, a slowly developing obstruction will not become evident until the lumen is practically closed. Cancer of the sigmoid and the rectum causes earlier symptoms of partial obstruction, with constipation alternating with diarrhea, lower abdominal crampy pains, and distension.

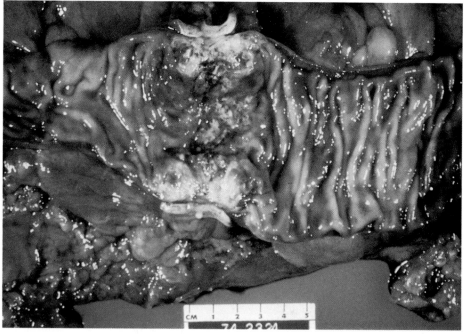

Figure 7–8 Colon cancer. (From WRS Group, with permission.)

DIAGNOSTIC, SYMPTOMATIC, AND THERAPEUTIC TERMS

Term	Meaning
aerophagia ă-ĕr-ō-FĂ-jē-ăh	swallowing air
anorexia ăn-ō-RĚK-sē-ă	loss of appetite
anorexia nervosa an-ō-RĚK-sē-ă nĕr-VŌ-să	eating disorder characterized by a refusal to maintain body weight appropriate for age and height; intense fear of gaining weight or becoming obese, which does not diminish as weight loss progresses and patient becomes emaciated. Psychiatric therapy is usually required if patient refuses to eat
appendicitis ă-pĕn-dĭ-SĪ-tĭs	inflammation of the appendix, usually due to obstruction or infection (Fig. 7–9)
ascites ă-SĪ-tēz	abnormal accumulation of serous (edematous) fluid in the abdomen or pleura. The condition may be associated with numerous disorders, including neoplastic and inflammatory disorders of the peritoneum; venous hypertension (high blood pressure) associated with cirrhosis of the liver and advanced congestive heart failure; and hyperaldosteronism with increased retention of sodium and water in the abdomen
borborygmus bŏr-bō-RĬG-mŭs	gurgling or splashing sound normally heard over the large intestine, caused by passage of gas through the liquid contents of the intestine
bulimia bū-LĬM-ē-ă	eating disorder characterized by binge eating followed by purging, use of laxatives or diuretics, strict dieting or fasting, or vigorous exercise in order to prevent weight gain, and persistent overconcern with body shape and weight
cachexia kă-KĔKS-ē-ă	a general lack of nutrition and wasting occurring in the course of a chronic disease or emotional disturbance
cholelithiasis kō-lē-lĭ-THĪ-ă-sĭs	condition characterized by the presence or formation of stones in the gallbladder (Fig. 7–10)

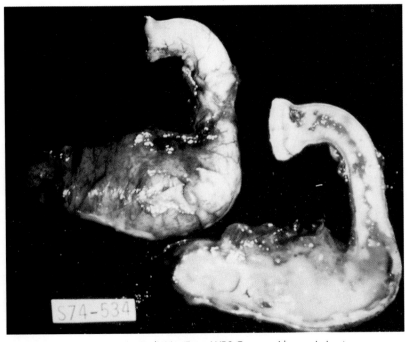

Figure 7–9   Appendicitis. (From WRS Group, with permission.)

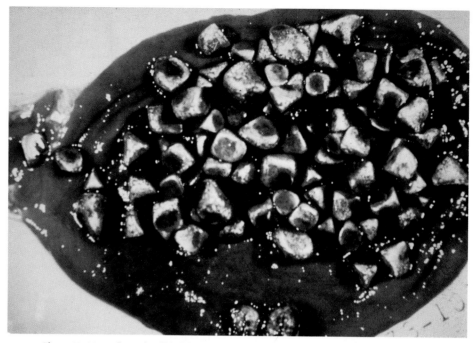

Figure 7–10 Inflamed gallbladder with gallstones. (From WRS Group, with permission.)

DIAGNOSTIC, SYMPTOMATIC, AND THERAPEUTIC TERMS (Continued)

Term	Meaning
cleft palate KLĔFT PĂL-ăt	a congenital fissure in the roof of the mouth forming a communicating passageway between the mouth and nasal cavities
Crohn's disease, granulomatous colitis, regional enteritis krōnz dĭ-ZĒZ, grăn-ū-LŎM-ă-tŭs kō-LĪ-tĭs, RĒ-jŭn-ăl ĕn-tĕr-Ī-tĭs	inflammatory condition of the intestinal tract, most commonly the ileum; distinguished from closely related bowel disorders by its inflammatory pattern
cirrhosis sĭr-RŌ-sĭs	liver disease with degeneration of liver cells
colic KŎL-ĭk	spasm in any hollow or tubular soft organ accompanied by pain, especially in the colon
deglutition dĕg-loo-TĬSH-ŭn	the act of swallowing
dysentery DĬS-ĕn-tĕr-ē	a term applied to a number of intestinal disorders, especially of the colon, characterized by inflammation of the mucous membrane
dyspepsia dĭs-PĔP-sē-ă	gastric indigestion or "upset stomach," usually referring to epigastric discomfort after meals
dysphagia dĭs-FĀ-jē-ă	inability or difficulty in swallowing; aphagia
eructation ĕ-rŭk-TĀ-shŭn	the act of belching; the raising of gas or a small quantity of acid from the stomach
fecalith FĒ-kă-lĭth	fecal concretion
flatus FLĀ-tŭs	gas or air expelled through the anus

DIAGNOSTIC, SYMPTOMATIC, AND THERAPEUTIC TERMS
(Continued)

Term	Meaning
gastroesophageal reflux disease (GERD) găs-trō-ĕ-sŏf-ă-JĒ-ăl RĒ-flŭks dĭ-ZĒZ	backflow of gastric contents into the esophagus caused by the regurgitation of HCl from the stomach into the esophagus; heartburn
halitosis hăl-ĭ-TŌ-sĭs	offensive or "bad" breath
hematemesis hĕm-ă-TĔM-ĕ-sĭs	vomiting blood
irritable bowel syndrome (IBS)	a chronic stress-related disease characterized by diarrhea, constipation, and pain associated with rhythmic contractions of the intestine. Mucous colitis; spastic colon.
leukoplakia loo-kō-PLĀ-kē-ă	white patches on the mucous membrane of the tongue or cheek, common in smokers and possibly a forerunner to cancer
malabsorption syndrome măl-ăb-SŌRP-shĕn SĬN-drōm	impaired absorption of nutrients from the intestinal tract, especially the small intestine
melena MĔL-ĕ-nă	black, tarry feces due to action of intestinal secretions on free blood
obstipation ŏb-stĭ-PĀ-shŭn	extreme constipation
peristalsis pĕr-ĭ-STĂL-sĭs	a progressive wavelike movement that occurs involuntarily in hollow tubes of the body, especially the alimentary canal
pyloric stenosis pī-LŎR-ĭk stĕ-NŌ-sĭs	narrowing of the gastric pylorus; may be due to excessive thickening of the circular muscle of the pylorus
regurgitation rē-gŭr-jĭ-TĀ-shŭn	a backward flowing, as in the return of solids or fluids to the mouth from the stomach or the backward flow of blood through a defective heart valve
steatorrhea stē-ă-tō-RĒ-ă	excessive amount of fat in the feces due to improper fat digestion (malabsorption)
visceroptosis vĭs-ĕr-ŏp-TŌ-sĭs	downward displacement of the viscera (internal organs enclosed within a cavity), especially the abdominal organs

DIAGNOSTIC PROCEDURES

Imaging Procedure	Description
barium enema, lower GI BĂ-rē-ŭm ĔN-ĕ-mă	enema using a liquid contrast medium, barium sulfate; retained in the lower GI tract during fluoroscopic and radiographic studies for diagnosing obstructions or other abnormalities of the colon
esophagram ē-SŎF-ă-grăm	radiological evaluation of the esophagus while administering a barium sulfate suspension under fluoroscopic guidance (also known as barium swallow)
cholecystography, gallbladder series kō-lē-sĭs-TŎG-ră-fē	radiographic images of the gallbladder after administration of a radiopaque contrast medium; used to evaluate the functioning of the gallbladder and to determine the presence of disease or gallstones
CT scan (liver, spleen)	visualization of the liver after a radioactive substance is injected intravenously (IV) and absorbed by the liver cells; used for diagnosing cysts, ruptures, tumors, abscesses, and other abnormalities

DIAGNOSTIC PROCEDURES (Continued)

Imaging Procedure	Description
endoscopic retrograde cholangiopancreatography (ERCP) ĕn-do-SKŌ-pĭk RĔT-rō-grăd ko-lăn-jē-ō-păn-krē-ă-TŎG-ră-fē	radiographic images of pancreas and bile ducts after IV injection of a radiopaque contrast medium
liver scan	injection of radioactive material capable of penetrating liver cells, followed by use of a special scanner to record the radiation emitted from the cells
sialography sī-ă-LŎG-ră-fē	radiological examination of the salivary glands and ducts after injection of a radiopaque contrast agent
sonography or ultrasonography sō-NŎG-ră-fē, ŭl-tră-sŏn-ŎG-ră-fē	ultrasound is used to produce an image or photograph of an organ or tissue. Ultrasonic echoes are recorded as they strike tissues of different densities
abdominal sonogram ăb-DŎM-ĭ-năl SŌ-nō-grăm	ultrasound imaging of the abdomen to detect diseases or deformities in digestive organs, such as the gallbladder, liver, and pancreas as well as vascular structures
upper GI	radiographic examination of upper GI tract after barium sulfate, a liquid contrast medium, is swallowed; used for diagnosing obstructions and other abnormalities of the esophagus, duodenum, and stomach

Endoscopic Procedure	Description
colonoscopy kō-lŏn-ŎS-kō-pē	visual examination of the colon using a colonoscope; may permit the removal of polyps, tissue for biopsy; used to confirm or establish a diagnosis
esophagogastroduodenoscopy (EGD) ē-sŏf-ă-gō-găs-trō-dū-ŏd-ĕ-NŎS-kō-pē	visual examination of the esophagus, stomach, and duodenum using an endoscope
esophagoscopy ē-sŏf-ă-GŎS-kō-pē	use of an esophagoscope for visual examination of or removal of a foreign object from the esophagus
gastroscopy găs-TRŎS-kō-pē	visual examination of the interior of the stomach using a gastroscope inserted through the mouth and esophagus
proctosigmoidoscopy, sigmoidoscopy prŏk-tō-sĭg-moy-DŎS-kō-pē, sĭg-moy-DŎS-kō-pē	visual examination of the rectum and sigmoid colon using a sigmoidoscope or proctoscope; may permit the removal of polyps, tissue for biopsy; used to confirm or establish a diagnosis

Laboratory Procedure	Description
alkaline phosphatase ĂL-kă-līn FŎS-fă-tās	blood level tests of this enzyme are used to determine various diseases associated with liver and bone disorders
aspiration biopsy cytology (ABC) ăs-pĭ-RĀ-shŭn BĪ-ŏp-sē sī-TŎL-ō-jē	microscopic study of cells obtained from superficial or internal lesions by suction through a fine needle; used primarily as a diagnostic procedure, usually to detect nuclear and cytoplasmic changes in tissue, especially those associated with cancer
fasting blood sugar (FBS)	measures blood glucose level after a 12-hour fast
glucose tolerance test (GTT) GLOO-kōs	a blood test involving glucose analysis after ingestion of a concentrated glucose dose; used to diagnose diabetes and hypoglycemia

DIAGNOSTIC PROCEDURES (Continued)

Laboratory Procedure	Description
liver biopsy BĪ-ŏp-sē	a diagnostic procedure in which a large-bore needle removes a core of liver tissue for histological examination
hepatitis panel	a series of tests including hepatitis B surface antigen (HbsAg), hepatitis B surface antibody (HbsAb), hepatitis B core antibody (HbcAb), hepatitis A antibody (Haab), and hepatitis C antibody; used to determine various forms of viral hepatitis
occult blood	a chemical test or microscopic examination for blood, especially in feces, that is not apparent on visual inspection; determines bleeding in GI disorders; helps to detect colon cancer (Fig. 7–8).
stool culture	microbiological procedure in which microorganisms in feces are grown on media or nutrient material

SURGICAL AND THERAPEUTIC PROCEDURES

Procedure	Description
anastomosis ă-năs-tō-MŌ-sĭs	surgical connection of two tubular structures
ileorectal ĭl-ē-ō-RĔK-tăl	surgical anastomosis of the ileum and rectum after total colectomy, as is sometimes performed in the treatment of ulcerative colitis
intestinal	establishment of a communication between two formerly distant portions of the intestine
biliary lithotripsy BĬL-ē-ār-ē LĬTH-ō-trĭp-sē	procedure that destroys gallstones using shock waves; gallstones pass out of the body painlessly in pulverized form
colostomy kō-LŎS-tō-mē	creation of an opening (mouth) of some portion of the colon through the abdominal wall to its outside surface, to divert fecal flow to a colostomy bag
pyloromyotomy pī-lō-rō-mī-ŎT-ō-mē	incision of the longitudinal and circular muscles of the pylorus, to treat hypertrophic pyloric stenosis

PHARMACOLOGY

Medication	Action
antacids	neutralize excess stomach acid and relieve gastritis and ulcer pain; also used to relieve indigestion and reflux esophagitis (heartburn) hiatal hernia
antidiarrheals	relieve diarrhea either by absorbing the excess fluids that cause diarrhea or by lessening intestinal motility (slowing the movement of fecal material through the intestine), allowing more time for absorption of water
antiflatulents	reduce the feeling of gassiness and bloating (flatulence) that accompanies indigestion. These agents facilitate the passing of gas by breaking down gas bubbles to a smaller size and by mildly stimulating intestinal motility
antiemetics, antinauseants	suppress nausea and vomiting, mainly by acting on brain control centers to stop nerve impulses; also used to control motion sickness and dizziness associated with inner ear infections. Some antihistamines and tranquilizers have antiemetic properties
antispasmodics	prevent or reduce smooth muscle spasms by acting on the automatic nervous system, thus relieving certain spastic conditions of the bowel

PHARMACOLOGY (Continued)

Medication	Action
cathartics, laxatives, purgatives	promote bowel movement or defecation or both: in smaller doses, they relieve constipation and are called laxatives; in larger doses, they evacuate the entire GI tract and are called purgatives (used before surgery or intestinal radiological examinations)
emetics	used to induce vomiting, especially in cases of poisoning

ABBREVIATIONS*

Abbreviations Related to Medication Time Schedules	Meaning
ac	before meals (ante cibum)
bid	twice a day
hs	at bedtime
NPO	nothing by mouth
pc, pp	after meals (postprandial)
PO	orally; by mouth
PRN	as required
qam, qm	every morning
qd	every day (qua que die)
qh	every hour
q2h	every 2 hours
qid	four times a day
qod	every other day
qpm, qn	every night
stat	immediately
tid	three times a day

Abbreviations Related to Diagnostic Tests	Meaning
ABC	aspiration biopsy cytology
alk phos	alkaline phosphatase
Ba	barium
BaE	barium enema
CT scan, CAT scan	computerized tomography scan
Dx	diagnosis
EGD	esophagogastroduodenoscopy
ERCP	endoscopic retrograde cholangiopancreatography
FBS	fasting blood sugar
GB	gallbladder
GTT	glucose tolerance test
IVC	intravenous cholangiography

ABBREVIATIONS* (Continued)

Abbreviations Related to Diagnostic Tests	Meaning
PUD	peptic ulcer disease
SGOT, SGPT	liver function enzyme tests
UGI	upper gastrointestinal tract (x-ray)

Other Abbreviations Related to the GI System	Meaning
BM	bowel movement
GERD	gastroesophageal reflux disorder
GI	gastrointestinal
HAV	hepatitis A virus
HBV	hepatitis B virus
IBS	irritable bowel syndrome
IV	intravenous
LLQ	left lower quadrant
LUQ	left upper quadrant
PE	physical examination
PMH	past medical history
RUQ	right upper quadrant

*Because many of these abbreviations deal with pharmacology and the administration of medication, they are not unique to the GI system.

MEDICAL RECORD

GI Evaluation

The patient's abdominal pain began 2 years ago when she first had intermittent, sharp epigastric pain. Each episode lasted 2 to 4 hours. Eventually she was diagnosed as having cholecystitis with cholelithiasis (see Fig. 7–10) and underwent cholecystectomy. Three to five large calcified stones were found.

Her postoperative course was uneventful until 4 months ago, when she began having continuous deep right-sided pain. This pain followed a crescendo pattern and peaked several weeks ago, at a time when family stress was also at its climax. Since then, the pain has been following a decrescendo pattern. It does not cause any nausea or vomiting, does not trigger any urge to defecate, and was not alleviated by passage of flatus. Her PMH is significant only for tonsillectomy, appendectomy, and the cholecystectomy. Her PE findings indicate that there was no hepatomegaly or splenomegaly. The rectal examination confirmed normal sphincter tone and heme-negative stool.

Impression   Abdominal pain. R/O hepatomegaly and splenomegaly.

Plan   Schedule a complete barium work-up for possible obstruction.

Worksheet 5 provides a dictionary and reading application and an analysis of this medical record.

WORSHEET 1

Use **esophag/o** *(esophagus) to build words meaning:*

1. pain in the esophagus _____

2. spasm of the esophagus _____

3. stricture or narrowing of the esophagus _____

Use **gastr/o** *(stomach) to build words meaning:*

4. inflammation of the stomach _____

5. pain in the stomach _____

6. disease of the stomach _____

7. enlargement of the stomach _____

Use **duoden/o** *(duodenum),* **jejun/o** *(jejunum),* **or ile/o** *(ileum) to build words meaning:*

8. relating to the duodenum _____

9. inflammation of the ileum _____

10. concerning the jejunum and ileum _____

Use **enter/o** *(small intestine) to build words meaning:*

11. inflammation of the small intestine _____

12. disease of the small intestine _____

Use **col/o** *(colon) to build words meaning:*

13. inflammation of the colon _____

14. visual examination of the colon _____

15. inflammation of the small intestine and colon _____

16. prolapse or downward displacement of the colon _____

17. disease of the colon _____

Use **proct/o** *(anus, rectum) or* **rect/o** *(rectum) to build words meaning:*

18. narrowing or constriction of the rectum _____

19. herniation of the rectum _____

20. paralysis of the anus (anal muscles) _____

Use chol/e (bile, gall) to build words meaning:

21. inflammation of the gallbladder _____

22. abnormal condition of a gallstone _____

Use hepat/o (liver) or pancreat/o (pancreas) to build words meaning:

23. tumor of the liver _____

24. enlargement of the liver _____

25. inflammation of the pancreas _____

WORKSHEET 2

Build a surgical term meaning:

1. excision of gums (tissue) _____

2. partial or complete excision of the tongue _____

3. repair of the esophagus _____

4. removal of part or all of the stomach _____

5. forming an opening between the stomach and jejunum _____

6. excision of (part of) the esophagus _____

7. forming an opening between the stomach, small intestine, and colon _____

8. repair of the intestine _____

9. fixation of the small intestine (to the abdominal wall) _____

10. suture of the bile duct _____

11. forming an opening into the colon _____

12. fixation of a movable liver (to the abdominal wall) _____

13. repair of the anus or rectum _____

14. removal of the gallbladder _____

15. repair of a bile duct _____

WORSHEET 3

■ ■ ■ ■ ■ ■ ■ ■ ■ ■ ■ ■ ■

Match the following words with the definitions in the numbered list.

anorexia   dysphagia   hematemesis
bulimia   dyspnea   melagra
cachexia   fecalith   melena
dyspepsia   halitosis   obstipation

1. _____ vomiting blood

2. _____ difficulty swallowing or inability to swallow

3. _____ fecal concretion

4. _____ "bad" breath

5. _____ loss of appetite

6. _____ poor digestion

7. _____ black stool

8. _____ a state of ill health, malnutrition, and wasting

9. _____ intractable constipation

10. _____ binging and purging

WORKSHEET 4

Match the following words with the definitions in the numbered list.

alkaline phosphatase	choledochoplasty	pc, pp
anastomosis	Crohn's disease	proctosigmoidoscopy
antacids	emetics	pyloromyotomy
antidiarrheals	FBS	qid
antiflatulents	gastroscopy	stat
bid	lower GI	stomatoplasty
cathartics	occult blood	upper GI
cholecystography		

1. _____ after meals

2. _____ fecal examination for blood that is not apparent on visual inspection; used to determine bleeding in GI disorders; helps detect colon cancer

3. _____ agents that produce vomiting

4. _____ twice a day

5. _____ surgical reconstruction of a bile duct

6. _____ an enema with a barium solution is administered while a series of radiographs are taken of the large intestine

7. _____ visual examination of the stomach

8. _____ surgical reconstruction of the mouth

9. _____ promote bowel movement and/or defecation

10. _____ surgical formation of a passage or opening between two hollow viscera or vessels

11. _____ radiographic images of the gallbladder after administration of a radiopaque contrast medium

12. _____ inflammatory condition of the intestinal tract, most commonly the ileum; distinguished from closely related bowel disorders by its inflammatory pattern

13. _____ reduce the feelings of gassiness and bloating caused by indigestion

14. _____ neutralize excess acid in the stomach and help to relieve gastritis and ulcer pain

15. _____ used to detect abnormalities of glucose metabolism

16. _____ blood level tests of this enzyme to determine various diseases associated with liver and bone disorders

17. _____ four times a day

18. _____ immediately

19. _____ endoscopic procedure for visualization of the rectosigmoid colon

20. _____ barium solution swallowed for a radiographic examination of the esophagus, stomach, and duodenum

WORKSHEET 5

Medical Record: GI Evaluation

Underline the following terms in the medical record (see p. 104). Use a medical dictionary and other resources to define the terms and to determine their pronunciation; then practice reading the medical record aloud.

appendectomy _____

cholecystectomy _____

cholecystitis _____

cholelithiasis _____

crescendo _____

decrescendo _____

defecate _____

epigastric _____

flatus _____

heme _____

hepatomegaly _____

PMH _____

sphincter _____

stool _____

tonsillectomy _____

Medical Record Evaluation: GI Evaluation

1. *While referring to Figure 7–3, describe where the gallbladder is located in relation to the liver.*

2. *Has the patient had any other surgeries?*

3. *If so, what were they?*

4. *How does her most recent postoperative episode of discomfort (pain) differ from the initial pain she described?*

WORSHEET 6

Label the following illustration. Check your answers by referring to Figure 7–1.

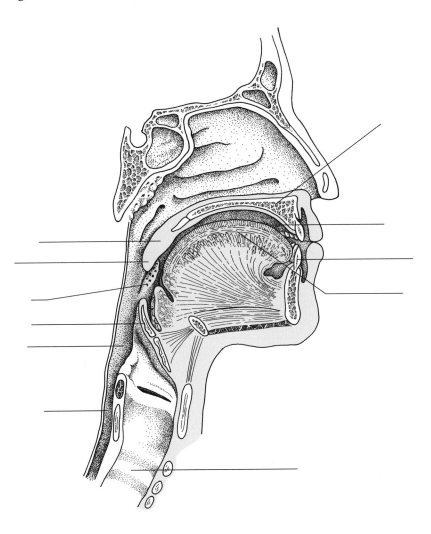

Epiglottis   Hard palate   Pharynx   Teeth   Tonsil   Uvula
Esophagus   Oral cavity   Soft palate Tongue   Trachea

WORKSHEET 7

■ ■ ■ ■ ■ ■ ■ ■ ■ ■ ■ ■ ■ ■

Label the following illustration. Check your answers by referring to Figure 7–3.

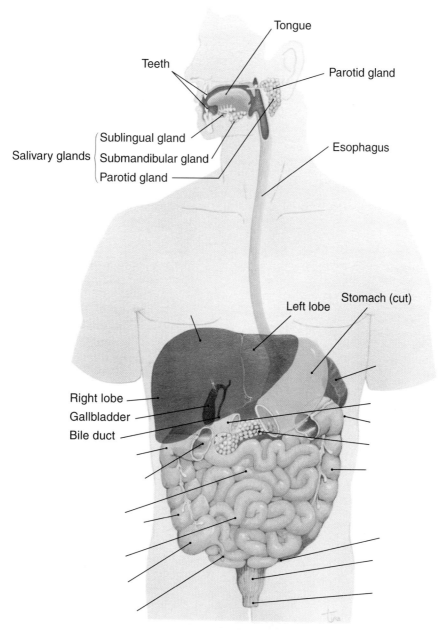

Anus	Descending colon	Jejunum	Sigmoid colon
Appendix	Duodenum	Liver	Spleen
Ascending colon	Hepatic flexure	Pancreas	Splenic flexure
Cecum	Ileum	Rectum	Transverse colon

Chapter 8

PREFIXES • ABBREVIATIONS • PRONUNCIA...

ROOTS • COMBINING FORMS • SUFFIXES

RESPIRATORY SYSTEM

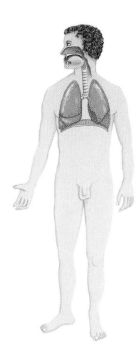

Chapter Outline

Student Objectives

Anatomy and Physiology
Internal Respiration
External Respiration
Respiratory System

Combining Forms

Suffixes

Prefixes

Pathology
Chronic Obstructive Pulmonary
 Disease
Influenza
Pleural Effusions
Tuberculosis
Bronchopneumonia
Cystic Fibrosis

Respiratory Distress Syndrome
Oncology
 Primary Pulmonary Cancer
**Diagnostic, Symptomatic,
 and Therapeutic Terms**
Diagnostic Procedures
Imaging Procedures
Endoscopic Procedures
Clinical Procedures
Laboratory Procedures
Surgical and Therapeutic Procedures
Pharmacology
Abbreviations
Medical Record
Respiratory Evaluation
Worksheets

Student Objectives

Upon completion of this chapter, you will be able to do the following:

1. List the major structures of the respiratory system and briefly describe the function of each.
2. Differentiate between external and internal respiration.
3. List the structures associated with the respiratory system and describe their function.
4. Describe the function of the diaphragm and intercostal muscles in the breathing process.
5. Identify combining forms, suffixes, and prefixes related to the respiratory system.
6. Identify and discuss pathology related to the respiratory system.
7. Identify diagnostic, symptomatic, and therapeutic terms related to the respiratory system.
8. Identify diagnostic procedures related to the respiratory system.
9. Identify surgical and therapeutic procedures related to the respiratory system.
10. Discuss pharmacology related to the treatment of respiratory disorders.
11. Identify abbreviations related to the respiratory system.
12. Demonstrate your knowledge of the chapter by completing the worksheets.

115

ANATOMY AND PHYSIOLOGY

The respiratory system consists of the organs that are responsible for the breathing process. Along with the cardiovascular system, it is responsible for the exchange of oxygen (O_2) and carbon dioxide (CO_2). The entire breathing process involves internal and external respiration.

Internal Respiration

All body cells require a continuous source of O_2 for metabolism. They also require a means for removing CO_2, a waste product produced as part of the metabolic process. These two needs are satisfied during a process called **internal respiration** or **cellular respiration**. Respiration involves an exchange of gases. Internal respiration involves the exchange of O_2 and CO_2. With internal respiration CO_2 leaves body cells and enters blood in surrounding capillaries. Meanwhile, O_2 from blood passes into cells. When the exchange is completed, blood flows from capillaries to the veins and finally returns to the heart.

External Respiration

External respiration consists of two separate, simultaneous activities:

- Ventilation, the exchange of air between the lungs and atmosphere that occurs in breathing
- Exchanging O_2 in the lungs with CO_2 in the pulmonary capillaries

Ventilation is the movement of air into and out of the lungs. It allows for the exchange of gases in the lungs with the gases found in the environment. During expiration (exhaling), CO_2 is expelled; during inspiration (inhaling), environmental air, rich in O_2, enters the lungs. Breathing is largely an involuntary activity brought about by nervous stimulation of the diaphragm and intercostal muscles.

Blood entering the pulmonary capillaries contains a high concentration of CO_2. As blood flows through the pulmonary capillaries, it gains O_2 from the lungs. Simultaneously, CO_2 diffuses from the blood and enters the lungs.

Respiratory System

As you read the following paragraphs, refer to Figure 8–1 to help you understand the anatomy and physiology of the respiratory system.

During the breathing process, air is drawn into the (1) **nasal cavity**. The nasal cavity is divided into a right and left side by a vertical partition called the nasal **septum**. The interior portion of the nasal cavity warms, moistens, and filters incoming air.

The receptors for the sense of smell are located in the nasal cavity. These receptors, called the **olfactory** neurons, are found among the epithelial cells lining the nasal tract and are covered with a layer of mucus. Because these receptors are located higher in the nasal passage than inhaled air normally reaches, a person must sniff or inhale deeply to identify weak odors.

Air passes from the nasal cavity to the pharynx, a muscular tube that serves as a passageway for food and air. It consists of three sections:

- The (2) **nasopharynx**, posterior to the nose
- The (3) **oropharynx**, posterior to the mouth
- The (4) **laryngopharynx**, superior to the larynx

Within the nasopharynx is a collection of lymphatic tissue known as (5) **adenoids**, or **pharyngeal tonsils**. The (6) **palatine tonsils**, more commonly known as tonsils, are located in the oropharynx. They protect the opening to the respiratory tract from microscopic organisms that may attempt entry by this route. The (7) **larynx** ("voice box"), found in the laryngopharynx, is responsible for sound production, or phonation. A leaf-shaped structure on top of the larynx,

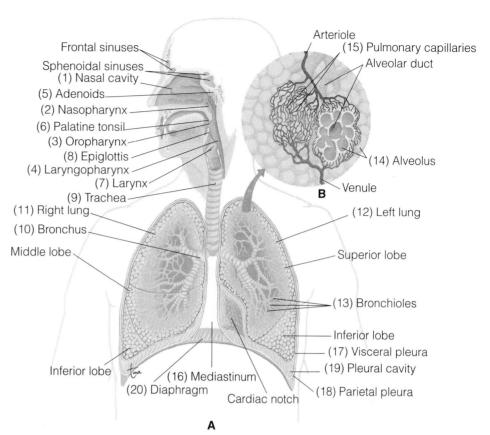

Frontal sinuses
Sphenoidal sinuses
(1) Nasal cavity
(5) Adenoids
(2) Nasopharynx
(6) Palatine tonsil
(3) Oropharynx
(8) Epiglottis
(4) Laryngopharynx
(7) Larynx
(9) Trachea
(11) Right lung
(10) Bronchus
Middle lobe

Arteriole
(15) Pulmonary capillaries
Alveolar duct
(14) Alveolus
Venule
B

(12) Left lung
Superior lobe
(13) Bronchioles
Inferior lobe
(17) Visceral pleura
(19) Pleural cavity
(18) Parietal pleura

Inferior lobe
(16) Mediastinum
(20) Diaphragm
Cardiac notch

A

Figure 8–1   Respiratory system. (*A*) Anterior view of the upper and lower respiratory tracts. (*B*) Microscopic view of alveoli and pulmonary capillaries. The colors represent the vessels, not the oxygen content of the blood. (Adapted from Scanlon, VC, and Sanders, T: Understanding Human Structure and Function. F.A. Davis, Philadelphia, 1997, p 268, with permission.)

the (8) **epiglottis**, seals off the air passage to the lungs during swallowing. This ensures that food or liquids do not obstruct the flow of air to the lungs. The larynx is a short passage that joins the pharynx with the (9) **trachea** (windpipe). The inner wall of the trachea is composed of a mucous membrane lining embedded with tiny hairs called cilia. This membrane traps incoming particles, and the cilia move the entrapped material upward into the pharynx. The trachea is composed of smooth muscle embedded with C-shaped cartilage rings, which provide rigidity to keep the air passage open. The trachea divides into two branches called (10) **bronchi** (singular, **bronchus**). One branch leads to the (11) **right lung** and the other to the (12) **left lung**. Like the trachea, bronchi contain C-shaped cartilage rings.

Each bronchus divides into smaller and smaller branches, eventually forming (13) **bronchioles**. Where bronchioles terminate, tiny air sacs called (14) **alveoli** (singular, **alveolus**) are formed. An alveolus resembles a small balloon because it expands and contracts with inflow and outflow of air. The (15) **pulmonary capillaries** lie adjacent to the thin tissue membranes of the alveoli. CO_2 diffuses from the blood within the pulmonary capillaries and enters the alveolar spaces. Simultaneously, O_2 from the alveoli diffuses into the blood. After the exchange of gases, blood returns to the heart, from which it is pumped to body tissues for internal respiration.

The lungs are divided into lobes: three lobes in the right lung and two lobes in the left lung. The space between the right and left lungs, called the (16) **mediastinum**, contains the heart, aorta, esophagus, and bronchi.

A serous membrane, the **pleura**, envelops the lungs and folds over to line the walls of the thoracic cavity. The innermost membrane lying next to the lung is the (17) **visceral pleura;** the outermost membrane, lining the thoracic cavity, is the (18) **parietal pleura**. Between these two membranes is the (19) **pleural cavity**. It contains a small amount of lubricating fluid, which permits the visceral pleura to glide smoothly over the parietal pleura during breathing.

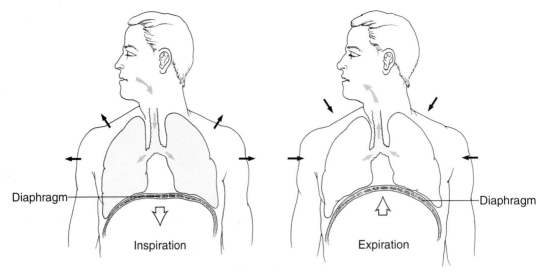

Figure 8–2   The diaphragm contracts and flattens during inhalation, then relaxes during exhalation.

Ventilation depends on a pressure differential between the atmosphere and chest cavity. A large muscular partition, the (20) **diaphragm**, lies between the chest and abdominal cavities. The diaphragm assists in changing the volume of the thoracic cavity in order to produce the needed pressure differential for ventilation. When the diaphragm contracts, it partially descends into the abdominal cavity, thus decreasing the pressure within the chest and drawing air into the lungs. When the diaphragm relaxes, it slowly re-enters the thoracic cavity, thus increasing the pressure within the chest (inspiration). As the pressure increases, air leaves the lungs (expiration). The **intercostal** muscles assist the diaphragm in changing the volume of the thoracic cavity by elevating and lowering the rib cage (Fig. 8–2).

COMBINING FORMS

Combining Form	Meaning	Example	Pronunciation
nas/o	nose	nas/al pertaining to	NĀ-zl
rhin/o		rhin/o/plasty surgical repair	RĪ-nō-plăs-tē
adenoid/o	adenoid	adenoid/ectomy excision, removal	ăd-ĕ-noyd-ĔK-tō-mē
tonsill/o	tonsils	tonsill/o/tome instrument to cut	tŏn-SĬL-ō-tōm
pharyng/o	pharynx, throat	pharyng/o/scope instrument to view or examine	făr-ĬN-gō-skōp
laryng/o	larynx (voice box)	laryng/o/plegia paralysis	lă-rĭng-gō-PLĒ-jē-ă

COMBINING FORMS (Continued)

Combining Form	Meaning	Example	Pronunciation
trache/o	trachea	trache/o/stomy forming an opening (mouth)	trā-kē-ŎS-tō-mē

bronchi/o
 	
bronch/o
	bronchus	bronchi/ectasis
		    expansion, dilation
		bronch/o/scope
		    instrument to view or examine
			brŏng-kē-ĔK-tă-sĭs
			
			BRŎNG-kă-skōp

pneum/o
 	
pneumon/o
	air, lung	pneum/o/cele
		    hernia, swelling
		pneumon/o/lysis
		    separation, destruction, loosening
			NŪ-mō-sēl
			
			nū-mō-NŎL-ĭ-sĭs

pulmon/o	lung	pulmon/ary pertaining to	PŬL-mō-nĕ-rē
lob/o	lobe	lob/ar pertaining to	LŌ-băr
alveol/o	alveolus	alveol/ar pertaining to	ăl-VĒ-ō-lăr
pleur/o	pleura	pleur/algia pain	ploo-RĂL-jē-a
phren/o	diaphragm, mind	phren/ectomy excision	frĕ-NĔK-tō-mē

pector/o
 	
steth/o
 	
thorac/o
	chest	pector/al
		    pertaining to
		steth/o/scope
		    instrument to view or examine
		thorac/o/centesis
		    puncture
			PĔK-tō-răl
			
			STĔTH-ō-skōp
			
			thō-răk-ō-sĕn-TĒ-sĭs

spir/o	breathe	spir/o/meter instrument for measuring	spī-RŎM-ĕt-ĕr
coni/o	dust	pneum/o/coni/osis air, lung abnormal condition	nū-mō-kō-nē-Ō-sĭs
anthrac/o	black, coal	anthrac/osis abnormal condition	ăn-thră-KŌ-sĭs
ox/o	oxygen (O_2)	hyp/ox/ emia decrease blood	hī-pŏk-SĒ-mē-ă
orth/o	straight	orth/o/pnea breathing	or-THŎP-nē-ă
atel/o	incomplete, imperfect	atel/ectasis dilation, expansion	ăt-ĕ-LĔK-tă-sĭs

SUFFIXES

Suffix	Meaning	Example	Pronunciation
-capnia	carbon dioxide (CO_2)	hyper/capnia excessive	hī-pĕr-KĂP-nē-ă
-osmia	smell	an/osmia lack of	ăn-ŎZ-mē-ă
-phonia	voice	dys/phonia difficult, painful	dĭs-FŌ-nē-ă
-pnea	breathing	eu/pnea good, normal	ūp-NĒ-ă
-ptysis	spitting	hem/o/ptysis blood	hē-MŎP-tĭ-sĭs
-thorax	chest	pneum/o/thorax air	nū-mō-THŌ-răks

PREFIXES

Prefix	Meaning	Example	Pronunciation
brady-	slow	brady/pnea breathing	brăd-ĭp-NĒ-ă
eu-	good, normal	eu/pnea breathing	ūp-NĒ-ă
tachy-	rapid	tachy/pnea breathing	tăk-ĭp-NĒ-ă

PATHOLOGY

Chronic Obstructive Pulmonary Disease

Chronic obstructive pulmonary disease (COPD), also called chronic obstructive lung disease (COLD), includes respiratory disorders characterized by a chronic partial obstruction of the air passages. The patient experiences difficulty in breathing (**dyspnea**) on exertion and often exhibits a chronic cough. The three major disorders included in COPD are asthma, chronic bronchitis, and emphysema.

Asthma produces periods of spasms in the bronchial passages. One important cause of asthma is exposure to allergens or irritants. Other causes include stress, cold, and exercise. Bronchospasms associated with asthma are often sudden and violent (**paroxysmal**), causing dyspnea. During recovery, coughing episodes produce large amounts of mucus (**productive cough**). Over a period of time, the epithelium of the bronchial passages thickens, making breathing difficult. Treatment includes agents that loosen and break down mucus (**mucolytics**) and medications that open up the bronchi (**bronchodilators**) by relaxing the smooth muscles of the bronchi.

Chronic bronchitis is an inflammation of the bronchi believed to be caused primarily by smoking and air pollution. Other agents such as viruses and bacteria, however, may also be responsible for the disorder. Because of its chronic nature, this type of bronchitis is characterized by swelling of the mucosa and a heavy, productive cough, often accompanied by chest pain.

Patients usually seek medical attention when they suffer exercise intolerance, wheezing, and short-ness of breath. Bronchodilators and medications that facilitate the removal of mucus (**expecto-rants**) help to widen the air passages. Steroids are often needed as the disease progresses.

Emphysema is a disease that causes alveoli to lose elasticity. The air sacs expand (**dilate**) but are unable to contract to their initial size. Residual air becomes trapped in the alveoli, resulting in a characteristic "barrel-chested" appearance. This disease is often found in combination with another respiratory disorder, such as asthma, tuberculosis, or chronic bronchitis. It is also asso-ciated with long-term heavy smoking. Emphysema sufferers often find it easier to breathe when sitting or standing erect (**orthopnea**). As the disease progresses, however, orthopnea is no longer effectual. Treatment for emphysema is similar to that for chronic bronchitis.

Influenza

Influenza (flu) is an acute infectious respiratory disease. Three major viral types are responsible: type A, type B, and type C. Type A and type B are of primary concern because they are often associated with worldwide epidemics (**pandemics**). Influenza type A epidemics occur about every 2 to 3 years; type B, about every 4 to 6 years. Both of these viruses mutate readily, and new vaccines must be developed in anticipation of their spread.

The onset of the flu is usually very rapid. The patient experiences fever, chills, headache, generalized muscle pain (myalgia), and loss of appetite. The patient is ill during the acute phase, but recovery occurs in about 7 to 10 days. Rarely does the flu virus cause death. Should death occur, it is frequently a result of a secondary pneumonia caused by a lower respiratory invasion by bacteria or viruses. Children should avoid using aspirin for relief of symptoms caused by viruses. An apparent relationship exists between Reye's syndrome and the use of aspirin by chil-dren 2 to 15 years of age to relieve symptoms caused by viral diseases.

Pleural Effusions

Pleural effusion is an excess of fluid in the pleural cavity. The pleural cavity normally contains only a small amount of lubricating fluid, but in many disorders this amount increases. These conditions include failure of the heart to pump adequate amounts of blood to body tissues (**con-gestive heart failure**), liver diseases associated with an accumulation of fluid in the abdominal and plural cavities (**ascites**), infectious lung diseases, and trauma.

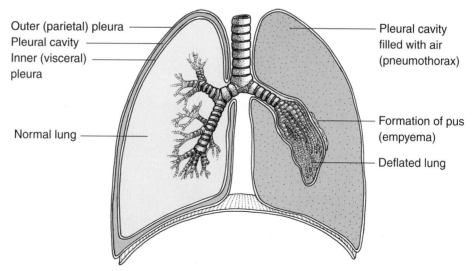

Figure 8–3   Pneumothorax is the presence of air in the pleural cavity, which can cause a lung to collapse. Empyema is the accumulation of pus in the cavity between the pleura and lung tissue.

Two noninvasive techniques used in the diagnosis of pleural effusion are listening to the sounds of the chest cavity with a stethoscope (**auscultation**) and gently tapping the chest with the fingers to determine the position, size, or consistency of the underlying structures (**percussion**). Different types of pleural effusions include pus in the pleural space (**empyema**), serum in the pleural space (**hydrothorax**), blood in the pleural space (**hemothorax**), air in the pleural space (**pneumothorax**) (Fig. 8–3), and a mixture of pus and air in the pleural space (**pyopneumothorax**). Depending on the amount and type of fluid, treatment may include surgical puncture of the chest (**thoracocentesis, thoracentesis**) to remove excess fluid. Sometimes chest tubes are inserted to facilitate removal of the fluid.

Tuberculosis

Tuberculosis (TB) is an infectious disease that afflicts more than 2.5 billion people worldwide. Although the number of U.S. citizens with the disease decreased by about 6 percent per year since 1953, over the last several years the trend has reversed, and a significant number of new cases are currently reported yearly. The increase in the disease is correlated with the increase of drug-resistant strains, the number of people with acquired immunodeficiency syndrome (AIDS), and those who are homeless or live in poverty. This disease is highly communicable.

Tuberculosis is spread by inhaling droplets of respiratory secretions (**aerosol transmission**) or particles of dry sputum containing the TB organism, which can remain alive (**viable**) and infectious for 6 to 8 months outside of the body. The first time the TB organism enters the body (**primary tuberculosis**), the disease develops slowly. It eventually produces focal lesions encased in small pockets called granulomas (**tubercles**). Usually the granulomas remain dormant for years, keeping the patient asymptomatic. When the immune system becomes impaired (**immunocompromised**) or when the patient is reintroduced to the bacterium, the full-blown disease may develop.

Although primarily a lung disease, TB can infect the bones, genital tract, meninges, and peritoneum. Many of the TB strains that infect AIDS patients are not responsive to standard medications (**drug resistant**), and treatment becomes a challenge.

Bronchopneumonia

The term **bronchopneumonia** refers to any inflammatory disease of the lungs. It may be caused by a variety of agents, including bacteria, viruses, diseases, chemicals, and other substances. Infectious pneumonias are primarily attributed to bacteria or viruses. A sometimes-fatal type of pneumonia is associated with influenza. Other potentially fatal pneumonias may result from food

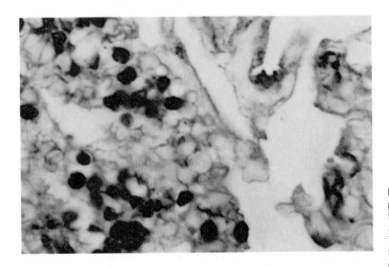

50μm

Figure 8–4 *Pneumocystis carinii* pneumonia. Darkly stained cysts in lung tissue of patient with *Pneumocystis carinii* pneumonia. (From Taber's Cyclopedic Medical Dictionary, ed 18. F.A. Davis, Philadelphia, 1997, p 1503, with permission.)

or liquid inhalation. Some pneumonias affect only a lobe of the lung (**lobar pneumonia**), whereas others affect both the right and left lungs (**bilateral** or "**double**" **pneumonia**). Chest pain, mucopurulent sputum, and spitting of blood (**hemoptysis**) are frequent symptoms of the disease. The lungs may undergo solidification (**consolidation**) because of a pathological engorgement.

Pneumocystis carinii pneumonia (PCP) is a particularly important disease associated with AIDS. Recent evidence suggests that it is caused by a fungus that resides in or on most people (**normal flora**) but causes no harm as long as the individual remains healthy. When the immune system becomes compromised, however, this organism becomes infectious (**opportunistic**). Diagnosis relies on examination of biopsied lung tissue (Fig. 8–4) or bronchial washings (**lavage**).

Cystic Fibrosis

Cystic fibrosis, a hereditary disorder, affects the exocrine glands. The disease causes widespread involvement (**systemic**), especially of the lungs, pancreas, and digestive tract. Mucus produced in an individual afflicted with cystic fibrosis is extremely thick (**viscous**) and blocks the bronchioles. Air becomes trapped in the lungs, but use of mists (**aerosols**) and postural drainage (Fig. 8–5) provides relief.

An important finding in cystic fibrosis is an increase in the amount of salt excreted in sweat. Although the disease is fatal, improved methods of treatment have extended life expectancy, and patient survival is approximately 30 years.

Respiratory Distress Syndrome

Respiratory distress syndrome (RDS) is most often caused by the absence or impairment in the production of a phospholipid substance of the lungs called **surfactant**. This substance aids in decreasing the surface tension of the alveoli. Lungs require surfactant in order to fill with air and expand (**compliance**). Lacking surfactant, the alveoli collapse and inhalation becomes extremely difficult.

When this condition is found in newborn infants, it is called **infant respiratory distress syndrome (IRDS)** or **hyaline membrane disease (HMD)**. IRDS is most frequently seen in premature infants or infants born to diabetic mothers. Before birth, lung tissue normally develops surfactant. If the amount of this substance is inadequate, clinical symptoms are noticeable immediately after birth, including blueness (**cyanosis**) of the extremities, rapid breathing (**tachypnea**), flaring of the nostrils (**nares**), intercostal retraction, and a characteristic grunt audible during exhalation. Radiography shows a membrane that has a ground-glass appearance (**hyaline membrane**). Although severe cases of IRDS result in death, some forms of therapy are effective.

Adult respiratory distress syndrome (ARDS) is caused by an impairment of surfactant production or by exposure to substances that remove surfactant from the lungs. Accidental inhalation of foreign substances, water, smoke, chemical fumes, and vomit is often the cause.

Oncology

Primary Pulmonary Cancer

Smoking is the leading cause of all types of lung cancers. The most common form of lung cancer in the United States is primary pulmonary cancer. The site most frequently involved is the epithelium of the bronchial passages; lung cancer located here is called bronchogenic carcinoma. In this type of cancer, the cells at the base of the epithelium (**basal cells**) divide repeatedly, until eventually the entire epithelium is involved. Within a short time the epithelium begins to invade the underlying tissues. Masses form and block air passages and alveoli, thereby reducing the surface area needed for gas exchange. Bronchogenic carcinoma spreads (**metastasizes**) rapidly to other areas of the body, frequently to lymph nodes, liver, bones, brain, or kidney. Surgery, radiation, and chemotherapy are common methods of treatment; however, lung cancer is difficult to control and survival rates are extremely low.

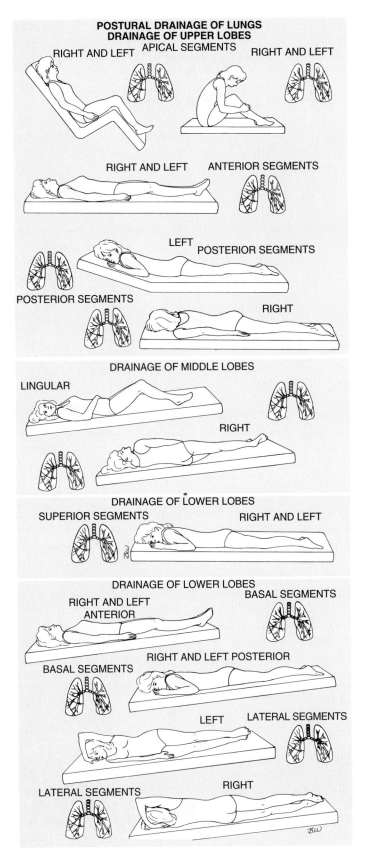

Figure 8–5 Positions for postural drainage of lungs. (From Taber's Cyclopedic Medical Dictionary, ed 18. F.A. Davis, Philadelphia, 1997, pp 1535–1536, with permission.)

DIAGNOSTIC, SYMPTOMATIC, AND THERAPEUTIC TERMS

Term	Meaning
acidosis ăs-ĭ-DŌ-sĭs	excessive acidity of body fluids, frequently associated with pulmonary insufficiency resulting in the retention of carbon dioxide
anosmia ăn-ŎZ-mē-ă	absence of the sense of smell
anoxia, hypoxia ăn-ŎK-sē-ă, hī-PŎK-sē-ă	absence or deficiency of O_2 in tissues
anoxemia, hypoxemia ăn-ŏk-SĒ-mē-ă, hī-pŏk-SĒ-mē-ă	absence or deficiency of O_2 in blood
asphyxia ăs-FĬK-sē-ă	condition in which there is insufficient O_2; literally means "without pulse"
atelectasis ăt-ĕ-LĔK-tă-sĭs	a collapsed or airless state of the lung, which may be acute or chronic, and may involve all or part of the lung. In fetal atelectasis the lungs fail to expand normally at birth
compliance kŏm-PLĪ-ăns	ease with which lung tissue can be stretched
coryza kŏ-RĪ-ză	head cold; upper respiratory infection (URI)
croup croop	condition resulting from an acute obstruction of the larynx caused by an allergen, foreign body, infection, or new growth; symptoms include resonant, barking cough; suffocative and difficult breathing; laryngeal spasm; and sometimes the formation of a membrane
Cheyne-Stokes respiration CHĀN-stōks	breathing characterized by fluctuation in the depth of respiration. The patient breathes deeply for a short time, then breathes very slightly, then not at all. This pattern occurs repeatedly. Cheyne-Stokes respiration is usually caused by diseases that affect the respiratory centers (e.g., heart failure or brain damage)
epiglottitis ĕp-ĭ-glŏt-Ī-tĭs	usually severe, life-threatening infection of the epiglottis and surrounding area that occurs most often in children between 2 and 12 years of age. In the classic form, a sudden onset of fever, dysphagia, inspiratory stridor, and severe respiratory distress occurs that often requires intubation or tracheostomy to open the obstructed airway
epistaxis ĕp-ĭ-STĂK-sĭs	nosebleed; nasal hemorrhage
mucus MŪ-kŭs	viscous fluid secreted by mucous membranes that communicate with the air
pertussis pĕr-TŬS-ĭs	whooping cough; acute infectious disease characterized by a "whoop"- sounding cough. Immunization of infants as part of the diphtheria-pertussis-tetanus (DPT) vaccine prevents contracting the disease
phlegm flĕm	abnormal amounts of mucus, especially expectorated from the mouth
pleurisy, pleuritis PLOOR-ĭ-sē, ploo-RĪ-tĭs	inflammation of the pleural membrane characterized by a stabbing pain that is intensified by coughing or deep breathing

DIAGNOSTIC, SYMPTOMATIC, AND THERAPEUTIC TERMS
(Continued)

Term	Meaning
pneumoconiosis, pneumoconioses (pl.) nū-mō-kō-nē-Ō-sĭs	respiratory disorder (usually occupational) caused by inhaling dust particles (e.g., anthracosis [coal dust], chalicosis [stone dust], siderosis [iron], asbestosis [asbestos])
postural drainage PŎS-tū-răl	positioning a patient so that gravity aids in the drainage of secretions from the bronchi and lobes of the lungs
pulmonary edema PŬL-mō-nĕ-rē ĕ-DĒ-mă	excessive fluid in the lungs that induces cough and dyspnea; common in left heart failure
pulmonary embolus PŬL-mō-nĕ-rē ĔM-bō-lŭs	a mass of undissolved matter (e.g., blood clot, tissue, air bubbles, bacteria) in the pulmonary arteries or its branches
rale, crackle răl, KRĂK-ĕl	abnormal respiratory sound heard on auscultation, caused by exudates, spasms, hyperplasia, or when air enters moisture-filled alveoli
rhonchus, rhonchi (pl.) RŎNG-kŭs, RŎNG-kī	rale or rattling in the throat, especially when it resembles snoring
sputum SPŪ-tŭm	pathological viscous fluid formed in the lower respiratory tract that often contains blood, pus, and bacteria
sudden infant death syndrome (SIDS)	the completely unexpected and unexplained death of an apparently well or virtually well infant. The most common cause of death between the second week and first year of life; crib death
stridor STRĪ-dor	abnormal sound caused by a spasm or swelling of the larynx
wheeze hwēz	a whistling or sighing sound resulting from narrowing of the lumen of the respiratory passageway that is noted by use of a stethoscope. It occurs in asthma, croup, hay fever, obstructive emphysema, and other obstructive respiratory conditions

DIAGNOSTIC PROCEDURES

Imaging Procedures	Description
bronchography bronğ-KŎG-ră-fē	radiological evaluation of the trachea and bronchi following administration of a radiopaque contrast medium
percutaneous transtracheal pĕr-kū-TĀ-nē-ŭs trăns-TRĀ-kē-ăl	radiographic imaging procedure of the bronchial tree after administration of a contrast medium directly into the trachea via a percutaneous puncture
chest radiographs RĀ-dē-ō-grăfs	series of x-ray images designed to evaluate the chest, heart, lungs, and rib cage
CT scan (thoracic) thō-RĂS-ĭk	provides a cross-sectional view of the chest, with or without an injected radiographic iodine contrast medium; used primarily to highlight blood vessels and tissue masses
lung profusion studies	imaging procedure that uses a radionucleotide to visualize the lung, especially in suspected pulmonary emboli

DIAGNOSTIC PROCEDURES (Continued)

Endoscopic Procedures	Description
bronchoscopy brŏng-KŎS-kō-pē	visual examination of the bronchi using a flexible bronchoscope inserted through the mouth and trachea into the bronchial tubes; used for suctioning, biopsy, removal of foreign bodies, and collection of fluid or sputum for examination and diagnosis
laryngoscopy lăr-ĭn-GŎS-kō-pē	visual examination of the larynx with a laryngoscope; may be viewed directly or indirectly by transmitting image of the larynx via a laryngeal mirror; used for performing biopsies, collecting sputum samples, identifying tumors, and accounting for changes in the voice
mediastinoscopy mē-dē-ăs-tĭ-NŎS-kō-pē	allows direct visualization of the mediastinal structures, heart, trachea, esophagus, bronchus, thymus, and lymph nodes; especially important in early diagnosis of bronchogenic carcinoma

Clinical Procedures	Description
pulmonary function studies	one of a number of tests used to determine the ability of the lungs to exchange O_2 and CO_2, including determining the ability of the alveolar capillary membrane to transport O_2 to the blood and to carry CO_2 from the blood into the expired air
spirometry spī-RŎM-ĕ-trē	measurement of lung capacity and flow including the time necessary for exhaling the total volume of inhaled air. This device produces a graphic record for the patient's chart
tuberculin test tū-BĔR-kū-lĭn	test to determine the presence of a tuberculosis infection based on a positive reaction of the subject to tuberculin. Common tests do not distinguish between active or inactive infection. Test is positive when area around the site is indurated
Mantoux măn-TŪ	intradermal injection of tuberculin

Laboratory Procedures	Description
arterial blood gases (ABGs)	assessment of partial pressure of oxygen (PaO_2) and carbon dioxide ($PaCO_2$) and determines acidity (pH) of an arterial blood sample. This test evaluates pulmonary gas exchange and is important in treating disturbances of acid-base balance
sputum culture SPŪ-tŭm	microbial test performed using a sputum sample; identifies disease-causing organisms of lower respiratory tract, especially those that cause pneumonias
sweat test	measurement of the amount of salt (sodium chloride) in sweat; used almost exclusively in children to confirm cystic fibrosis
throat culture	test used to identify pathogens, especially group A streptococci. It is important to treat streptococcal infections, as they may lead to serious secondary disorders

SURGICAL AND THERAPEUTIC PROCEDURES

Procedures	Description
antral irrigation (lavage) ĂN-trăl	washing or irrigation of the sinuses in patients who are not responding to treatment
rhinoplasty RĪ-nō-plăs-tē	cosmetic surgery that corrects deformities of the external nose; may be performed when nose is too long, too wide, humped, or projects too far away from the face
pleurectomy, decortication ploor-ĔK-tō-mē, dē-kŏr-tĭ-KĀ-shŭn	excision of part of the pleura
pneumonectomy nū-mō-NĔK-tō-mē	excision of a lung or lobe of the lung
resection	a partial excision of a bone or other structure
segmental, lung	removal of one or more lung segments (a bronchiole and its alveoli)
submucosal	removal of tissue below the mucosa, especially excision of cartilaginous tissue beneath the mucosal tissue of the nose
thoracentesis, thoracocentesis thō-ră-sĕn-TĒ-sĭs, thō-răk-ō-sĕn-TĒ-sĭs	surgical puncture and drainage of pleural cavity

PHARMACOLOGY

Medication	Action
antihistamines	counteract the effects of histamines, which cause nasal passage swelling and inflammation; primary agents used to relieve allergic rhinitis (hay fever) symptoms
antitussives	suppress coughing
bronchodilators	cause dilation of the bronchi, thereby "opening up" the breathing passages
decongestants	reduce congestion or swelling, especially in the nasal passages, by constricting blood vessels and limiting blood flow to the area
expectorants	facilitate the removal of secretions from the lungs, bronchi, and trachea
mucolytics	liquefy or break down tenacious, "sticky" mucus so that it can be coughed up more easily

ABBREVIATIONS

Diagnostic and Symptomatic	Meaning
ABGs	arterial blood gases
AP	anteroposterior
ARDS	adult respiratory distress syndrome
COPD	chronic obstructive pulmonary disease
CPR	cardiopulmonary resuscitation
CXR	chest x-ray film; chest radiograph
FEF	forced expiratory flow
FEV	forced expiratory volume
FVC	forced vital capacity
HMD	hyaline membrane disease
Hx	history
IPPB	intermittent positive-pressure breathing

ABBREVIATIONS (Continued)

Diagnostic and Symptomatic	Meaning
IRDS	infant respiratory distress syndrome
PA	posteroanterior
PCP	*Pneumocystis carinii* pneumonia
PFT	pulmonary function tests
PND	paroxysmal nocturnal dyspnea
RD	respiratory disease
RDS	respiratory distress syndrome
SOB	shortness of breath
T&A	tonsillectomy and adenoidectomy
TB	tuberculosis
TPR	temperature, pulse, and respiration
URI	upper respiratory infection
VC	vital capacity

Laboratory	Meaning
AFB	acid-fast bacillus (TB organism)
CO$_2$	carbon dioxide
O$_2$	oxygen

MEDICAL RECORD

Respiratory Evaluation

History of Present Illness   This 49-year-old man with known history of COPD is admitted because of exacerbation of SOB over the past few days. Patient was a heavy smoker and states that he quit smoking for a short while but now smokes three to four cigarettes a day. He has a Hx of difficult breathing, high blood pressure, COPD, and peripheral vascular disease. He underwent triple bypass surgery in 19XX. PE indicates scattered bilateral wheezes and rhonchi heard anteriorly and posteriorly.

Compared with a portable chest film from 4/17/XX, deterioration since the previous study is noted that most likely indicates interstitial vascular congestion. Some superimposed inflammatory change cannot be excluded. There may also be some pleural reactive change.

Dx   (1) Acute exacerbation of chronic obstructive pulmonary disease; (2) congestive heart failure; (3) hypertension; (4) peripheral vascular disease.

Worksheet 5 provides a dictionary and reading application and an analysis of this medical record.

WORKSHEET 1

Use rhin/o *(nose) to build a medical word meaning:*

1. disease of the nose _____

2. inflammation of the (mucous membranes of the) nose _____

3. discharge from the nose _____

Use laryng/o *(larynx or "voice box") to build a medical word meaning:*

4. inflammation of the larynx _____

5. visual examination of the larynx _____

6. spasm of the larynx _____

7. stricture or narrowing of the larynx _____

8. pertaining to the larynx and the trachea _____

9. disease of the larynx _____

Use bronch/o *or* bronchi/o *(bronchus) to build a medical word meaning:*

10. instrument to view the bronchus _____

11. inflammation of the bronchus _____

12. dilation or expansion of the bronchus _____

13. spasm of the bronchus _____

14. disease of the bronchus _____

Use pneumon/o *or* pneum/o *(air, lung) to build a medical word meaning:*

15. inflammation of the lungs _____

16. x-ray of the lungs _____

Use thorac/o *(chest) to build a medical word meaning:*

17. pertaining to the chest _____

18. pain in the muscles of the chest _____

Use the suffix -pnea *(breathing) to build a medical word meaning:*

19. difficult or painful breathing _____

20. breathing in a straight (upright) position _____

21. not breathing (temporary) _____

22. good, normal breathing _____

23. slow breathing _____

Use the suffix -thorax (chest) to build a medical word meaning:

24. air in the chest _____

25. blood in the chest _____

WORKSHEET 2

■ ■ ■ ■ ■ ■ ■ ■ ■ ■ ■ ■ ■

Build a surgical term meaning:

1. forming an opening in the larynx _____

2. puncture of the lung _____

3. excision of a lobe (of the lung) _____

4. surgical repair of the nose _____

5. puncture of the chest _____

6. suture of the larynx _____

7. fixation of the lung (to the thoracic wall) _____

8. surgical repair of the bronchus _____

9. forming an opening in the trachea _____

10. excision of (part of) the pleura _____

WORKSHEET 3

■ ■ ■ ■ ■ ■ ■ ■ ■ ■ ■ ■ ■

Match the following medical terms with the definitions in the numbered list.

anosmia	compliance	pertussis
anoxemia	coryza	rales, crackles
atelectasis	epistaxis	sputum
Cheyne-Stokes respiration	mucus	stridor

1. _____ pathological fluid formed in the lungs or bronchi

2. _____ abnormal respiratory sounds heard in auscultation, indicating pathology

3. _____ ease with which lung tissue can be stretched

4. _____ viscous fluid secreted by mucous membranes

5. _____ whooping cough

6. _____ irregular breathing characterized by alteration in depth of respiration and apnea

7. _____ lack of sense of smell

8. _____ absence of or decrease in O_2 in the blood

9. _____ abnormal sound caused by a spasm or swelling of the larynx or a bronchus

10. _____ head cold; upper respiratory infection

WORKSHEET 4

■ ■ ■ ■ ■ ■ ■ ■ ■ ■ ■ ■ ■ ■ ■

Select a term that best describes the statements that follow.

antihistamines	bronchoscopy	hemoptysis
antitussives	COPD	Mantoux test
antral irrigation	CT scan (thoracic)	mucolytics
AP	CXR	spirometry
arterial blood gases	decongestants	sweat test
bronchography	FEV	thoracentesis

1. _____ measurement of lung capacity and flow including the time necessary for exhaling the total volume of inhaled air

2. _____ x-ray films of the bronchial tree following intratracheal injection of a contrast medium

3. _____ sequence of radiographs, each representing a "slice" of the lung at different depths

4. _____ washing of the sinuses in patients who are not responding to treatment

5. _____ anteroposterior

6. _____ chronic obstructive pulmonary disease

7. _____ prevent or relieve coughing

8. _____ primary agents used to relieve discomfort associated with allergic rhinitis, which block the action of histamines

9. _____ liquefy "sticky" mucus so that it can be coughed up more readily

10. _____ assesses the PaO_2 and $PaCO_2$ levels of arterial blood in order to evaluate and manage acid-base disturbances

11. _____ puncture of the chest to remove fluids

12. _____ measures the amount of salt for diagnosis of cystic fibrosis

13. _____ interdermal test used to detect the presence of tuberculosis infection

14. _____ chest x-ray examination; chest radiograph

15. _____ forced expiratory volume

WORKSHEET 5

. . . .

MEDICAL RECORD: RESPIRATORY EVALUATION

Underline the following terms in the medical record (see p. 129). Use a medical dictionary and other resources to define the terms and to determine their pronunciation; then practice reading the medical record aloud.

bilateral _____

COPD _____

Dx _____

exacerbation _____

Hx _____

inflammatory _____

interstitial vascular congestion _____

PE _____

peripheral vascular disease _____

pleural _____

rhonchi _____

SOB _____

MEDICAL RECORD EVALUATION: RESPIRATORY EVALUATION

1. *What symptom caused the patient to seek medical help?*

2. *What was the patient's previous history?*

3. *What were the findings of the physical examination?*

4. *What changes were noted from the previous film?*

5. *What is the present Dx?*

6. *What new diagnosis was made that did not appear in the previous medical history?*

7. *What is the abbreviation for congestive heart failure?*

WORKSHEET 6

■ ■ ■ ■ ■ ■ ■ ■ ■ ■ ■ ■ ■ ■ ■

Label the structures indicated on the following diagram. To check your answers, refer to Figure 8–1.

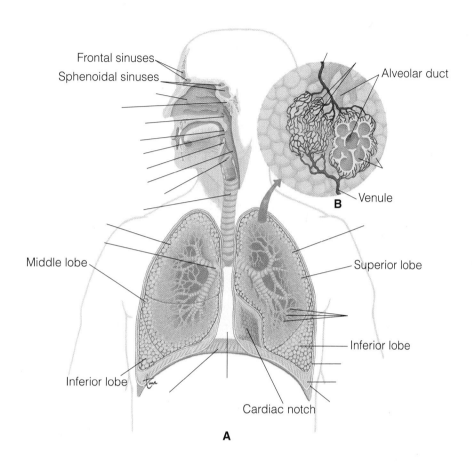

Frontal sinuses

Sphenoidal sinuses

Alveolar duct

Venule

B

Middle lobe

Superior lobe

Inferior lobe

Inferior lobe

Cardiac notch

A

Adenoids	Epiglottis	Nasal cavity	Pleural cavity
Alveolus	Laryngopharynx	Nasopharynx	Pulmonary capillaries
Arteriole	Larynx	Oropharynx	Right lung
Bronchioles	Left lung	Palatine tonsil	Trachea
Bronchus	Mediastinum	Parietal pleura	Visceral pleura
Diaphragm			

Chapter 9

CARDIOVASCULAR SYSTEM

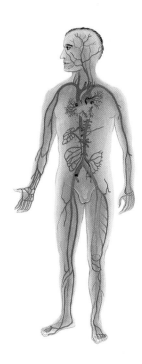

Chapter Outline

Student Objectives

Anatomy and Physiology
Vascular System
  Arteries
  Capillaries
  Veins
Heart
Conduction System of the Heart
Blood Pressure
Fetal Circulation

Combining Forms

Suffixes

Prefixes

Pathology
Atherosclerosis
Coronary Artery Disease

Infective Endocarditis
Varicose Veins
Oncology

**Diagnostic, Symptomatic,
  and Therapeutic Terms**

Diagnostic Procedures
Imaging Procedures
Clinical Procedures
Laboratory Procedures

Surgical and Therapeutic Procedures

Pharmacology

Abbreviations

Medical Record
Acute Myocardial Infarction

Worksheets

Student Objectives

Upon completion of this chapter, you will be able to do the following:

1. List and describe the structure and function of three types of blood vessels.

2. List and describe the major structures and functions of the heart.

3. Differentiate between systemic and pulmonary circulation.

4. Define systolic and diastolic blood pressures.

5. Discuss the function of the conduction system of the heart.

6. List the structures, in sequential order, through which electrical current passes during the cardiac cycle.

7. Identify the combining forms, suffixes, and prefixes related to the cardiovascular system.

8. Identify and discuss pathology related to the cardiovascular system.

Student Objectives (Continued)

9. Identify diagnostic, symptomatic, and therapeutic terms related to the cardiovascular system.

10. Identify diagnostic procedures related to the cardiovascular system.

11. Identify surgical and therapeutic procedures related to the cardiovascular system.

12. Discuss pharmacology related to the treatment of cardiovascular disorders.

13. Define abbreviations related to the cardiovascular system.

14. Demonstrate your knowledge of the chapter by completing the worksheets.

ANATOMY AND PHYSIOLOGY

The cardiovascular system is composed of the heart and blood vessels. The heart is a hollow muscular organ lying in the mediastinum, the center of the thoracic cavity located between the lungs. It pumps blood to body cells through a vast network of blood vessels. Blood returns to the heart, again through blood vessels, to begin the cycle again.

The body is composed of trillions of cells, all requiring a constant supply of food and other vital products for survival. As they metabolize food for energy, they produce waste products. Therefore, cells also require a means of removing accumulated waste products. Because body cells are not always located near the source of the products they need and are not always near the organs necessary for elimination of waste, they require a transportation system. The cardiovascular system, in conjunction with the blood and lymphatic systems (discussed in Chap. 10), is responsible for transportation of products to and from body cells.

Vascular System

Three major types of vessels, **arteries**, **capillaries**, and **veins**, carry blood throughout the body. Each type of vessel differs in structure, depending on its function. Figure 9–1 illustrates the structures that comprise the vascular system. Refer to this figure as you read the following.

Arteries

Arteries carry blood from the heart to body tissues and organs. Blood is propelled through arteries by the pumping action of the heart. Consequently, arterial walls are thick and muscular and capable of expanding to accommodate the surge of blood that results when the heart contracts. The surge of blood felt in the arteries when blood is pumped from the heart is referred to as a **pulse**. Because of the pressure against arterial walls associated with the pumping action of the heart, a cut or severed artery may lead to profuse bleeding.

Arterial blood (except for that found in the pulmonary artery) contains a high concentration of oxygen (O_2). It appears bright red and is said to be **oxygenated**. Oxygenated blood travels to smaller vessels called **arterioles** (little arteries) and finally to the smallest vessels, the **capillaries**.

Capillaries

Capillaries are microscopic vessels that join the arterial system with the venous system. Although seemingly the most insignificant of the three vessel types because of their microscopic size, capillaries are functionally the most important. Capillary walls are composed of a single layer of cells. The thinness of their walls and differences in pressure make it possible for substances, including gases, to pass quite readily into and out of the vessels. Consequently, the primary function of the vascular system, that of providing cells with vital products and removal of waste products, occurs

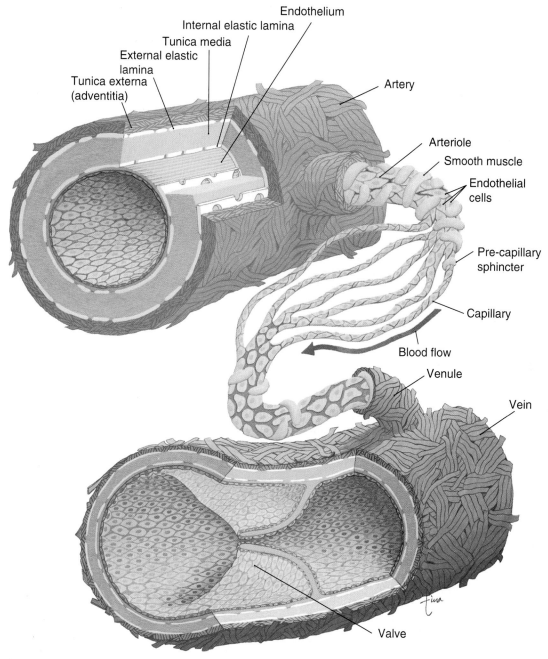

Figure 9–1 Structure of an artery, arteriole, capillary network, venule, and vein. (From Scanlon, VC, and Sanders, T: Understanding Human Structure and Function. F.A. Davis, Philadelphia, 1997, p 226, with permission.)

at the capillary level. The vast number of capillaries makes their combined diameter so great that blood flows through them very slowly. The pulse that was present in the arteries can no longer be detected in the capillaries. The slow movement of blood through capillaries allows sufficient time for delivery of vital products and removal of waste from the surrounding tissues.

Veins

Veins return blood to the heart. They are formed from smaller vessels called **venules** (little veins), which develop from the union of capillaries. Because the extensive network of capillaries throughout the body absorbs the propelling pressure exerted by the heart, blood in veins use other methods to return to the heart, including:

- Skeletal muscle contraction
- Gravity
- Respiratory activity
- Valves

Valves are small structures within veins that prevent the backflow of blood. Valves are especially important for returning blood from the legs to the heart because blood must travel a long distance against the force of gravity to reach the heart.

Blood carried in the veins (except for the blood in the pulmonary veins) contains a low concentration of O_2 (deoxygenated) with a corresponding high concentration of carbon dioxide (CO_2). Deoxygenated blood takes on a characteristic purple color. It continuously circulates to the lungs, so that CO_2 can be expelled.

Heart

The heart has three distinct tissue layers and is contained in a sac called the **pericardium**.

- The **endocardium**, a serous membrane that lines the four chambers of the heart and its valves and is continuous with the arteries and veins
- The **myocardium**, the muscular layer of the heart
- The **epicardium**, the outermost layer of the heart

As you read the following material, refer to Figure 9–2 to identify the internal and external structures of the heart and major vessels.

The heart is divided into four chambers: (1) **right atrium**, (2) **right ventricle**, (3) **left atrium**, and (4) **left ventricle**. The two upper chambers, the atria, collect blood; the two lower chambers, the ventricles, pump blood from the heart. The right side of the heart provides for the oxygenation of blood (pulmonary circulation), and the left side is responsible for the transportation of blood to body systems (systemic circulation).

Deoxygenated blood returns to the heart by way of two large veins: the (5) **superior vena cava**, which collects and carries blood from the upper part of the body; and the (6) **inferior vena cava**, which collects and carries blood from the lower part of the body. The superior and inferior venae cavae (singular, vena cava) deposit deoxygenated blood into the upper right chamber of the heart, the right atrium. From the right atrium, blood passes through the (7) **tricuspid valve** to the right ventricle. During contraction of the ventricle, the tricuspid valve prevents a backflow of blood to the right atrium. When the heart contracts, blood leaves the right ventricle by way of the (8) **left pulmonary artery** and (9) **right pulmonary artery** and travels to the lungs. The (10) **pulmonary semilunar valve** (or pulmonary valve) prevents a backflow of blood into the right ventricle. In the lungs, the pulmonary artery branches into millions of capillaries, each lying close to an alveolus. Here, CO_2 in the blood is replaced by O_2 that has been drawn into the lungs during inhalation.

Pulmonary capillaries unite to form four pulmonary veins, two (11) **right pulmonary veins** and two (12) **left pulmonary veins**, the vessels that carry oxygenated blood back to the heart. Pulmonary veins deposit blood in the left atrium. From here, blood passes through the (13) **mitral (bicuspid) valve** to the left ventricle. Upon contraction of the heart, the oxygenated blood leaves the left ventricle through the largest artery of the body, the (14) **aorta**. Within the aorta is a valve called the (15) **aortic semilunar valve** that permits blood to flow in only one direction—from the left ventricle to the aorta. The aorta branches into many smaller arteries that carry blood to all parts of the body. Some arteries derive their names from the organs or areas of the body that they vascularize. For example, the splenic artery vascularizes the spleen, and the renal arteries vascularize the kidneys.

It is important to recognize that O_2, present in the blood passing through the chambers of the heart, cannot be used by the myocardium. Instead, an arterial system composed of the coronary

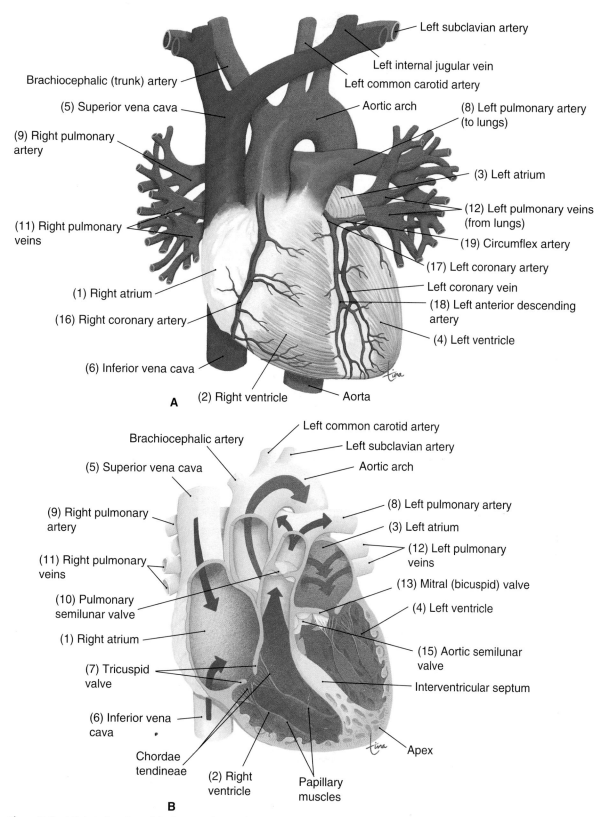

Figure 9–2   (*A*) Anterior view of the heart and major blood vessels. (*B*) Frontal section of the heart in anterior view showing internal structures. (From Scanlon, VC, and Sanders, T: Understanding Human Structure and Function. F.A. Davis, Philadelphia, 1997, p 213, with permission.)

arteries branches from the aorta and provides the myocardium with its own blood supply. These arteries lie over the top of the heart much as a crown fits over a head, hence the name **coronary** (pertaining to a crown). The artery vascularizing the right side of the heart is the (16) **right coronary artery**. The artery vascularizing the left side of the heart is the (17) **left coronary artery**. It divides into the (18) **left anterior descending artery** and the (19) **circumflex artery**. If blood flow in the coronary arteries is diminished, myocardial damage may result. When severe damage occurs, part of the heart muscle may die.

Conduction System of the Heart

Within the heart is specialized cardiac tissue known as **conductive tissue**. Its sole function is the initiation and propagation of contraction impulses. It consists of four masses of highly specialized cells. Refer to Figure 9–3 to identify the following structures:

- (1) **Sinoatrial (SA) node**
- (2) **Atrioventricular (AV) node**
- (3) **Bundle of His** (AV bundle)
- (4) **Purkinje fibers**

The SA node, located in the upper portion of the right atrium, possesses its own intrinsic rhythm. Without being stimulated by external nerves, it has the ability to initiate and propagate each heartbeat, thereby setting the basic pace for the cardiac rate. For this reason, the SA node is commonly known as the **pacemaker** of the heart. Cardiac rate may be altered by impulses from the autonomic nervous system. Such an arrangement allows outside influences to accelerate or decelerate the heart rate. For example, during physical exertion the heart beats faster, and during rest it beats slower.

Each electrical impulse discharged by the SA node is transmitted to the AV node, causing the atria to contract. The AV node is located at the base of the right atrium. From this point, a tract of conduction fibers called the bundle of His, composed of a right and left branch, relays the impulse to the Purkinje fibers. These fibers extend up the ventricle walls. The Purkinje fibers transmit the impulse to both the right and left ventricles, causing them to contract. Blood is now forced from the heart through the pulmonary artery and aorta.

In summary, the sequence of the four structures responsible for conduction of a contraction impulse is as follows:

SA node → AV node → bundle of His → Purkinje fibers

Impulse transmission through the conduction system generates weak electrical currents that can be detected on the surface of the body. These electrical impulses can be recorded on an instrument called an **electrocardiograph**. The needle deflection of the electrocardiograph produces waves or peaks designated by the letters P, Q, R, S, and T, each of which is associated with a specific electrical event. The P wave is the depolarization (contraction) of the atria, and the QRS complex is the depolarization (contraction) of the ventricles. The T wave, which appears a short time later, is the repolarization (recovery) of the ventricles.

Blood Pressure

Blood pressure measures the force exerted by blood against the arterial walls during two phases of a heartbeat: the contraction phase, called **systole**, when the blood is forced out of the heart; and the relaxation phase, called **diastole**, when the ventricles are filling with blood. Systole is the maximum force exerted by blood against the arterial walls; diastole, the weakest. These measurements are recorded as two figures separated by a diagonal line; the systolic pressure is given first, followed by the diastolic pressure. For instance, blood pressure may be recorded as 120/80 bpm; in this example, 120 is the systolic pressure, 80 the diastolic pressure.

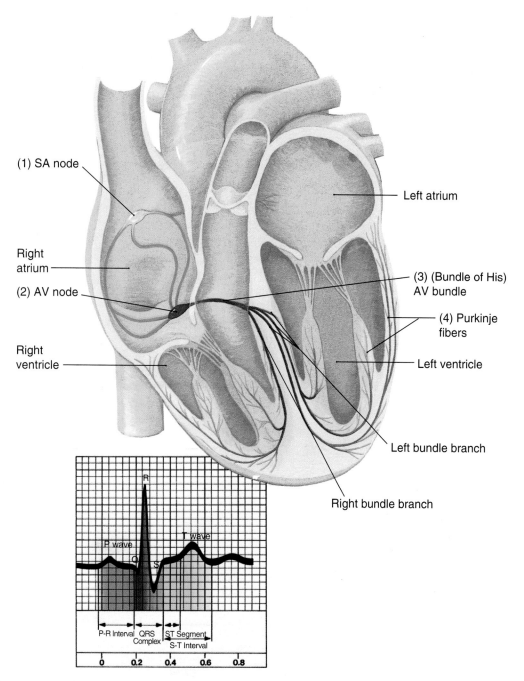

Figure 9–3   Conduction pathway of the heart. Anterior view of the interior of the heart. The electrocardiogram tracing is of one normal heartbeat. (From Scanlon, VC, and Sanders, T: Understanding Human Structure and Function. F.A. Davis, Philadelphia, 1997, p 217, with permission.)

Several factors influence blood pressure:

- Resistance of blood flow in blood vessels
- Pumping action of the heart
- Viscosity or thickness of blood
- Elasticity of arteries
- Quantity of blood in the vascular system

Elevated blood pressure is called **hypertension**; decreased blood pressure is called **hypotension**.

Fetal Circulation

Blood circulation through a fetus is by necessity different from that of a newborn infant. Respiration, the procurement of nutrients, and the elimination of metabolic wastes occur through the maternal blood instead of through the organs of the fetus. The capillary exchange between the maternal and fetal circulation occurs within the placenta. This remarkable structure includes part of the mother's uterus during pregnancy and is discharged following delivery as the afterbirth. Refer to Figure 9–4 to identify the major structures in fetal circulation.

The (1) **umbilical cord**, containing (2) two **arteries**, carries deoxygenated blood from the fetus to the (3) **placenta**. After oxygenation in the placenta, blood returns to the fetus via the (4) **umbilical vein**. Most of the blood in the umbilical vein enters the (5) **inferior vena cava** through the (6) **ductus venosus**, where it is delivered to the (7) **right atrium**. Some of this blood passes to the (8) **right ventricle**, but most of it passes through a small opening in the atrial septum called the (9) **foramen ovale**, which closes shortly after birth.

An additional structure found in the fetal circulatory system is the (10) **ductus arteriosus**. This structure shunts most blood out of the pulmonary arteries, causing it to flow into the aorta, thus bypassing the nonfunctional lungs of the fetus.

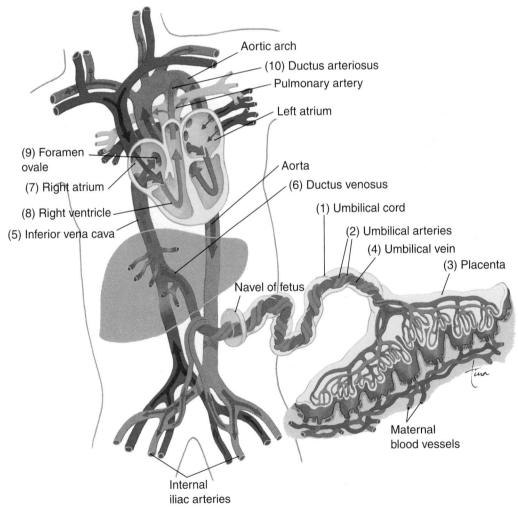

Figure 9–4 Fetal circulation. Fetal heart and blood vessels are shown on the left. Arrows depict the direction of blood flow. The placenta and umbilical blood vessels are shown on the right. (From Scanlon, VC, and Sanders, T: Understanding Human Structure and Function. F.A. Davis, Philadelphia, 1997, p 238, with permission.)

COMBINING FORMS

Combining Form	Meaning	Example	Pronunciation
angi/o	vessel	angi/o/rrhaphy suture	an-jē-OR-ă-fē
vas/o		vas/o/spasm involuntary contraction, twitching	VĂS-ō-spăzm
aort/o	aorta	aort/o/stenosis stricture, narrowing	ā-or-tō-stĕn-Ō-sĭs
arteri/o	artery	arteri/al pertaining to	ăr-TĔR-ĭ-ăl
arteriol/o	arteriole	arteriol/itis inflammation	ăr-tĕr-ē-ō-LĪ-tĭs
ather/o	fatty plaque	ather/o/scler/ osis hardening abnormal condition	ăth-ĕr-ō-sklĕ-RŌ-sĭs
atri/o	atrium	atri/o/tome instrument to cut	Ā-trē-ō-tōm
cardi/o	heart	cardi/o/megaly enlargement	kăr-dē-ō-MĔG-ă-lē
hemangi/o	blood vessel	hemangi/oma tumor	hē-MĂN-jē-ō-mă
phleb/o	vein	phleb/o/tomy incision, cut into	flĕ-BŎT-ō-mē
ven/o		ven/ous pertaining to	VĒ-nŭs
thromb/o	blood clot	thromb/o/lysis destruction, separation, loosening	thrŏm-BŎL-ĭ-sĭs
sphygm/o	pulse	sphygm/o/meter instrument for measuring	sfĭg-MŎM-ĕt-ĕr

SUFFIXES

Suffix	Meaning	Example	Pronunciation
-gram	record, a writing	angi/o/gram vessel	ĂN-jē-ō-grăm
-graph	instrument for recording	electr/o/ cardi/o/graph electricity heart	ē-lĕk-trō-KĂR-dē-ō-grăf

PREFIXES

Prefix	Meaning	Example	Pronunciation
endo-	within	endo/arter/ itis artery inflammation	ĕn-dō-ăr-tĕr-Ĭ-tĭs
extra-	outside	extra/atri/ al atrium pertaining to	ĔKS-tră-Ā-trē-ăl
peri-	around	peri/card/ itis heart inflammation	pĕr-ĭ-kăr-DĬ-tĭs
trans-	across, through	trans/sept/ al septum pertaining to	trăns-SĔP-tăl

PATHOLOGY

Atherosclerosis

Atherosclerosis, a form of arteriosclerosis, is a degenerative vascular disorder where fatty plaque (**atheromas**) accumulates in the innermost lining of the arteries (**tunica intima**) (Fig. 9–5). Plaque builds up over the years and hardens (**scleroses**). One of the major risk factors for developing atherosclerosis is an elevated cholesterol level (**hypercholesterolemia**). Other major risk factors include age, family history, smoking, hypertension, and diabetes. With atherosclerosis, vascular elasticity is lost and the vascular channel (**lumen**) narrows. As atheromas increase in size, they impede the flow of blood, leading to O_2 deficiency in surrounding tissues (**ischemia**). Ulcerations often occur on the surface of the plaque, leading to clot formation (**thrombosis**) and, ultimately, total blockage (**occlusion**) of the vessel. When a thrombus dislodges, it is called an embolus. Emboli that travel in venous circulation may cause death. Emboli that travel in arterial circulation frequently lodge in a capillary bed and cause a localized infarct. Sometimes plaque weakens the vessel wall to such an extent that it forms a bulge (**aneurysm**) that may rupture.

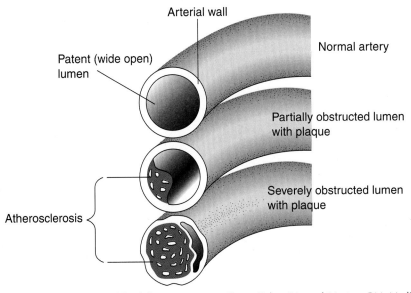

Figure 9–5 Atherosclerosis obstructing blood flow in an artery. (From Gylys, BA, and Masters, RM: Medical Terminology Simplified: A Programmed Learning Approach by Body Systems, ed 2. F.A. Davis, Philadelphia, 1998, p 398, with permission.)

Atheromas may form in the abdominal aorta; in the coronary, cerebral, and renal arteries; and in the major arteries of the legs (**femoral arteries**). Removal of the innermost layer of the artery (**endarterectomy**), especially in the carotid or femoral arteries, is a common method of treatment.

Coronary Artery Disease

Any disease that interferes with the ability of coronary arteries to deliver sufficient blood to the heart muscle is referred to as **coronary artery disease (CAD)**. The usual cause of CAD, however, is arteriosclerosis. About 20 percent of the total cardiac output is needed to supply the O_2 requirements of the heart muscle. When coronary arteries are unable to deliver this amount, localized areas of the heart experience ischemia. Myocardial ischemia causes a suffocating chest pain (**angina pectoris** or **angina**) and difficulty in breathing (**dyspnea**). When pain cannot be controlled with medication, a small piece of vein, usually from the leg (**saphenous vein**), is used to bypass the obstruction. One end of the graft vessel is sutured to the aorta and the other end to the coronary artery below the blocked area (**anastomosis**). This re-establishes blood flow to the heart muscle. A less invasive treatment for an obstructed coronary artery is a technique in which a small deflated balloon is placed at the site of the occlusion and then inflated to compress the plaque against the arterial wall (**angioplasty; percutaneous transluminal coronary angioplasty [PTCA]**) (Fig. 9–6). Some of the latest techniques involve using lasers and ultrasound to remove plaque.

Coronary artery disease may ultimately produce an acute myocardial infarction (MI). In this life-threatening condition, blood supply to part of the heart is totally suppressed, causing necrosis of the heart muscle (**myocardial infarction**) (Fig. 9–7). The clinical signs and symptoms of an acute MI include intense angina, profuse sweating (**diaphoresis**), paleness (**pallor**), and dyspnea. An arrhythmic heartbeat, accompanied by either a rapid heart action (**tachycardia**) or a slow heart action (**bradycardia**), may also accompany MI.

As the heart muscle undergoes necrotic changes, several enzymes are released, including **glutamic oxaloacetic transaminase (GOT)** (also called **aspartate transaminase [AST]**), **creatine phosphokinase (CPK)** (also called **creatine kinase [CK]**), and **lactate dehydrogenase (LD)**. The rapid elevation of these enzymes helps differentiate MI from pericarditis, aortic aneurysm, and acute pulmonary embolism.

ARTERIAL BALLOON ANGIOPLASTY

1. UNINFLATED BALLOON CATHETER IN ARTERY

PLAQUE

2. TOTAL INFLATION OF BALLOON CATHETER

DILATED VESSEL

3. CATHETER IS DEFLATED AND REMOVED.

4. PROCEDURE COMPLETED. DIAMETER OF LUMEN HAS BEEN INCREASED.

Figure 9–6   Arterial balloon angioplasty. (From Taber's Cyclopedic Medical Dictionary, ed 18. F.A. Davis, Philadelphia, 1997, p 108, with permission.)

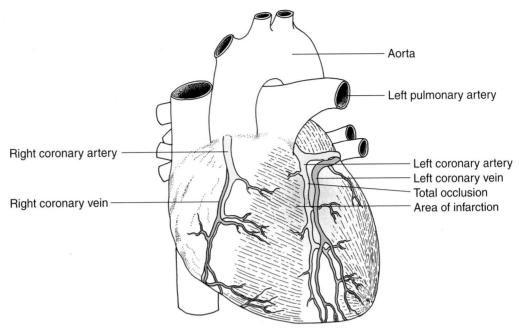

Figure 9–7 Myocardial infarction.

Infective Endocarditis

Infection of the inner layer of the heart and, often, of the valves is called **infective endocarditis**. Either bacteria or, less commonly, fungi are the usual causes. The infecting organisms become embedded in blood clots **(thrombi)** and form small masses **(vegetations)** that collect on the leaflets of the valves. Degeneration and scarring of the valves or the cords attached to the valves lead to a backflow of blood **(regurgitation)**.

Birth **(congenital)** defects or some infections, especially those associated with scarlet fever or rheumatic fever, may produce valve scarring. When this occurs, there may be a narrowing of the valves **(stenosis)** or an inability of the valves to close properly **(insufficiency)**. Although medications may prove helpful, heart surgery frequently is the only recourse. Whenever possible, the original valve is repaired **(valvotomy** or **commissurotomy)**, but more often it is replaced with an artificial device.

Patients who have had open heart surgery, rheumatic fever, scarlet fever, or valvular disease are susceptible to endocarditis. Thus, they are given antibiotic treatment before undergoing invasive procedures **(prophylactic treatment)** such as tooth removal, root canal procedures, and other minor surgeries.

Varicose Veins

Varicose veins develop when the valves of the veins are damaged **(incompetent)** and fail to prevent the backflow of blood in the vein. Although found in almost any part of the body, they are most common in the esophagus **(varices)**, anus **(hemorrhoids)**, and legs. Blood accumulates in flabby areas of the vein, and excess fluid eventually seeps from the vein, causing swelling in surrounding tissues **(edema)**.

Varicose veins of the legs can result from a congenital weakness of the valves, pregnancy, occupations that require standing for long periods of time, injury **(trauma)**, or inflammation of the vein wall **(phlebitis)**. In phlebitis, there is usually pain and tenderness. A cordlike mass may develop under the skin but diminishes as the disease subsides. If infection occurs in a deep vein and involves the inner layer of vein tissue, clots may form **(thrombophlebitis)**. A more serious condition may develop when a thrombus breaks loose from a vein wall and begins to travel in

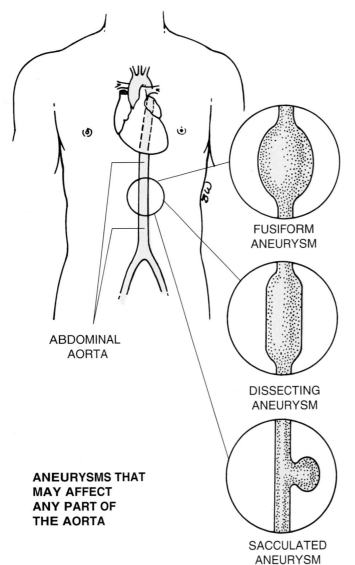

FUSIFORM
ANEURYSM

ABDOMINAL
AORTA

DISSECTING
ANEURYSM

ANEURYSMS THAT
MAY AFFECT
ANY PART OF
THE AORTA

SACCULATED
ANEURYSM

Figure 9–8 Aortic aneurysms. (From Taber's Cyclopedic Medical Dictionary, ed 18. F.A. Davis, Philadelphia, 1997, p 102, with permission.)

DIAGNOSTIC, SYMPTOMATIC, AND THERAPEUTIC TERMS
(Continued)

Term	Meaning
fibrillation fĭ-brĭl-Ā-shŭn	quivering or spontaneous muscle contractions, especially of the heart, causing ineffectual contractions; often may be corrected with a defibrillator
hemostasis hē-mō-STĀ-sĭs	arrest of bleeding or circulation
hyperlipidemia hī-pĕr-lĭp-ĭ-DĒ-mē-ă	excessive amounts of lipids (cholesterol, phospholipids, and triglycerides) in the blood
hypertension hī-pĕr-TĔN-shŭn	condition that is present when, on several separate occasions, blood pressure registers higher than normal
infarct ĭn-FĂRCT	area of tissue that undergoes necrosis following cessation of blood supply
ischemia ĭs-KĒ-mē-ă	local and temporary deficiency of blood supply because of circulatory obstruction

the vascular system. Any masses, including blood clots, that move within the vascular s
known as **emboli** (singular, **embolus**). Death may result if an embolus lodges in a vi
Emboli may be removed directly by excision (**embolectomy**) or may be dissolved (**thror**
using medications.

Treatment of mild cases of varicose veins includes rest periods, during which th
elevated, and use of elastic stockings. In extreme cases, the affected vein is tied (**lig;**
removed (**stripped**).

Oncology

The most common primary tumor of the heart is composed of mucous connective tis
oma); however, these tend not to be malignant. Some myxomas originate in the endoc
the heart chambers, but most arise in the left atrium. Occasionally they interfere with n
function and cause a decrease in exercise tolerance, difficulty in breathing (**dyspnea**),
lungs (**pulmonary edema**), and systemic disturbances including joint pain (**arthralgia**
of discomfort and uneasiness (**malaise**), and anemia. These tumors are usually idei
located by two-dimensional echocardiography. The tumor should be removed
surgically.

Most malignant tumors of the heart are the result of a malignancy in another
body (**primary tumor**) that has spread (**metastasized**) to the heart. The type usu
originates as a darkly pigmented mole or tumor (**malignant melanoma**) of the skin. Ott
sites of malignancy that metastasize to the heart are bone marrow and lymphatic tissue.
of the metastatic tumor of the heart involves treating the primary tumor.

DIAGNOSTIC, SYMPTOMATIC, AND THERAPEUTIC TERMS

Term	Meaning
Adams-Stokes syndrome	altered state of consciousness due to decreased blood flow to the
aneurysm ĂN-ū-rĭzm	localized abnormal dilation of a vessel, usually an artery (Fig. 9–8
arrest ă-RĔST	the condition of being stopped or bringing to a stop
cardiac KĂR-dē-ăk	a loss of effective cardiac function, which results in cessation of circulation; may be due to asystole in which there is no observabl myocardiac activity or to ventricular fibrillation
circulatory SĔR-kū-lă-tor-ē	cessation of the circulation of blood as a result of ventricular stan fibrillation
arrhythmia ă-RĬTH-mē-ă	irregularity in heart action
bruit, murmur brwē or broot	soft blowing sound heard on auscultation; may result from vibrati associated with the movement of blood, valvular action, or both
cardiomyopathy kăr-dē-ō-mī-ŎP-ă-thē	any disease of heart muscle not caused by an impairment of coror circulation and ischemia; may be caused by viral infections, metal disorders, or general systemic disease
coarctation kō-ărk-TĀ-shŭn	narrowing of a vessel, especially the aorta
congestive heart failure (CHF)	failure of the heart to supply an adequate amount of blood to tiss organs; most commonly caused by impaired coronary blood flow
embolus, emboli (pl) ĔM-bō-lŭs	mass of undissolved matter (foreign object, air, gas, tissue, throml circulating in blood or lymphatic channels until it becomes lodge vessel

DIAGNOSTIC, SYMPTOMATIC, AND THERAPEUTIC TERMS
(Continued)

Term	Meaning
mitral valve prolapse (MVP) MĪ-trăl, PRŌ-lăps	common and occasionally serious condition in which the leaflets of the mitral valve prolapse into the left atrium during systole; may cause nonanginal chest pain, palpitations, dyspnea, and fatigue
patent PĂ-tĕnt	open, unobstructed, or not closed (e.g., a patent artery)
patent ductus arteriosus PĂ-tĕnt DŬK-tŭs ăr-tē-rē-Ō-sŭs	failure of the ductus arteriosus to close after birth
tetralogy of Fallot tĕ-TRĂL-ō-jē, făl-Ō	congenital anomaly consisting of four elements: (1) pulmonary artery stenosis; (2) interventricular septal defect; (3) transposition of the aorta, so that both ventricles empty into the aorta; (4) right ventricular hypertrophy caused by increased workload of the right ventricle
thrombus, thrombi (pl) THRŎM-bŭs	blood clot that obstructs a vessel

DIAGNOSTIC PROCEDURES

Imaging Procedure	Description
aortography ā-or-TŎG-ră-fē	radiological examination of the aorta and its branches following the injection of a radiographic contrast medium via a catheter
cardiac catheterization KĂR-dē-ăk kăth-ĕ-tĕr-ĭ-ZĀ-shŭn	passage of a catheter into the heart through a vein or artery to evaluate valve function, septal defects, congenital anomalies, blood supply, or myocardial function (Fig. 9–9)
coronary angiography KOR-ō-nă-rē ăn-jē-ŎG-ră-fē	radiological examination of the blood vessels of and around the heart
echocardiography ĕk-ō-kăr-dē-ŎG-ră-fē	noninvasive diagnostic method that uses ultrasound to visualize internal cardiac structures and produce images of the heart. A transducer is placed on the chest to direct ultra-high-frequency sound waves toward cardiac structures. Reflected echoes are then converted to electrical impulses and displayed on a screen
doppler DŎP-lĕr	noninvasive adaptation of ultrasound technology in which blood flow velocity is assessed in different areas of the heart. Sound waves strike moving red blood cells and are reflected back to a recording device that graphically records blood flow
phonocardiography fō-nō-kăr-dē-ŎG-ră-fē	provides a graphic display of heart sounds during the cardiac cycle. Transducer sends ultrasonic pulses through the chest wall, and the echoes are converted into images on a monitor to assess overall cardiac performance. An electrocardiograph is simultaneously displayed to provide a reference point for each of the sounds and their duration
subtraction angiography sŭb-TRĂK-shĕn ăn-jē-ŎG-ră-fē	imaging technique used to display soft-tissue structures such as blood vessels without the confusing overlay of bone images
venography vē-NŎG-ră-fē	radiography of a vein after injection of a contrast medium; incomplete filling of a vein indicates obstruction

CENTRAL VENOUS CATHETER

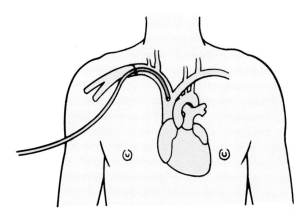

CATHETER (LINE) ENTERING VEIN

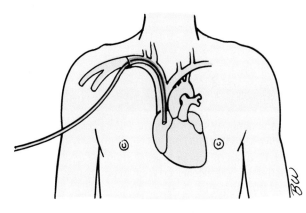

CATHETER TIP IN PLACE IN
RIGHT ATRIUM

Figure 9–9 Central venous catheter. (From Taber's Cyclopedic Medical Dictionary, ed 18. F.A. Davis, Philadelphia, 1997, p 332, with permission.)

DIAGNOSTIC PROCEDURES (Continued)

Clinical Procedure	Description
electrocardiogram (ECG, EKG) ē-lĕk-trō-KĂR-dē-ō-grăm	graphic record that shows the spread of electrical excitation to different parts of the heart; aids in diagnosing abnormal heart rhythms and myocardial damage
Holter monitor test HŎL-tĕr	ECG taken with a small portable recording system capable of storing up to 24 hours of ECG tracings; particularly useful in obtaining a cardiac arrhythmia record that would be missed during an ECG of only a few minutes' duration
stress test	ECG taken under controlled exercise stress conditions; may show abnormal ECG tracings that do not appear during an ECG taken when the patient is resting

DIAGNOSTIC PROCEDURES (Continued)

Laboratory Procedure	Description
cardiac enzyme studies KĂR-dē-ăk ĔN-zīm	blood test that assesses the concentration of three cardiac enzymes: glutamic oxaloacetic transaminase (GOT) (also called aspartate transaminase [AST]), CPK (also called creatine kinase [CK]), and LD (also called lactate dehydrogenase), which are released by necrotic heart tissue. Each enzyme rises, peaks, and declines at predictable times after MI. These levels, along with a clinical evaluation and an ECG, help to establish a diagnosis and extent of an MI
lipid profile LĬP-ĭd	panel of tests (glucose, total lipids, total cholesterol, triglycerides, phospholipids, and lipoprotein electrophoresis) used to assess risk factors of ischemic heart disease

SURGICAL AND THERAPEUTIC PROCEDURES

Procedures	Description
angioplasty ĂN-jē-ō-plăs-tē	a procedure that alters a vessel, either by surgery or by dilation of the vessel using a balloon catheter
percutaneous transluminal coronary angioplasty (PTCA) pĕr-kū-TĀ-nē-ŭs trăns-LŪ-mĭ-năl KOR-ō-nă-rē	dilation of an occluded vessel by use of a balloon catheter under fluoroscopic guidance. The catheter is inserted transcutaneously, and the balloon is inflated, thereby dilating the narrowed vessel
anastomosis ă-năs-tō-MŌ-sĭs	end-to-end union or joining of two vessels to provide an alternate pathway for the flow of blood
arterial ăr-TĒ-rē-ăl	end-to-end union or joining of two arteries or two separate segments of the same artery to ensure a blood supply to the capillaries of that organ
atherectomy ăth-ĕr-ĔK-tō-mē	removal of material from an occluded vessel by using a specially designed radiological catheter
biopsy BĪ-ŏp-sē	removal and examination of a small piece of tissue for diagnostic purposes
arterial ăr-TĒ-rē-ăl	removal and examination of a segment of an arterial vessel wall to confirm inflammation of the vessel wall, or arteritis, a type of vasculitis
thrombolysis thrŏm-BŎL-ĭ-sĭs	destruction of a blood clot
intravascular ĭn-tră-VĂS-kū-lăr	infusion of a thrombolytic agent into a vessel to dissolve a blood clot
ligation and stripping lī-GĀ-shŭn	tying a varicose vein followed by removal of the affected segment
pericardiocentesis pĕr-ĭ-kăr-dē-ō-sĕn-TĒ-sĭs	puncturing of the pericardium to remove fluid in order to test for protein, sugar, and enzymes or to determine the causative organism of pericarditis
phlebotomy, venipuncture flē-BŎT-ō-mē, VĔN-ĭ-pŭnk-chŭr	incision of a vein to remove blood or introduce fluids or medications
valvotomy, mitral commissurotomy văl-VŎT-ō-mē, MĪ-trăl kŏm-ĭ-shŭr-ŌT-ō-mē	incision of a mitral valve to increase the size of the opening; used in treating mitral stenosis
infusion ĭn-FŪ-zhŭn	introduction of fluid into the body
vasoconstrictor văs-ō-kŏn-STRĬK-tor	infusion of a vasoconstrictor such as vasopressin via a radiological catheter to reduce blood flow to a lesion

PHARMACOLOGY

Medication	Action
antianginals	relieves angina pectoris by expanding the blood vessels of the heart; most common drug in this category is nitroglycerin
antihypertensives	agents used to lower blood pressure
beta-adrenergic blocking agents, beta blockers	agents used to relieve cardiac arrhythmias, angina pectoris, post-MI hypertension, and migraine headaches
calcium channel blockers	agents that selectively block the flow or entry of calcium into cells; used to treat angina pectoris, some arrhythmias, and some forms of hypertension
diuretics	agents that reduce body fluid volume by stimulating urine flow; considered first step in management of hypertension
heparin	anticoagulant produced by liver cells and found in tissues; used in preventing and treating thrombosis and embolism
inotropics, cardiotonics	agents that alter the force of heart's contraction; used to treat cardiac arrhythmias and cardiac failure
tissue plasminogen activators (TPA)	used to dissolve blood clots responsible for MIs. If administered promptly (about 3 hours), it considerably decreases the chances of death
vasodilators	drugs to expand blood vessels; used to treat angina pectoris and hypertension
peripheral	agents used to expand blood vessels in the extremities and decrease blood pressure; also used to treat poor peripheral circulation and reduce pain caused by atherosclerosis

ABBREVIATIONS

Abbreviation	Meaning
ACG	angiocardiography
AF	atrial fibrillation
AS	aortic stenosis
ASD	atrial septal defect
ASHD	arteriosclerotic heart disease
BBB	bundle branch block
BP	blood pressure
CAD	coronary artery disease
CC	cardiac catheterization
CCU	coronary care unit
CHD	coronary heart disease
CHF	congestive heart failure
CPR	cardiopulmonary resuscitation
CV	cardiovascular
DVT	deep vein thrombosis
ECG, EKG	electrocardiogram
ECHO	echocardiogram
ICU	intensive care unit
MI	myocardial infarction, mitral insufficiency
MS	mitral stenosis

ABBREVIATIONS (Continued)

Abbreviation	Meaning
MVP	mitral valve prolapse
P	pulse, phosphorus
PAT	paroxysmal atrial tachycardia
PTCA	percutaneous transluminal coronary angioplasty
PVCs	premature ventricular contractions
SA	sinoatrial (node)
SK	streptokinase
TPA, tPA	tissue plasminogen activator
VSD	ventricular septal defect
VT	ventricular tachycardia

Laboratory	Meaning
AST	aspartate transaminase
CK	creatine kinase
CPK	creatine phosphokinase
GOT	glutamic oxaloacetic transaminase
HDL	high-density lipoprotein
LD	lactate dehydrogenase
LDL	low-density lipoprotein
VLDL	very-low-density lipoprotein

MEDICAL RECORD

Acute Myocardial Infarction

History of Present Illness   The patient is a 68-year-old woman hospitalized for acute anterior myocardial infarction. She had a history of sudden onset of chest pain. Approximately 2 hours before hospitalization she had severe substernal pain with radiation to the back. ECG showed evidence of abnormalities. She was given streptokinase and treated with heparin at 800 U/hr. She will be evaluated with a partial thromboplastin time and cardiac enzymes in the morning.

The patient had been seen in 19XX, with a history of an inferior MI in approximately 19XX or 19XX, but she was stable and underwent a treadmill test, the results of which showed no ischemia and she had no chest pain. Her records confirmed an MI with enzyme elevation and evidence of a previous inferior MI.

At this time the patient is stable, is in the CCU, and will be given appropriate follow-up and supportive care.

Impression   Acute lateral anterior MI and old, healed inferior MI.

Worksheet 5 provides a dictionary and reading application and an analysis of this medical record.

WORKSHEET 1

Use ather/o *(fatty plaque)* to build a medical word meaning:

1. a tumor of fatty plaque _____

2. condition of hardening of fatty plaque _____

Use phleb/o *(vein)* to build a medical word meaning:

3. inflammation of a vein _____

4. hardening of a vein (wall) _____

5. abnormal condition of a blood clot in a vein _____

Use ven/o *(vein)* to build a medical word meaning:

6. abnormal condition of hardening of a vein _____

7. spasm of a vein _____

8. pertaining to a vein _____

9. narrowing of a vein _____

Use cardi/o *(heart)* to build a medical word meaning:

10. enlargement of the heart _____

11. inflammation of the inner (lining) heart _____

12. inflammation of the epicardium _____

13. pertaining to the heart and lung _____

14. pertaining to heart (and blood) vessels _____

15. inflammation of the heart muscle _____

16. disease of the heart muscle _____

Use arteri/o *(artery)* to build a medical word meaning:

17. condition of hardening of the artery _____

18. spasm of the artery _____

19. rupture of an artery _____

20. pertaining to an artery _____

WORKSHEET 2

Build a surgical term meaning:

1. incision of the heart _____

2. puncture of the heart _____

3. fixation of a vein (in varicocele) _____

4. suture of an artery _____

5. (partial) excision of the pericardium _____

6. incision of a vein _____

7. surgical repair of an artery _____

8. surgical repair of a vessel _____

9. removal of an embolus _____

10. suture of a vein _____

WORKSHEET 3

■ ■ ■ ■ ■ ■ ■ ■ ■ ■ ■ ■ ■

Match the following words with the definitions in the numbered list.

Adams-Stokes syndrome	fibrillations	infarct
aneurysm	hyperlipidemia	ischemia
cardiac arrest	hypertension	patent
coarctation	hypotension	tetralogy of Fallot

1. _____ narrowing of a vessel, especially the aorta

2. _____ a loss of effective cardiac function, which results in cessation of circulation

3. _____ high blood pressure

4. _____ altered state of consciousness because of decreased blood flow to the brain

5. _____ open, unobstructed

6. _____ congenital birth defect affecting the cardiovascular system

7. _____ local and temporary deficiency in blood supply

8. _____ quivering or spontaneous muscle contractions, especially in the heart

9. _____ excessive amounts of lipids in the blood

10. _____ local abnormal dilation of a vessel, usually an artery

WORKSHEET 4

■ ■ ■ ■ ■ ■ ■ ■ ■ ■ ■ ■ ■ ■

Select the word that best describes the statements that follow.

antianginals	echocardiography	MS
arterial biopsy	electrocardiography (ECG, EKG)	pericardiocentesis
arterial anastomosis	Holter monitor	phlebotomy, venipuncture
beta blockers	inotropics, cardiotonics	phonocardiography
cardiac enzyme studies	ligation and stripping	stress test
diuretics	MI	vasodilators

1. _____ procedure that uses ultrasound to assess the structure of the heart

2. _____ procedure that graphically records the heart's electrical impulses on a paper strip

3. _____ puncturing the pericardium to remove fluid in order to test for protein, sugar, and LD or to determine the causative organism of pericarditis

4. _____ mitral stenosis

5. _____ medication to relieve chest pain

6. _____ drugs that affect the force of muscular contraction of the heart

7. _____ series of blood tests that establish a diagnosis and extent of MI

8. _____ incision of a vein to remove blood or introduce fluids or medications

9. _____ reduces heart workload by blocking the activity of epinephrine and norepinephrine

10. _____ measures the efficiency of the heart when subjected to a predetermined exercise

11. _____ specialized microphone records and graphically displays the sounds of the heart to assess abnormal acoustic events

12. _____ myocardial infarction

13. _____ tying off of a varicose vein, followed by removal of the affected segment

14. _____ end-to-end union of two different arteries or two separate segments of the same artery

15. _____ excision of a specimen of an arterial vessel wall for examination and testing

WORKSHEET 5

■ ■ ■ ■ ■ ■ ■ ■ ■ ■ ■ ■ ■

MEDICAL RECORD: ACUTE MYOCARDIAL INFARCTION

Underline the following terms in the medical record (see p. 155). Use a medical dictionary and other resources to define the terms and to determine their pronunciation; then practice reading the medical record aloud.

acute _____

cardiac enzymes _____

CCU _____

ECG _____

enzyme elevation _____

heparin _____

infarction _____

ischemia _____

lateral _____

myocardial _____

partial thromboplastin time _____

streptokinase _____

substernal pain _____

treadmill _____

MEDICAL RECORD EVALUATION: ACUTE MYOCARDIAL INFARCTION

1. *How long had the patient experienced chest pain before she was seen in the hospital?*

2. *Did she have a previous history of chest pain?*

3. *What are the cardiac enzymes that are tested to confirm the diagnosis of MI?*

4. *Initially, what medications were administered to stabilize the patient?*

5. *During the current admission, what part of the heart was damaged?*

6. *Was the location of damage to the heart for this admission the same as for the initial MI?*

WORKSHEET 6

Label the structures indicated on the following diagram. Check your answers by referring to Figure 9–2A.

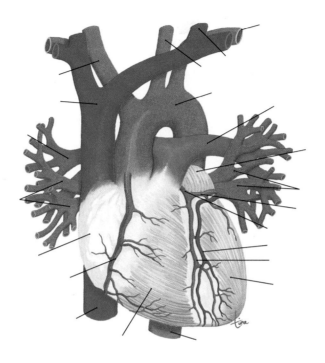

Aorta	Left common carotid artery	Left ventricle
Aortic arch	Left coronary artery	Right atrium
Brachiocephalic (trunk) artery	Left coronary vein	Right coronary artery
Circumflex artery	Left internal jugular vein	Right pulmonary artery
Inferior vena cava	Left pulmonary artery	Right pulmonary veins
Left anterior descending artery	Left pulmonary veins	Right ventricle
Left atrium	Left subclavian artery	Superior vena cava

WORKSHEET 7

■ ■ ■ ■ ■ ■ ■ ■ ■ ■ ■ ■

Label the structures on the following diagram. Check your answers by referring to Figure 9–2B.

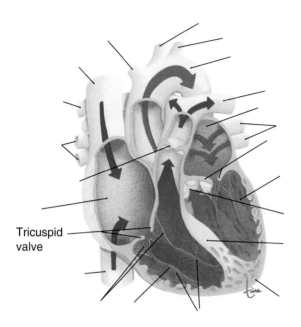

Tricuspid valve

Aortic arch	Left atrium	Papillary muscles
Aortic semilunar valve	Left common carotid artery	Pulmonary semilunar valve
Apex	Left pulmonary artery	Right atrium
Brachiocephalic artery	Left pulmonary veins	Right pulmonary artery
Chordae tendineae	Left subclavian artery	Right pulmonary veins
Inferior vena cava	Left ventricle	Right ventricle
Interventricular septum	Mitral (bicuspid) valve	Superior vena cava

BLOOD, LYMPH, AND IMMUNE SYSTEMS

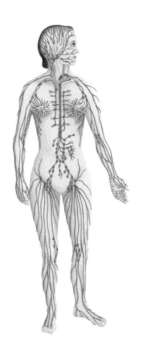

Chapter Outline

Student Objectives

Anatomy and Physiology
Blood
   Red Blood Cells (Erythrocytes)
   White Blood Cells (Leukocytes)
   Platelets
   Plasma
Lymph System
Immune System
   Blood Groups

Combining Forms

Suffixes

Prefixes

Pathology
Anemias
Acquired Immunodeficiency
   Syndrome (AIDS)
Autoimmune Diseases
Edema

Hemophilia
Infectious Mononucleosis
Allergy
Oncology
   Leukemia
   Hodgkin's Disease
   Kaposi's Sarcoma

**Diagnostic, Symptomatic,
  and Therapeutic Terms**

Diagnostic Procedures
Imaging Procedures
Laboratory Procedures

Surgical and Therapeutic Procedures

Pharmacology

Abbreviations

Medical Record
Therapeutic Plasmapheresis

Worksheets

Student Objectives

Upon completion of this chapter, you will be able to do the following:

1. Describe the appearance and function of blood cells.

2. List the components of blood plasma, and briefly explain the function of plasma.

3. Describe the functions of the lymphatic system, and explain the relationship between plasma and lymph.

4. Describe the immune system, and explain its importance in body protection.

5. List the two major white blood cells associated with immunity, and describe their function.

Student Objectives (Continued)

6. List the major blood groups, and give their agglutinogen and agglutinin.

7. Identify combining forms, suffixes, and prefixes related to the blood, lymph, and immune systems.

8. Identify and discuss pathology related to the blood, lymph, and immune systems.

9. Identify diagnostic, symptomatic, and therapeutic terms related to blood, lymph, and immune systems.

10. Identify diagnostic procedures related to blood, lymph, and immune systems.

11. Identify surgical and therapeutic procedures related to blood, lymph, and immune systems.

12. Discuss pharmacology related to the treatment of blood, lymph, and immune disorders.

13. Define abbreviations related to blood, lymph, and immune systems.

14. Demonstrate your knowledge of the chapter by completing the worksheets.

ANATOMY AND PHYSIOLOGY

Blood, lymph, and the immune systems share common structures and functions. Blood and lymph are specialized tissues of the body. Both are composed of cells suspended in a liquid medium, and both play a vital role in defending the body against infection. As body defenders, they work together with the immune system. Because blood and lymph have the ability to move throughout the entire body, they provide a transportation system for body cells.

Blood

Blood is composed of a liquid medium called plasma and a solid portion that consists of three major types of blood cells: red blood cells (RBCs) (**erythrocytes**), white blood cells (WBCs) (**leukocytes**), and platelets (**thrombocytes**). Most blood cells in adults are formed in the bone marrow (**myelogenic**) tissue of the skull, ribs, sternum, vertebrae, and pelvis, as well as at the ends of the long bones of the arms and legs, but some WBCs originate in lymphatic tissue.

Blood cells develop from an undifferentiated cell, the **hemocytoblast**, also called a stem cell (Fig. 10–1). The development and maturation of different blood cells is called **hematopoiesis** or **hemopoiesis**. Red blood cell development is called **erythropoiesis**, white blood cell development **leukopoiesis**, and platelet development **thrombopoiesis**. When blood cells are mature, they enter the circulatory system.

Although blood comprises only about 8 percent of all body tissues, it is essential to life. Blood provides a transportation system for all body tissues and functions in protecting against invasion by foreign substances by maintaining the cells responsible for specific immunity (Fig. 10–2).

Red Blood Cells (Erythrocytes)

RBCs are the most numerous of the circulating blood cells. During erythropoiesis, they develop a specialized iron-containing compound called **hemoglobin**, which gives them their red color. Hemoglobin carries oxygen (O_2) to body tissues, where it is exchanged for carbon dioxide (CO_2). The millions of hemoglobin molecules in each of the trillions of RBCs attest to the magnitude of the job they perform. During erythropoiesis, the red blood cell decreases in size. Just before maturity, the nucleus passes from the cell. It leaves behind a small fragment of nuclear material that resembles a fine, lacy net, which gives this cell its name, **reticulocyte**. Eventually, all of the nuclear material disappears and the mature erythrocyte enters the circulatory system.

Red blood cells (erythrocytes) live about 120 days and then rupture, releasing hemoglobin and cell fragments. Hemoglobin breaks down into **hemosiderin**, an iron compound, and several

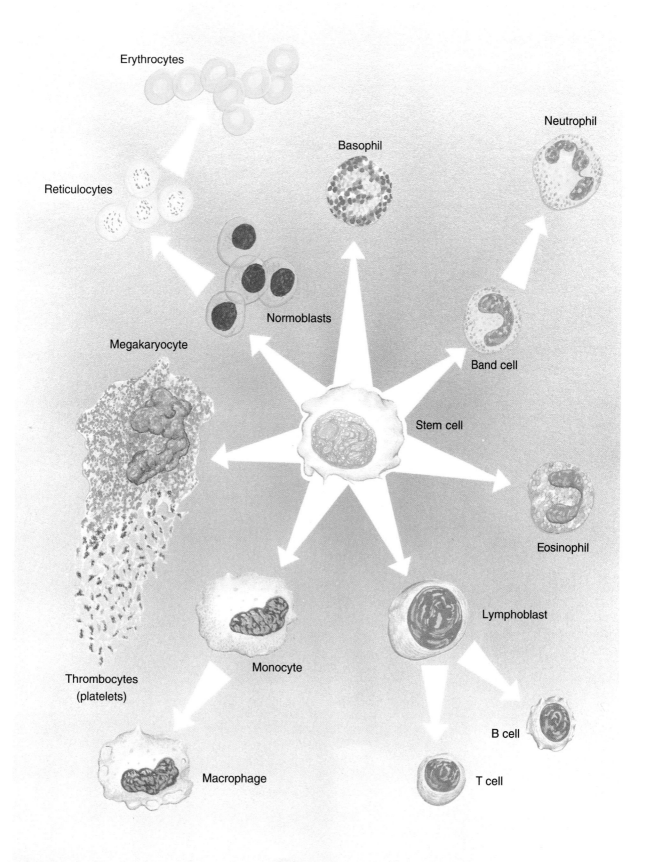

Erythrocytes

Reticulocytes

Normoblasts

Megakaryocyte

Thrombocytes
(platelets)

Monocyte

Macrophage

Basophil

Neutrophil

Band cell

Stem cell

Eosinophil

Lymphoblast

B cell

T cell

Figure 10–1 Hematopoiesis. Stem cells, which are found in red bone marrow and in lymphatic tissue, are the precursor cells for all the types of blood cells. (From Scanlon, VC, and Sanders, T: Understanding Human Structure and Function. F.A. Davis, Philadelphia, 1997, p 199, with permission.)

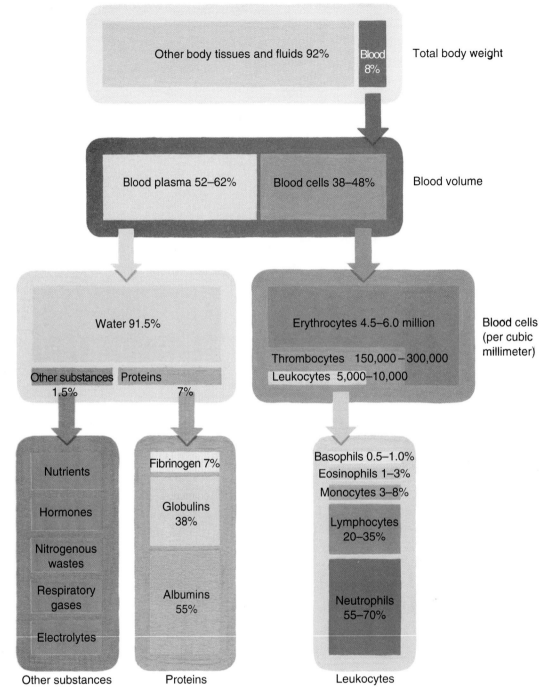

Figure 10–2 Components of blood and their relationship to other body tissues. (From Scanlon, VC, and Sanders, T: Understanding Human Structure and Function. F.A. Davis, Philadelphia, 1997, p 178, with permission.)

bile pigments. Most hemosiderin returns to the bone marrow and is reused to manufacture new blood cells. The liver eventually excretes bile pigments.

White Blood Cells (Leukocytes)

The chief function of WBCs is to protect the body against invasion by bacteria and foreign substances. Unlike RBCs, which remain exclusively in the vascular system, WBCs pass through capillary walls. They wander through tissue spaces to infection sites, where they destroy harmful substances and produce substances that aid in tissue repair.

Table 10–1   PROTECTION PROVIDED BY WHITE BLOOD CELLS

Granulocytes		Mononuclear Leukocytes	
Cell	**Activity**	**Cell**	**Activity**
neutrophils	phagocytic	monocytes	phagocytic
eosinophils	detoxification	lymphocytes	immunologic
basophils	release of substances	B cells	humoral immunity
	that increase circulation	T cells	cellular immunity

WBCs are divided into two categories, depending on whether they have granules in their cytoplasm: **granulocytes** (those with granules) and **agranulocytes** (those without granules). Because agranulocytes are also characterized by having a single-lobed nucleus, they are more frequently called **mononuclear leukocytes**. Both of these categories are subdivided, as shown in Table 10–1.

Granulocytes   Granulocytes are formed in red bone marrow from stem cells, which give rise to **myeloblasts**. Myeloblasts develop into neutrophils, eosinophils, and basophils. These names are derived from the type of dye that stains their cytoplasmic granules when a blood smear is stained in the laboratory. In addition to the presence of granules, these cells are further characterized by a nucleus that is composed of several lobes in their mature form; hence, these cells are also called **polymorphonuclear** cells.

The neutrophil, the most numerous of the circulating white cells, is very motile and highly phagocytic, permitting it to ingest and devour bacteria and other particulate matter. Eosinophils and basophils, although capable of phagocytosis, rarely display this activity.

Eosinophils protect the body by releasing many substances capable of neutralizing toxic compounds, especially of a chemical nature. Eosinophils increase in number during allergic reactions and animal parasite infestations.

Basophils release **histamines** and **heparin** when tissue is damaged. Histamines initiate inflammation, thereby increasing blood flow. This brings additional blood cells to damaged tissue for repair and healing. Heparin acts on blood vessels in the area of damaged tissue by preventing blood from clotting.

Mononuclear Leukocytes   Mononuclear leukocytes, also called agranulocytes, include **monocytes** and **lymphocytes**. In early development, monocytes and lymphocytes migrate from the bone marrow and enter the lymphatic system, where they change and mature. Monocytes are called macrophages when they exit the vascular system to begin their phagocytic activities. Macrophages and lymphocytes are chief players in a mode of body defense called specific immunity (Fig. 10–3).

Platelets

The smallest formed elements of blood are platelets, sometimes called thrombocytes. They initiate blood clotting when injury occurs.

Blood clotting is not a single reaction, but rather a chain of interlinked reactions. At least 13 separate steps are involved, but these steps can be combined into three major reactions, as shown here.

- Thromboplastin may be either released by traumatized tissue at the injury site or formed when platelets rupture. Thromboplastin and other blood clotting factors combine with calcium ions to form prothrombin activator.
- Prothrombin activator reacts with prothrombin and calcium ions to form thrombin.
- Thrombin converts the soluble blood protein fibrinogen to fibrin. Fibrin, a threadlike insoluble protein, forms a meshwork entangling blood cells and platelets. This jellylike mass of protein, blood cells, and platelets is known as a blood clot.

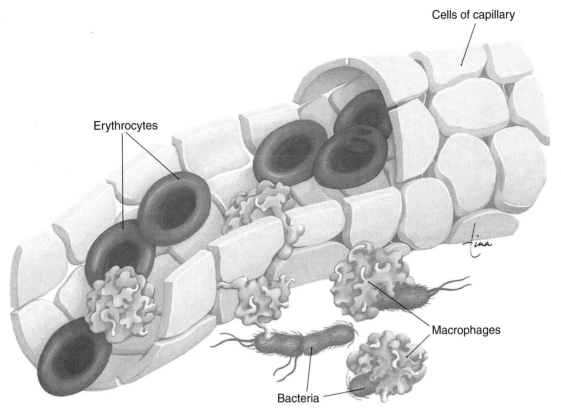

Figure 10–3   White blood cell leaving a capillary to destroy pathogens in surrounding tissue. (From Scanlon, VC, and Sanders, T: Essentials of Anatomy and Physiology, ed. 2. F.A. Davis, Philadelphia, 1995, p 252, with permission.)

Plasma

Plasma is the liquid portion of the blood in which blood cells are suspended. It is composed of about 92 percent water and contains the plasma proteins (albumins, globulins, and fibrinogen), gases, nutrients, salts, hormones, and excretory products. Plasma makes possible the chemical communication between all body cells by carrying these products to all parts of the body. When free of blood cells, plasma is a thin, almost colorless fluid.

Blood serum is a product of blood plasma. It differs from plasma in that it does not contain fibrinogen. When a blood sample is placed in a test tube and permitted to clot, the resulting clear fluid that remains after the removal of the clot from the test tube is serum. The formation of the clot has removed fibrinogen from the plasma.

Lymph System

The lymphatic system consists of a fluid called lymph and a network of transporting structures called lymph vessels, lymph nodes, spleen, thymus, and tonsils. The primary function of the lymphatic system is to drain fluid from tissue spaces and return it to the blood (Fig. 10–4). Other functions provided by the lymphatic system include transporting materials (nutrients, hormones, and oxygen) to body cells and carrying waste products from body tissues back to the bloodstream. It also transports lipids away from the digestive organs. Finally, it aids in the control of infection by providing lymphocytes and monocytes, the cells associated with the specific immune response.

Lymph originates from blood plasma. As whole blood circulates through capillaries, a small amount of plasma seeps out of these thin-walled vessels. This fluid, now called interstitial fluid, or tissue fluid, resembles plasma, except that it contains less protein. Interstitial fluid nourishes and cleanses the body tissues through which it circulates. It also collects cellular debris, bacteria,

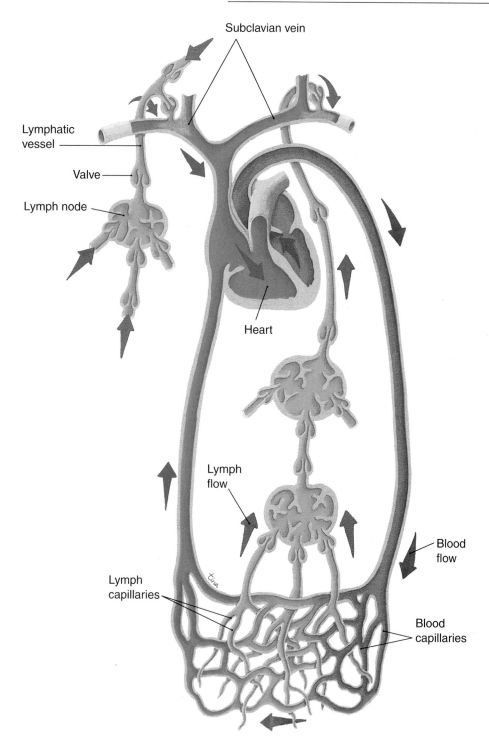

Subclavian vein

Lymphatic
vessel

Valve

Lymph node

Heart

Lymph
flow

Blood
flow

Lymph
capillaries

Blood
capillaries

Figure 10–4 Relationship of lymphatic vessels to the cardiovascular system. Lymph capillaries collect tissue fluid, which is returned to the blood. The arrows indicate the flow of blood and lymph. (From Scanlon, VC, and Sanders, T: Understanding Human Structure and Function. F.A. Davis, Philadelphia, 1997, p 248, with permission.)

and particulate matter. Eventually, interstitial fluid either returns to blood capillaries or enters blind-ended vessels called lymph capillaries (Fig. 10–5). Once it enters a lymph capillary it is called lymph. Lymph passes from lymph capillaries to larger vessels and finally to lymph nodes, which serve as depositories for cellular debris. As lymph passes through the nodes, it is filtered and replenished with lymphocytes and antibodies. Bacteria and debris are phagocytized by mac-

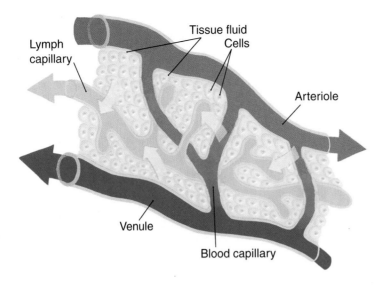

Figure 10–5 Dead-end lymph capillaries found in tissue spaces. Arrows indicate the flow of blood, lymph, and tissue fluid. (From Scanlon, VC, and Sanders, T: Understanding Human Structure and Function. F.A. Davis, Philadelphia, 1997, p 249, with permission.)

rophages that line the nodes (Fig. 10–6). When a local infection exists, the number of bacteria entering a node is so great that the node frequently enlarges and becomes tender.

Figure 10–7 illustrates lymphatic circulation. Lymph vessels from the right chest and arm join the right lymphatic duct. This duct drains into the right subclavian vein, a major vessel in the cardiovascular system. Lymph from all other parts of the body enters the thoracic duct and drains into the left subclavian vein. Lymph is redeposited into the circulating blood and becomes plasma. This cycle repeats itself.

The three organs associated with the lymphatic system are the spleen, thymus gland, and tonsils. Like lymph nodes, the spleen acts as a filter for lymph. Phagocytic cells within the spleen lining remove cellular debris, bacteria, parasites, and other infectious agents, thereby cleansing the lymph. The spleen also destroys old RBCs and serves as a repository for healthy blood cells that are placed into circulation when needed.

The thymus gland is located in the mediastinum, the upper part of the chest. It partially controls the immune system. The thymus changes lymphocytes to T cells, which provide a specific type of immunity called cellular immunity.

Tonsils are masses of lymphatic tissue located in the pharynx. They act as a filter to protect the upper respiratory structures from invasion by pathogens. They also aid in the development of WBCs.

Immune System

Throughout life, one is exposed to an infinite number and variety of organisms and other substances capable of causing disease or even death. However, most people suffer only a few diseases throughout their lives because of numerous body defenses, called resistance. The most complex of the resistance mechanisms of the body in both structure and function is the **specific immune system**, also called the **acquired immune system**. This system develops throughout life as a result of exposure to one disease after another.

With each exposure, the immune system identifies the invader, musters a unique response that destroys it, and then retreats with a memory of both the invader and the method of destruction. In the event of a second encounter by the same invader at a later time, the immune system is armed and ready to destroy it before it can cause disease. Such an invader is called an **antigen**.

The WBCs responsible for the immune response include monocytes and lymphocytes. After a brief stay in the vascular system, monocytes enter tissue spaces and become highly phagocytic. As such, they are called **macrophages**. In this form, they consume large numbers of bacteria and other antigens. They process these substances and place their antigenic property on their cell

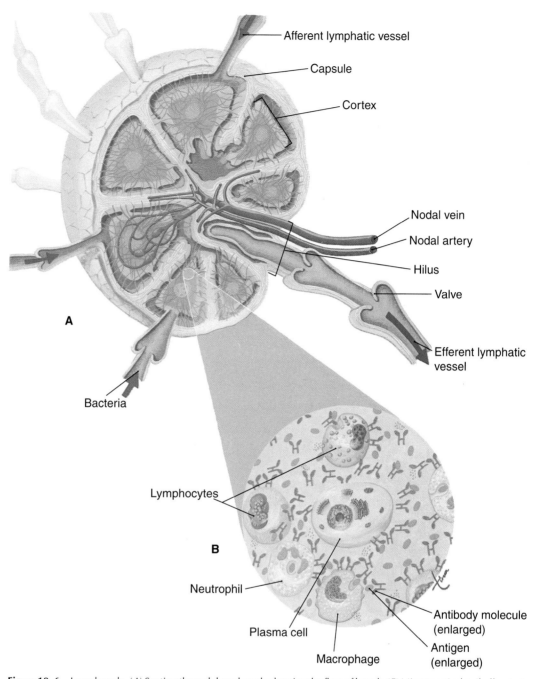

Figure 10–6   Lymph node. (*A*) Section through lymph node showing the flow of lymph. (*B*) Microscopic detail of bacteria being destroyed within the lymph node. (From Scanlon, VC, and Sanders, T: Understanding Human Structure and Function. F.A. Davis, Philadelphia, 1997, p 251, with permission.)

surface, thereby becoming antigen-presenting cells (APCs). The APC awaits an encounter with a competent specialized lymphocyte to initiate the specific immune response.

Two types of lymphocytes function in the immune response: **T lymphocytes (T cells)** and **B lymphocytes (B cells)**. B cells mature in bone marrow, and T cells mature in the thymus gland. T cells use one mode of attack called **cellular immunity**; B cells use another called **humoral immunity**. T cells determine a specific weakness in the cellular membrane of the **antigen** and use this weakness as a point of attack to destroy the antigen. B cells produce a clone of cells called **plasma cells** that produce proteins called **antibodies**. Antibodies enter the circulatory system and travel throughout the body in plasma, tissue fluid, and lymph. When antibodies encounter

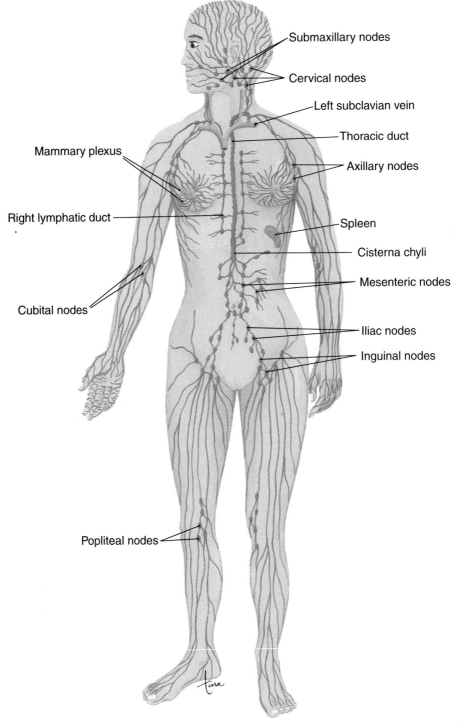

Figure 10–7   System of lymph vessels and the major groups of lymph nodes. Lymph is returned to the blood in the right and left subclavian veins. (From Scanlon, VC, and Sanders, T: Understanding Human Structure and Function. F.A. Davis, Philadelphia, 1997, p 250, with permission.)

their unique antigen, they destroy it, neutralize it, or render it harmless. All such reactions are highly specific; that is, the antibody will react only against the antigen that caused its formation, a characteristic called specificity.

The characteristic of specificity is used in clinical diagnosis. If a patient has antibodies to a given disease, the patient currently has the disease, or had the disease, or had an immunizing

Table 10–2   AGGLUTINOGENS AND AGGLUTININS
OF THE ABO SYSTEM

Blood Type	Agglutinogen (RBC Antigen)	Agglutinin (Plasma Antibody)
type A	A	anti-B
type B	B	anti-A
type AB	A and B	none
type O	none	anti-A and anti-B

vaccination to the disease. Tuberculosis testing and roseola testing are two tests that rely on the presence or absence of antibodies to determine immune status due to prior exposure.

There are several different types of T cells, one of which is the helper T cell. This cell is essential to the proper functioning of the entire immune response. If the helper T cell is unavailable to participate in the immune response, the immune system essentially shuts down and the patient becomes a victim of even the most harmless organisms and eventually dies.

A memory component in the immune system allows an immediate disposal of the same antigen if it is encountered again. Memory cells are produced by B and T cells during the initial exposure to an antigen. These memory cells migrate to and remain in lymphoid tissue. In the event of future exposures to the same antigen, memory cells "recall" how they previously disposed of the antigen and repeat the process. Disposing of the antigen during the second and all subsequent exposures is extremely rapid and much more effective than it was during the first exposure.

Blood Groups

Human blood is divided into four groups based on the presence or absence of blood antigens (**agglutinogens**) on the surface of RBCs. Because these blood antigens do not cause the formation of antibodies within the individual in whom they are found, they are called isoantigens. Four blood groups, A, B, AB, and O, are identified by the presence or absence of these agglutinogens. Type A blood has A antigen; type B blood, B antigen; type AB blood, both A and B antigens; and type O has neither A nor B antigens. In each of these four blood groups, the plasma does not contain the antibody (**agglutinin**) against the antigen that is present on the RBCs. Rather, the plasma contains the opposite antibodies. These antibodies occur naturally; that is, they are present although there has been no exposure to the antigen (Table 10–2).

In addition to the blood groups just listed, there are numerous other antigens that may be present on RBCs. One such antigen includes the Rh blood group (factor). This particular factor may cause hemolytic disease of the newborn (HDN) because of an incompatibility between maternal and fetal blood.

Although hematologists have identified more than 300 different blood antigens, most of these are not highly antigenic and do not cause concern in pregnancy or transfusions.

COMBINING FORMS

Combining Form	Meaning	Example	Pronunciation
aden/o	gland	aden/o/pathy disease	ăd-ĕ-NŎP-ă-thē
blast/o	embryonic cell	erythr/o/blast/osis red abnormal condition	ĕ-rĭth-rō-blăs-TŌ-sĭs
chrom/o	color	hypo/chrom/ic decrease pertaining to	hī-pō-KRŌM-ĭk

COMBINING FORMS (Continued)

Combining Form	Meaning	Example	Pronunciation
eosin/o	dawn (rose colored)	eosin/o/phil 　　　　attraction to	ē-ō-SĬN-ō-fĭl
erythr/o	red	erythr/o/cyte 　　　　cell	ē-RĬTH-rō-sīt
granul/o	granule	granul/o/cyte 　　　　cell	GRĂN-ū-lō-sīt
hem/o	blood	hem/o/lysis 　　　　destruction	hē-MŎL-ĭ-sĭs
hemat/o		hemat/oma 　　　　tumor	hē-mă-TŌ-mă
immun/o	safe	immun/o/logist 　　　　specialist in the study	ĭm-ū-NŎL-ō-jĭst
kary/o	nucleus	kary/o/lysis 　　　　destruction	kăr-ē-ŎL-ĭ-sĭs
nucle/o		nucle/ar 　　　　pertaining to	NŪ-klē-ăr
leuk/o	white	leuk/emia 　　　　blood	loo-KĒ-mē-ă
lymph/o	lymph	lymph/oma 　　　　tumor	lĭm-FŌ-mă
morph/o	shape	morph/o/logy 　　　　study of	mor-FŎL-ō-jē
myel/o	bone marrow, spinal cord	myel/oid 　　　　resembling	MĪ-ĕ-loyd
phag/o	swallowing, eating	phag/o/cyte 　　　　cell	FĂG-ō-sīt
poikil/o	varied, irregular	poikil/o/cyte 　　　　cell	POY-kĭl-ō-sīt
reticul/o	net, mesh	reticul/o/cyte 　　　　cell	rĕ-TĬK-ū-lō-sīt
sider/o	iron	hem/o/sider/osis blood　　　abnormal condition	hē-mō-sĭd-ĕr-Ō-sĭs
splen/o	spleen	splen/o/megaly 　　　　enlargement	splē-nō-MĔG-ă-lē
thromb/o	blood clot	thromb/o/lysis 　　　　destruction	thrŏm-BŎL-ĭ-sĭs
thym/o	thymus	thym/ectomy 　　　　excision	thī-MĔK-tō-mē

SUFFIXES

Suffix	Meaning	Example	Pronunciation
-blast	embryonic cell	myel/o/blast bone marrow	MĪ-ĕl-ō-blăst
-emia	blood condition	an/emia without	ă-NĒ-mē-ă
-globin	protein	hem/o/globin blood	hē-mō-GLŌ-bĭn
-osis	abnormal condition, abnormal increase (when used with blood cells)	erythr/o/cyt/osis red cell	ĕ-rĭth-rō-sī-TŌ-sĭs
-penia	decrease, deficiency	leuk/o/cyt/o/penia white cell	loo-kō-sī-tō-PĒ-nē-ă
-phil	attraction to (for)	eosin/o/phil eosin (dye)	ē-ŏ-SĬN-ō-fĭl
-phoresis	borne, carried	electr/o/phoresis electricity	ē-lĕk-trō-fō-RĒ-sĭs
-poiesis	formation, production	hem/o/poiesis blood	hē-mō-poy-Ē-sĭs
-stasis	standing still	hem/o/stasis blood	hē-mō-STĀ-sĭs

PREFIXES

Prefix	Meaning	Example	Pronunciation
a-	without, not	a/granul/o/cyte granule cell	ă-GRĂN-ū-lō-sīt
aniso-	unequal, dissimilar	aniso/cyt/ osis cell abnormal condition	ăn-ī-sō-sī-TŌ-sĭs
hetero-	different	hetero/phil attraction to	HĔT-ĕr-ō-fĭl
homo-	same	homo/graft transplant	HŌ-mō-grăft
iso-	same, equal	iso/chrom/ic color pertaining to	Ī-sō-KRŌ-mĭk
macro-	large	macro/cyt/ ic cell pertaining to	măk-rō-SĬ-tĭk
micro-	small	micro/cyt/ osis cell abnormal increase	mī-krō-sī-TŌ-sĭs
mono-	one	mono/cyte cell	MŎN-ō-sīt
poly-	many, much	poly/morph/o/nucle/ ar shape nucleus pertaining to	pŏl-ē-mor-fō-NŪ-klē-ăr

PATHOLOGY

Anemias

Anemia is any condition in which the oxygen-carrying capacity of blood is reduced. It is not a disease but rather a symptom of various diseases. It is caused when there is a decrease in the number of circulating RBCs (**erythropenia**), a decrease in the amount of hemoglobin (**hypochromasia**) within them, or a decrease in the volume of packed erythrocytes (**hematocrit**).

Anemias are identified according to their etiology or by the appearance of the red cells. In healthy individuals, RBCs fall within a normal reference range as to size (**normocytic**) and amount of hemoglobin (**normochromic**). Variations from these normal values include RBCs that are excessively large (**macrocytic**) or excessively small (**microcytic**) or have decreased amounts of hemoglobin (**hypochromic**). Some of the causes of anemias include excessive blood loss, excessive blood cell destruction, decreased blood formation, and faulty hemoglobin production. Table 10–3 summarizes various types of anemias. The signs and symptoms associated with most anemias include difficulty in breathing (**dyspnea**), weakness, rapid heartbeat (**tachycardia**), paleness (**pallor**), low blood pressure (**hypotension**), and often a slight fever.

Acquired Immunodeficiency Syndrome (AIDS)

AIDS is a transmissible infectious disease caused by the human immunodeficiency virus (HIV), which slowly destroys the immune system. Eventually the immune system becomes so weak

Table 10–3   COMMON ANEMIAS

Types and Causes of Various Common Anemias

Aplastic anemia (hypoplastic anemia): This form of anemia is associated with bone marrow failure. It is often a result of exposure to cytotoxic agents, radiation, hepatitis virus, and certain medications. However, most are idiopathic. Because there is suppression of the bone marrow, the numbers of WBCs and platelets are also diminished. This serious form of anemia may be fatal.

Hemolytic anemia: Hemolytic anemia is caused by the destruction of RBCs before the end of their normal life span. Erythroblastosis and sickle cell anemia are two disorders that cause hemolytic anemias. Hemolytic anemia is associated with jaundice because there is an increase in bilirubin in the blood.

Hemorrhage: This form of anemia is found in acute blood loss, such as trauma, and childbirth or chronic blood loss (e.g., bleeding ulcers). If the underlying order is corrected, hemoglobin levels return to normal.

Iron-deficiency anemia: Iron-deficiency anemia is caused by a greater demand on stored iron than can be supplied, often as a result of inadequate dietary iron intake or malabsorption of iron. This is the most common type of anemia worldwide.

Folic acid deficiency anemia: This anemia is caused by insufficient folic acid intake because of poor diet, impaired absorption, prolonged drug therapy, or increased requirements as a result of pregnancy or rapid growth as seen in children. Treatment consists of increasing folic acid in the diet or eliminating contributing causes.

Pernicious anemia: This form of anemia is associated with low levels of vitamin B_{12} in peripheral RBCs. It is chronic and progressive and found mostly in people older than 50 years of age. The stomach does not have "intrinsic factor"; therefore, vitamin B_{12} cannot be absorbed. The anemia is treated with B_{12} injections.

Sickle cell anemia: This anemia is the most common genetic disorder among people of African descent. It is caused by a defect in the gene responsible for hemoglobin synthesis. The RBC changes from its normal shape and forms crescents and other irregular shapes that cannot enter capillaries when O_2 levels are low. As a result, the patient experiences severe pain and internal bleeding. Sickle cell anemia is a recessive genetic disease. If the patient has only one gene for the trait, he or she is a carrier and does not manifest the disease.

(**compromised**) that in the final stage of the disease, the patient falls victim to disorders that usually do not affect healthy individuals.

Transmission of HIV occurs primarily through the exchange of body fluids—mostly blood, semen, and vaginal secretions. The virus attacks the most important cell in the immune system, the helper T cell. Once infected by HIV, the helper T cell becomes a "mini-factory" for the replication of the virus. The incubation time from exposure to manifesting the signs and symptoms of AIDS may be quite long, usually about 7 to 10 years. Antibodies to the disease begin to appear in the blood (**seroconversion**) about 3 months after exposure. Although these antibodies are ineffective in destroying HIV, they are useful in serological tests used to diagnose the infection.

Eventually the entire immune system is affected and no longer functions. Gradually the patient begins to display the symptoms of AIDS: swollen lymph glands (**lymphadenopathy**), malaise, fever, night sweats, and weight loss. Infections caused by organisms that are normally considered harmless (**opportunistic infections**) become established in the patient. Kaposi's sarcoma, a neoplastic disorder, and *Pneumocystis carinii* pneumonia (PCP) are two very important diseases associated with AIDS. The immune system ultimately fails, and the patient dies. There is no effective treatment, nor are vaccines available. Controlling the spread of the disease depends on avoiding behaviors that cause its spread.

Autoimmune Diseases

Failure of the body to distinguish accurately between what is self and what is nonself leads to a phenomenon called **autoimmunity**. In this abnormal immunologic response, the body produces antibodies against antigens found on its own cells. The antibodies attack the antigens to such an extent that they cause tissue injury. Types of autoimmune disorders range from those that affect only a single organ to those that affect many organs and tissues (**multisystemic**).

Myasthenia gravis is an autoimmune disorder that affects the neuromuscular junction. Muscles of the limbs and eyes and those affecting speech and swallowing are usually involved. Other autoimmune diseases include **rheumatoid arthritis, idiopathic thrombocytopenic purpura (ITP), vasculitis,** and **systemic lupus erythematosus (SLE)**. Treatment consists of attempting to reach a balance between suppressing the immune response in order to avoid tissue damage and still maintaining the immune mechanism sufficiently to protect against disease. Administration of steroids is often the chosen treatment. Most autoimmune diseases have periods of flare-ups (**exacerbations**) and remissions (**latent periods**).

Edema

Edema is an abnormal accumulation of fluids in the intercellular spaces of the body. One of the major conditions that cause edema is a decrease in the blood protein level (**hypoproteinemia**). This lowers osmotic pressure within the blood. Consequently, large amounts of plasma pass out of blood vessels and into the surrounding tissues. Other causes of edema include poor lymph drainage, increased capillary permeability, and congestive heart failure.

Edema limited to a specific area (**localized edema**) may be relieved by elevation of that body part and application of cold packs. Systemic edema may be treated with medications that promote urination (**diuretics**).

Closely associated with edema is a condition called **ascites**, in which fluid collects within the peritoneal or pleural cavity. The chief causes of ascites are interference in venous return during cardiac disease, obstruction of lymphatic flow, disturbances in electrolyte balance, and liver disease.

Hemophilia

Hemophilia is a hereditary disorder in which the blood clotting mechanism is impaired. It results from the failure of prothrombin to form thrombin. The disease is sex-linked and found most often in men. Women are the carriers of the trait but generally do not have symptoms of the disease.

Patients with hemophilia lack factor VIII (**antihemophilic factor [AHF]**), an essential blood clotting factor. The amount and site of bleeding depend on the degree of deficiency. Mild symptoms include nosebleeds, easy bruising, and bleeding from the gums. Severe symptoms produce areas of blood seepage (**hematomas**) deep within muscles. If blood enters joints (**hemarthrosis**), it is associated with pain and possible permanent deformity. Uncontrolled bleeding any place in the body may lead to shock and death.

Infectious Mononucleosis

One of the acute infections caused by the Epstein-Barr virus (EBV) is **infectious mononucleosis**. It is found mostly in young adults and appears in greater frequency in early spring and early fall. Sore throat, fever, and enlarged cervical lymph nodes characterize this disease. Other signs and symptoms include gum infection (**gingivitis**), headache, tiredness, loss of appetite (**anorexia**), and general malaise. Occasionally, the liver and spleen enlarge (**hepatomegaly** and **splenomegaly**). Less common clinical findings include hemolytic anemia with jaundice, thrombocytopenia, and occasionally a ruptured spleen (**splenorrhexis**). Recovery usually ensures a lasting immunity.

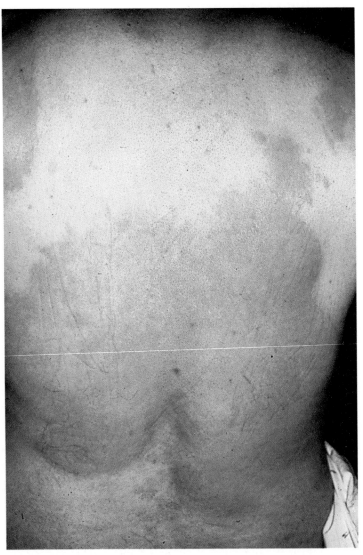

Figure 10–8   Urticaria (hives). These huge wheals occurred on a patient allergic to penicillin. (From Reeves, JRT, and Maibach, HI: Clinical Dermatology Illustrated: A Regional Approach, ed. 3. MacLennan & Petty, Roseberry, Australia, 1998 [distributed by F.A. Davis, Philadelphia], with permission.)

Allergy

An allergy is an acquired abnormal immune response. It requires an initial exposure to an antigen (**allergen**) that causes an allergic response (**sensitization**). Subsequent exposures to the allergen produce increasing allergic reactions that cause a broad range of inflammatory changes. One common manifestation is hives (**urticaria**) (Fig. 10–8). Other manifestations include eczema, allergic rhinitis, coryza, asthma, and, in the extreme, anaphylactic shock, a life-threatening situation. The offending allergens are identified by allergy sensitivity tests. Usually small scratches are made on the patient's back, and a liquid suspension of the allergen is introduced into the scratch. If antibodies to the allergen are present in the patient, the scratch becomes red, swollen, and hardened (**indurated**).

Desensitization involves repeated injections of a dilute solution containing the allergen. The initial concentration of the solution is too weak to cause symptoms. Additional exposure to higher concentrations promotes tolerance of the allergen.

Oncology

Leukemia

The major oncological disorder of the blood-forming organs is leukemia. With this condition, malignant cells replace healthy bone marrow cells. The disease may generally be categorized as to the type of leukocyte population affected—that is, granulocytic (**myelogenous**) or lymphocytic. The overgrowth (**proliferation**) of malignant cells may be either chronic or acute. In acute leukemias, the cells are highly embryonic (**blastic**) and the disease is more severe. In chronic leukemias, the cells are more mature and the disease is less severe. All forms of leukemias, if left untreated, are usually fatal.

The most common type of leukemia in adults is **acute myelogenous leukemia (AML)**. The survival rate with this type of leukemia, even with very aggressive treatment, is poor, and most individuals die within 1 year after diagnosis.

Acute lymphocytic leukemia (ALL) is primarily a disease of children. Some predisposing factors associated with acute forms of leukemia are ionizing radiation, viruses, genetic predisposition, and chemicals. **Chronic myelogenous leukemia (CML)** is associated with a unique chromosome called the Philadelphia chromosome. The age of onset of CML is usually between 40 and 50 years old. **Chronic lymphocytic leukemia (CLL)** is found primarily in patients older than 50 years of age.

Hodgkin's Disease

Hodgkin's disease is a malignant disease that primarily affects the lymph nodes (**lymphadenopathy**). However, the spleen, gastrointestinal tract, liver, or bone marrow may also be involved.

Hodgkin's disease usually begins with a painless enlargement of lymph nodes, usually on one side of the neck. Other symptoms include itching (**pruritus**), weight loss, progressive anemia, and fever. If nodes in the neck become excessively large, they may press on the trachea, causing difficulty in breathing (**dyspnea**), or on the esophagus, causing difficulty in swallowing (**dysphagia**).

Radiation and chemotherapy are important methods of controlling the disease. Newer methods of treatment include bone marrow transplants.

Kaposi's Sarcoma

Kaposi's sarcoma, a malignancy associated with AIDS, is often fatal because the tumors metastasize to various organs. The lesions emerge as purplish-brown macules and develop into plaques and nodules. The lesions initially appear over the lower extremities and tend to spread symmetrically over the upper body, particularly the face and oral mucosa.

DIAGNOSTIC, SYMPTOMATIC, AND THERAPEUTIC TERMS

Term	Meaning
anisocytosis ăn-ī-sō-sī-TŌ-sĭs	condition of marked variation in size of erythrocytes
antibody ĂN-tĭ-bŏd-ē	immunoglobulin produced by B lymphocytes in response to the presence of an antigen
antigen ĂN-tĭ-jĕn	a substance that stimulates the formation of antibodies when placed in an immunocompetent individual
ascites ă-SĪ-tēz	collection of serous fluid in the peritoneal and pleural cavity
dyscrasia dĭs-KRĂ-zē-ă	a morbid condition, usually referring to an imbalance of component elements; any abnormal or pathological condition of the blood
graft versus host reaction (GVHR) grăft	pathological reaction between the host and grafted tissue, resulting in rejection of a transplanted tissue
hemolysis hē-MŎL-ĭ-sĭs	destruction of RBCs with a release of hemoglobin that diffuses into the surrounding fluid
hemostasis hē-mō-STĂ-sĭs	arrest of bleeding or circulation
lymphadenopathy lĭm-făd-ĕ-NŎP-ă-thē	disease of the lymph nodes
lymphosarcoma lĭm-fō-săr-KŌ-mă	malignant neoplastic disorder of lymphatic tissue, not related to Hodgkin's disease
septicemia sĕp-tĭ-SĒ-mē-ă	presence of pathogenic bacteria in blood, characterized by chills and fever, purpuric pustules, and abscesses. If left untreated, may lead to shock and death
serology sē-RŎL-ō-jē	study of blood serum, especially antigen-antibody reactions

DIAGNOSTIC PROCEDURES

Imaging Procedure	Description
lymphadenography lĭm-făd-ĕ-NŎG-ră-fē	radiographic examination of lymph glands after injection of radiopaque material
lymphangiogram lĭm-FĂN-jē-ō-grăm	radiographic examination of a lymph vessel
splenography splē-NŎG-ră-fē	radiographic image of the spleen

Laboratory Procedure	Description
activated partial thromboplastin time (APTT) thrŏm-bō-PLĂS-tĭn	this test screens for deficiencies of some clotting factors; valuable for preoperative screening for bleeding tendencies
blood culture	test to determine the presence of pathogens in the bloodstream
complete blood cell (CBC) count	series of tests that include hemoglobin, hematocrit, red and white blood cell counts, differential WBC count, RBC indices, and RBC and WBC morphology

DIAGNOSTIC PROCEDURES (Continued)

Laboratory Procedure	Description
differential count	enumerates the distribution of WBCs in a stained blood smear. The different kinds of WBCs are counted and reported as a percentage of the total examined. Because the differential values change considerably in pathology, this test is often used as a first step to diagnose a disease
erythrocyte sedimentation rate (ESR; sed rate)	measures the distance RBCs settle when whole blood is placed in narrow tube. The sedimentation rate increases in inflammatory diseases, cancer, and pregnancy, and decreases in liver disease
hemoglobin (Hgb, Hb) hē-mō-GLŌ-bĭn	measurement of the amount of hemoglobin found in whole blood (decreases in anemia; increases in dehydration, polycythemia vera, and thrombocytopenia purpura)
hematocrit (Hct, crit) hē-MĂT-ō-krĭt	measurement of the percentage of packed RBCs in a whole blood sample
Monospot	serological test performed on a blood sample to detect the presence of a nonspecific antibody called the heterophile antibody that is present in the serum of patients with infectious mononucleosis
prothrombin time (PT, pro time)	evaluates portions of coagulation system and indirectly measures prothrombin; commonly used to manage patients undergoing anticoagulant therapy
RBC indices	mathematical evaluation of RBCs by providing the approximate size, volume, and concentration of hemoglobin in an average RBC
Schilling test	definitive test for pernicious anemia; assesses the absorption of radioactive vitamin B_{12} by the gastrointestinal system (in pernicious anemia, B_{12} is not absorbed and passes in the stool)

SURGICAL AND THERAPEUTIC PROCEDURES

Procedure	Description
aspiration ăs-pĭ-RĀ-shŭn	drawing in or out by suction
bone marrow	removal of a bone marrow specimen for examination and diagnosis, using a surgical aspirating needle
lymphangiectomy lĭm-făn-jē-ĔK-tō-mē	removal of a lymph vessel
splenolaparotomy splē-nō-lăp-ă-RŎT-ō-mē	incision through the abdominal wall into the spleen
transfusion	the injecting of blood or blood components into the bloodstream
autologous aw-TŎL-ō-gŭs	transfusion prepared from the recipient's own blood
homologous hō-MŎL-ō-gŭs	transfusion prepared from another individual whose blood is compatible with that of the recipient
transplantation	the grafting of living tissue from its normal position to another site or from one person to another
bone marrow (autologous) aw-TŎl-ō-gŭs	harvesting, freezing (cryopreserving), and reinfusing of the patient's own bone marrow; used to treat bone marrow hypoplasia following cancer therapy
bone marrow (homologous) hō-MŎL-ō-gŭs	transplantation of bone marrow from one individual to another; used for treating aplastic anemia and immunodeficiency disorders

PHARMACOLOGY

Medication	Action
anticoagulants	agents that inhibit or delay the clotting process; used to prevent clots from forming in blood vessels of patients predisposed to this condition, and to preserve stored whole blood and blood products. These agents have no effect on blood clots that have already formed
fibrinolytics	agents that trigger the body to produce plasmin, an enzyme that dissolves clots; used to treat acute pulmonary embolism and, occasionally, deep vein thromboses
hemostatics	drugs, medicines, or blood components that serve to stop bleeding
immunosuppressive agents	substances that suppress or interfere with the immune response; used to control autoimmune disease or enhance the chances for survival of a foreign tissue graft or transplant
vaccines	a suspension of infectious agents, or some part of them, given for the purpose of establishing immunity to an infectious disease

ABBREVIATIONS

Diagnostic and Symptomatic	Meaning
AHF	antihemophilic factor VIII
AHG	antihemophilic globulin factor VIII
AIDS	acquired immunodeficiency syndrome
ALL	acute lymphocytic leukemia
AML	acute myelogenous leukemia
CDC	Centers for Disease Control
CLL	chronic lymphocytic leukemia
CML	chronic myelogenous leukemia
EBV	Epstein-Barr virus
HDN	hemolytic disease of the newborn
HIV	human immunodeficiency virus
Ig	immunoglobulin
ITP	idiopathic thrombocytopenia purpura
PA	pernicious anemia
PCP	*Pneumocystis carinii* pneumonia
SLE	systemic lupus erythematosus

Laboratory	Meaning
AC	anticoagulant
APTT	activated partial thromboplastin time
baso	basophil
CBC	complete blood count
CO_2	carbon dioxide
diff	(white cell) differential blood count
eos, eosin	eosinophil
ESR; SR, sed rate	erythrocyte sedimentation rate; sedimentation rate

ABBREVIATIONS (Continued)

Laboratory	Meaning
HCT, Hct	hematocrit
HGB, Hgb, Hb	hemoglobin
lymphs	lymphocytes
MCH	mean corpuscular hemoglobin
MCHC	mean corpuscular hemoglobin concentration
MCV	mean corpuscular volume
mL, ml	milliliter; 0.001 liter
O_2	oxygen
PCV	packed cell volume (hematocrit)
PMN, seg, poly	polymorphonuclear neutrophil
PTT	partial thromboplastin time
PT, pro time	prothrombin time
RBC	red blood cell
WBC	white blood cell

MEDICAL RECORD

Therapeutic Plasmapheresis

Procedure   Therapeutic plasmapheresis.

Diagnosis   Thrombotic thrombocytopenic purpura and hemolytic uremic syndrome.

Technique   Plasmapheresis was carried out in the patient's room on 4 West. A Cobe Spectra machine was used. The patient tolerated the procedure well and her vital signs remained stable. Hemodialysis nurse, Angie Greco, RN, attended the patient. The following figures represent the amount of plasma removed and the infusion of plasma and other fluids. The procedure was begun at 1350 hours and ended at 1540 hours. Hgb, 12.5; Hct, 42.6; WBC count, 9.1; platelets, 133; estimated total blood volume, 3648 mL; estimated plasma volume, 2116 mL; plasma removed, 3106 mL; AC infused, 712 mL; saline rinse back, 195 mL. Fresh frozen plasma infused, 1946 mL. Total volume infused, 2853 mL. Net volume lost, −253 mL.

Comment   The patient's blood pressure dropped slightly to 90 systolic, but returned to normal when the procedure was slowed. She tolerated the procedure extremely well. She seemed a bit more alert and less confused today.

Plans   The plans are to perform the next therapeutic plasmapheresis on Saturday, 9/25/XX and again next week on Tuesday and Friday.

Worksheet 5 provides a dictionary and reading application and an analysis of this medical record.

WORKSHEET 1

▪ ▪ ▪ ▪ ▪ ▪ ▪ ▪ ▪ ▪ ▪ ▪ ▪

Use the suffix **-osis** *(abnormal increase) to build a medical word meaning:*

1. abnormal increase in RBCs _____

2. abnormal increase in WBCs _____

3. abnormal increase in granulocytes _____

4. abnormal increase in thrombocytes _____

5. abnormal increase in lymphocytes _____

6. abnormal increase in reticulocytes _____

Use the suffix **-penia** *(deficiency, decrease) to build a medical word meaning:*

7. decrease in RBCs _____

8. decrease in WBCs _____

9. decrease in platelets _____

10. decrease in granulocytes _____

11. decrease in lymphocytes _____

Use the suffix **-poiesis** *(production or formation) to build a medical word meaning:*

12. production of blood _____

13. production of red cells _____

14. production of white cells _____

15. production of lymphocytes _____

Use **immun/o** *(protection, safety, immunity) to build a medical word meaning:*

16. specialist in the study of immunity _____

17. study of immunity _____

Use **splen/o** *(spleen) to build a medical word meaning:*

18. herniation of the spleen _____

19. inflammation of the spleen _____

20. destruction of the spleen _____

WORKSHEET 2

■ ■ ■ ■ ■ ■ ■ ■ ■ ■ ■ ■ ■ ■

Build a surgical word meaning:

1. excision of the spleen _____

2. incision of the spleen _____

3. removal of the thymus _____

4. destruction of the thymus _____

5. incision of the spleen through the abdominal wall _____

6. fixation of (a displaced) spleen _____

WORKSHEET 3

■ ■ ■ ■ ■ ■ ■ ■ ■ ■ ■ ■ ■ ■

Match the following words with the definitions in the numbered list.

anisocytosis	dyscrasia	lymphosarcoma
antibody	hemolysis	microcytosis
antigen	hemostasis	septicemia
ascites	lymphadenopathy	serology

1. _____ study of antigen-antibody reactions

2. _____ a substance that stimulates the formation of antibodies

3. _____ destruction of erythrocytes with the release of hemoglobin

4. _____ arrest of bleeding or circulation

5. _____ presence of pathogenic bacteria in blood

6. _____ immunoglobulin produced by B-cell lymphocytes in response to the presence of an antigen

7. _____ malignant neoplastic disorder of lymphatic tissue, unrelated to Hodgkin's disease

8. _____ any blood abnormality

9. _____ collection of serous fluid in the peritoneal cavity

10. _____ disease of lymph nodes

WORKSHEET 4

▪ ▪ ▪ ▪ ▪ ▪ ▪ ▪ ▪ ▪ ▪ ▪

Match the following words to the statements in the numbered list:

anticoagulants   fibrinolytics   Monospot
aspiration   hematocrit   poly, seg
CBC   hemoglobin   prothrombin time
differential count   hemostatics   splenography
EBV   Im   transfusion
ESR   Ig   transplantation

1. _____ substances that control blood flow

2. _____ test that assesses the amount of iron-containing pigment in RBCs

3. _____ measurement of the distance RBCs settle when placed in a narrow tube

4. _____ volume of packed RBCs expressed as a percentage of whole blood

5. _____ immunoglobulin

6. _____ polymorphonuclear neutrophil

7. _____ injecting of blood or blood components into the bloodstream

8. _____ nonspecific test for the presence of the heterophile antibody, present in patients with infectious mononucleosis

9. _____ drawing in or out by suction

10. _____ series of blood tests that includes WBC, RBC, diff, Hgb, Hct, RBC indices, and RBC and WBC morphology

11. _____ trigger the body to produce plasmin, an enzyme that dissolves clots

12. _____ agents that delay or inhibit clotting

13. _____ time required for blood to clot in a tube after the addition of calcium

14. _____ Epstein-Barr virus

15. _____ radiographic examination of the spleen

WORKSHEET 5

. . . .

MEDICAL RECORD: THERAPEUTIC PLASMAPHERESIS

Underline the following terms in the medical record (see p. 183). Use a medical dictionary and other resources to define the terms and to determine their pronunciation; then practice reading the medical record aloud.

hemodialysis _____

hemolytic uremic syndrome _____

Hgb _____

Hct _____

infusion _____

mL _____

plasma _____

plasmapheresis _____

platelets _____

purpura _____

saline _____

systolic _____

therapeutic _____

thrombocytopenic _____

vital signs _____

WBC _____

MEDICAL RECORD EVALUATION: THERAPEUTIC PLASMAPHERESIS

1. *What is the name of the dialysis machine used to perform the plasmapheresis?*

2. *What vital sign showed a slight abnormality but returned to normal when the procedure was slowed down?*

3. *If 250 mL is the equivalent of 1 cup, approximately how many cups of plasma were removed?*

4. *What was the net volume loss?*

5. *Were the Hgb, Hct, WBC count, and platelets within the reference range?*

6. *How long did the procedure take?*

MUSCULOSKELETAL SYSTEM

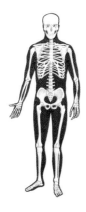
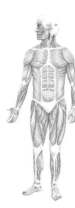

Chapter Outline

Student Objectives

Anatomy and Physiology
Skeletal System
  Functions
  Structure and Types of Bones
  Divisions of the Skeletal System:
    Axial and Appendicular
    Skeleton
  Projections and Depressions
    in Bones
  Joints or Articulations
Muscles
Attachments

Combining Forms
Skeletal System
  Bones of Upper Extremities
  Bones of Lower Extremities
  Other Combining Forms
Muscular System

Suffixes

Pathology
Bones
  Fractures
  Osteoporosis
  Spinal Disorders
Joints
Muscles
Oncology

**Diagnostic, Symptomatic,
  and Therapeutic Terms**

Diagnostic Procedures
Imaging Procedures

Surgical and Therapeutic Procedures

Pharmacology

Abbreviations

Medical Record
Radiographic Consultation:
  Injury of Left Wrist and Hand

Worksheets

Student Objectives

Upon completion of this chapter, you will be able to do the following:

1. Describe the functions of the skeletal system.
2. Locate and identify the major bones of the body.
3. Identify two main divisions of the skeletal system.
4. List four types of bones.
5. Explain the function of the vertebral column.
6. Identify the bones of the five regions of the vertebral column.

Student Objectives (Continued)

7. Describe the function of the thorax, and list five parts that compose its skeletal framework.

8. List three classifications of joints, and describe their function.

9. Explain the purpose of bone markings.

10. Describe three types of bone projections and depressions.

11. Identify five common types of fractures.

12. List three functions of muscles.

13. Identify combining forms, suffixes, and prefixes related to the musculoskeletal system.

14. Identify and discuss pathology related to the musculoskeletal system.

15. Identify diagnostic, symptomatic, and therapeutic terms related to the musculoskeletal system.

16. Identify diagnostic procedures related to the musculoskeletal system.

17. Discuss pharmacology related to the treatment of musculoskeletal disorders.

18. Define abbreviations related to the musculoskeletal system.

19. Demonstrate your knowledge of the musculoskeletal system by completing the worksheets.

ANATOMY AND PHYSIOLOGY

The musculoskeletal system consists of bones, joints, and muscles. Bones perform mechanical functions of support, protection, and body movement and metabolic functions of **hematopoiesis** (production of blood cells) and mineral storage. Muscle tissue is composed of contractile cells or fibers that affect movement of an organ or body part.

Skeletal System

Functions

Together with other soft tissue, many vital organs are enclosed and protected from injury by bones. For example, the bones of the skull protect the brain; the rib cage protects heart and lungs. Besides **support** and **protection**, the skeletal system includes a number of other important functions. **Movement** is possible because bones provide points of attachment for muscles, tendons, and ligaments. Bone marrow, found within the larger bones, is responsible for hematopoiesis, continuously producing millions of blood cells to replace those that have been destroyed. Bones serve as a **storehouse for minerals**, particularly phosphorus and calcium. When the body experiences a need for a certain mineral, such as calcium during pregnancy, it is withdrawn from the bones.

Structure and Types of Bones

The four principal types of bones are long bones, short bones, flat bones, and irregular bones.

    Long bones are found in the extremities of the body (e.g., legs, arms, and fingers). Figure 11–1 shows the parts of a long bone.

- The (1) **diaphysis** is the shaft or long, main portion of a bone. On each end of the diaphysis is (2) an **epiphysis** (plural: epiphyses), whose somewhat bulbous shape provides space for muscle and ligament attachments.

- In long bones, the bone shaft, or diaphysis, consists of (3) **compact bone** forming a cylinder that surrounds a central canal called the (4) **medullary cavity**. This medullary cavity or

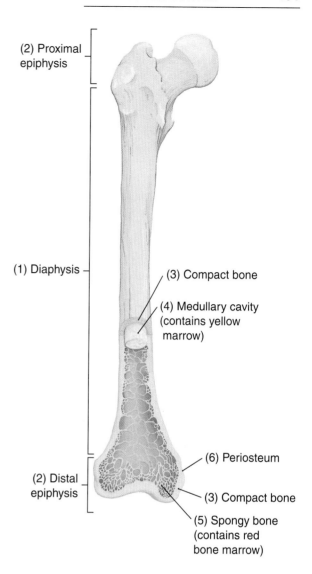

(2) Proximal epiphysis

(1) Diaphysis

(3) Compact bone

(4) Medullary cavity (contains yellow marrow)

(6) Periosteum

(2) Distal epiphysis

(3) Compact bone

(5) Spongy bone (contains red bone marrow)

Figure 11–1 Longitudinal section of a typical long bone (femur). (Adapted from Scanlon, VC, and Sanders, T: Understanding Human Structure and Function. F.A. Davis, Philadelphia, 1997, p 84, with permission.)

marrow cavity contains fatty yellow marrow in adults and consists primarily of fat cells and a few scattered blood cells.

- The epiphyses are made up largely of (5) **spongy bone** surrounded by a layer of compact bone. Red bone marrow is found within the porous chamber of spongy bone. This marrow is richly supplied with blood and consists of immature and mature blood cells in various stages of development. In an adult, the production of red blood cells (**erythropoiesis**) occurs in red bone marrow. Red bone marrow is also responsible for the formation of white blood cells (**leukopoiesis)** and platelets.

- The (6) **periosteum**, a dense white fibrous membrane, covers the remaining surface of the bone. It contains numerous blood and lymph vessels and nerves. In growing bones, the inner layer contains the bone-forming cells, called **osteoblasts**. Because blood vessels and osteoblasts are located here, the periosteum provides a means for bone repair and general bone nutrition. It also serves as a point of attachment for muscles, ligaments, and tendons.

Short bones are somewhat cubed-shaped. They consist of a core of spongy bone, also known as **cancellous** bone, which is enclosed in a thin layer of compact tissue (e.g., bones of the ankles, wrists, and toes).

Irregular bones include the bones that cannot be grouped under the previous headings because of their complex shapes (e.g., bones of the middle ear, vertebrae). **Flat bones** are exactly what their name suggests. They provide broad surfaces for muscular attachment or protection for internal organs (e.g., bones of the skull, shoulder blades, and sternum).

Divisions of the Skeletal System: Axial and Appendicular Skeleton

The axial and appendicular portions of the human skeleton are composed of 206 bones. Only the major bones are identified in Figure 11–2.

The **axial skeleton** consists of the bones of the skull, thorax, and vertebral column. These bones contribute to the formation of body cavities and provide protection for internal organs.

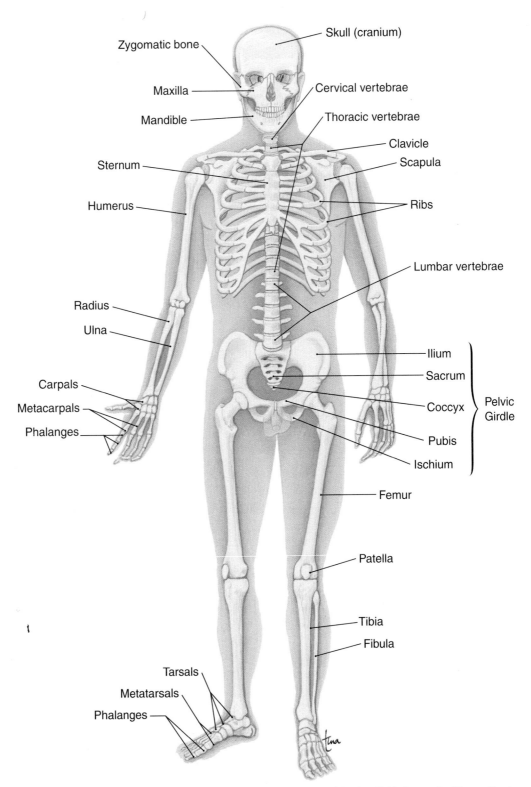

Figure 11–2   Anterior view of the skeleton. (Adapted from Scanlon, VC, and Sanders, T: Understanding Human Structure and Function. F.A. Davis, Philadelphia, 1997, p 89, with permission.)

The **appendicular skeleton** consists of the bones of the shoulder, the upper extremities, the hips, and the lower extremities. They attach to the axial skeleton as appendages.

Vertebral Column   The vertebral column of the adult is composed of 26 bones called vertebrae (singular, vertebra). The vertebral column supports the body and provides a protective bony canal for the spinal cord. As you read the following material, refer to Figure 11–3.

Five regions of bones comprise the vertebral column. Each region derives its name from its location within the spinal column. The seven (1) **cervical vertebrae** form the skeletal framework of the neck. The first cervical vertebra, the (2) **atlas**, supports the skull. The second cervical vertebra, the (3) **axis**, makes possible the rotation of the skull on the neck. Under the seventh cervical vertebra are twelve (4) **thoracic or dorsal vertebrae**, which support the chest and serve as a point of articulation for the ribs. The next five vertebrae, the (5) **lumbar vertebrae**, are situated in the lower back area and carry most of the weight of the torso. Below this area, the five sacral vertebrae are fused into a single bone in the adult and are referred to as the (6) **sacrum**. The tail of the vertebral column consists of four or five fragmented vertebrae fused together, referred to as the (7) **coccyx**.

Vertebrae are separated by flat, round structures, the (8) **intervertebral disks**, which are composed of a fibrocartilaginous substance with a gelatinous mass in the center (nucleus pulposus). When disk material protrudes into the neural canal, pressure on the adjacent nerve root causes pain. This condition is referred to as herniation of an intervertebral disk, **herniated nucleus pulposus (HNP)**, ruptured disk, or slipped disk.

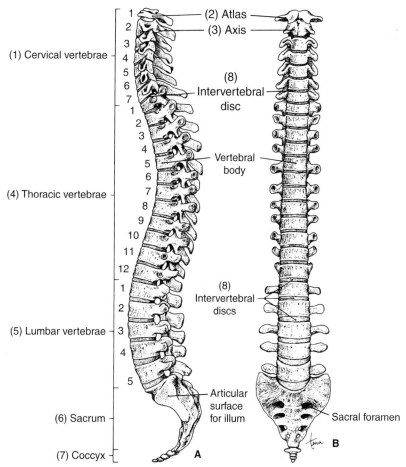

Figure 11–3   Vertebral column. (*A*) Lateral view of left side. (*B*) Anterior view. (Adapted from Scanlon, VC, and Sanders, T: Understanding Human Structure and Function. F.A. Davis, Philadelphia, 1997, p 95, with permission.)

Thorax   Two important internal organs of the thorax (chest) are the heart and lungs. Together with other soft tissue, the internal organs are enclosed and protected by the thorax. As you read the following paragraph, refer to Figure 11–4A.

The ribs, the (1) **sternum** (chest plate), and the thoracic vertebrae form the skeletal framework of the rib cage. There are 12 pairs of ribs, each pair is attached posteriorly to a thoracic vertebra. The (2) **true ribs** are the first seven pairs of ribs. These are attached directly to the sternum by a strip of (3) **costal cartilage**. The costal cartilage of the next five pairs of ribs is not fastened directly to the sternum. These are known as (4) **false ribs**. The last two pairs of false ribs are not joined, even indirectly, to the sternum but attach posteriorly to the thoracic vertebrae and are known as (5) **floating ribs**.

Pelvic (Hip) Girdle   The **pelvic (hip) girdle**, a basin-shaped structure along with its associated ligaments, supports the weight of the body from the vertebral column. It also supports the sigmoid colon, the rectum, the urinary bladder, and other soft organs of the abdominopelvic cavity. The pelvic girdle also provides a point of attachment for the legs, as shown in Figure 11–4B.

Male and female pelves differ considerably in size and shape. Some of the differences are attributable to the function of the female pelvis during the stages of childbearing. The female pelvis is shallower than the male pelvis but wider in every direction. The female pelvis not only supports the enlarged uterus as the fetus matures but also provides a large opening to allow the infant to pass through during birth.

Refer to Figure 11–4B as you read the following material.

Both the female and male pelves (singular: pelvis) are divided into the (1) **ilium**, (2) **ischium**, and (3) **pubis**. These are fused together in the adult to form a single bone called the innominate

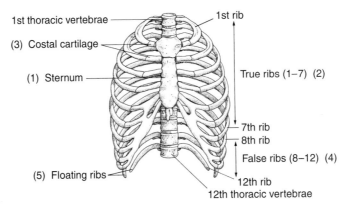

Figure 11–4A   The thorax.

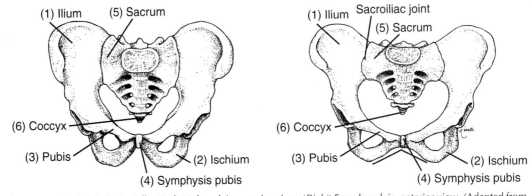

Figure 11–4B   Pelvic (hip) girdle. (*Left*) Male pelvis, anterior view. (*Right*) Female pelvis, anterior view. (Adapted from Scanlon, VC, and Sanders, T: Understanding Human Structure and Function. F.A. Davis, Philadelphia, 1997, p 100, with permission.)

bone. Nevertheless, the individual names are retained in order to identify the respective areas of the hip bone. The bladder is located behind the (4) **symphysis pubis;** the rectum is in the curve of the (5) **sacrum** and (6) **coccyx.** In the female, the uterus, fallopian tubes, ovaries, and vagina are located between the bladder and the rectum.

Projections and Depressions in Bones

Surfaces of bones have both projections and depressions to provide attachments for muscles, to join one bone to another, or to furnish cavities and pathways for nerve and blood supplies. A projection from a bone is called a **process.** Various types of projections, or processes, are evident in bones. Processes may be rounded, sharp, narrow, or have a large ridge, called a **crest. Depressions** are cavities or openings in a bone. There are several distinct types. The anatomical terms for the most common types of projections and depressions are summarized in Table 11–1.

Joints or Articulations

To allow for body movements, bones must have surfaces that join together **(articulate).** These articulating surfaces form joints that have various degrees of mobility. Some are freely movable **(diarthroses),** others are only slightly movable **(amphiarthroses),** and the remaining are totally immovable **(synarthroses).** All three types are necessary for smooth, coordinated body movements.

Joints that are freely movable (diarthrosis) are called synovial joints. The ends of the bones that comprise these joints are encased in a sleevelike extension of the periosteum called the **joint capsule.** This capsule binds the articulating bones to each other. In most synovial joints the capsule is strengthened by ligaments (fibrous bands, or sheets, of connective tissues) that lash the bones together, providing additional strength to the joint capsule.

A membrane called the **synovial membrane** surrounds the inside of the capsule. It secretes a fluid **(synovial fluid)** that lubricates the entire joint capsule. The ends of each of the bones are covered with a smooth layer of cartilage that serves as a cushion.

Muscles

All muscles, through contraction, provide the body with motion or body posture. The less apparent motions provided by muscles are the passage and elimination of food through the digestive

Table 11–1   PROJECTIONS AND DEPRESSIONS

	Description	Example
Projection		
Condyle	Rounded articulating knob	Condyle of the humerus
Trochanter	Massive process found only on the femur	Greater trochanter of the femur
Tubercle	Small, rounded process	Tubercle of the femur
Tuberosity	Large, rounded process	Tuberosity of the humerus
Depression		
Foramen	Rounded opening through a bone to accommodate blood vessels and nerves	Foramen of the skull through which cranial nerves pass
Fossa	Flattened or shallow basin	Axillary (armpit)
Sulcus	Groove, slight depression, or fissure	Deep furrows in the brain
Sinus	Cavity or hollow space in a bone	Frontal sinus

system, propulsion of blood through the arteries, and contraction of the bladder to eliminate urine.

There are three types of muscle tissue in the body: skeletal, cardiac, and smooth. **Skeletal muscles**, also called **voluntary** or **striated muscles**, are muscles whose action is controlled by will. Some examples of voluntary muscles are the muscles that move the eyeballs, tongue, and bones. Except for cardiac muscle, all striated muscles are voluntary.

Cardiac muscle makes up most of the wall of the heart. Like skeletal muscle, cardiac muscle is striated; unlike skeletal muscle, it experiences rhythmic involuntary contractions.

Smooth muscles (involuntary or **visceral muscles)** are muscles whose action is not controlled by will. They are found principally in the visceral organs, the walls of arteries, the walls of respiratory passages, and in the urinary and reproductive ducts. The contraction of smooth muscle is under autonomic (involuntary) nervous control.

Figure 11–5 and Table 11–2 show the actions performed by muscles. Most are in pairs and provide opposing functions (antagonists).

Attachments

Muscles attach to bones either by fleshy or fibrous attachments. In **fleshy attachments**, muscle fibers arise directly from bone. These fibers distribute force over wide areas, but a fleshy attachment is weaker than a fibrous attachment. In **fibrous attachments**, the connective tissue of the

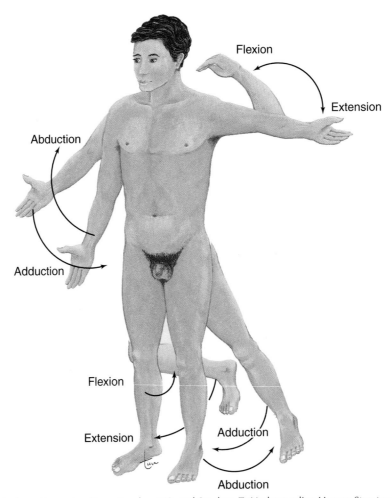

Figure 11–5 Actions of muscles. (From Scanlon, VC, and Sanders, T: Understanding Human Structure and Function. F.A. Davis, Philadelphia, 1997, p 117, with permission.)

Table 11–2   ACTIONS OF MUSCLES*

Motion	Action
Flexion } Extension }	Decreases the angle of a joint Increases the angle of a joint
Adduction } Abduction }	Moves closer to the midline Moves away from the midline
Pronation } Supination }	Turns the palm down Turns the palm up
Dorsiflexion } Plantar flexion }	Elevates the foot Lowers the foot (points the toes)
Rotation	Moves a bone around its longitudinal axis

*Most are grouped in pairs of antagonistic functions.

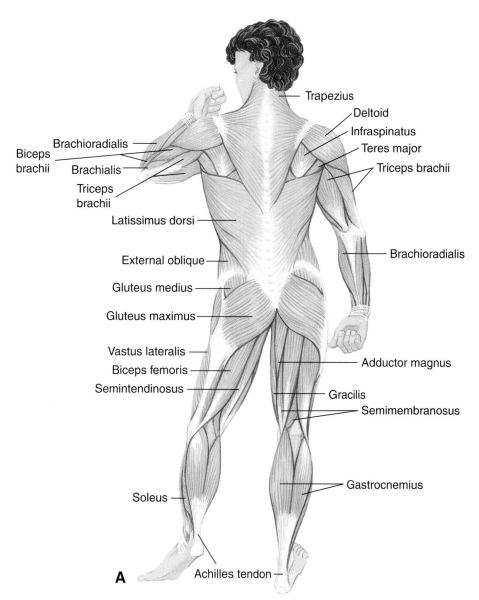

Figure 11–6   (*A*) Posterior and (*B*) anterior views of the muscles. (From Scanlon, VC, and Sanders, T: Understanding Human Structure and Function. F.A. Davis, Philadelphia, 1997, pp 118–119, with permission.)

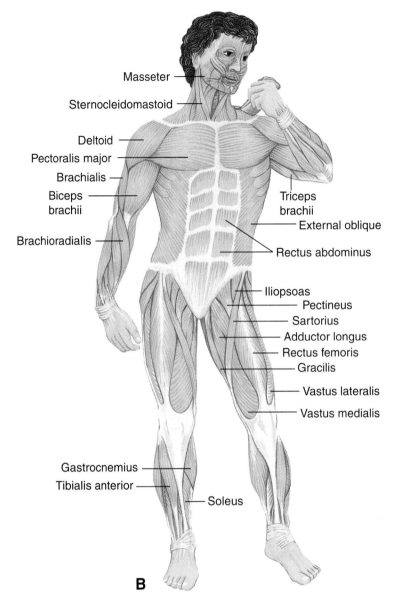

Masseter

Sternocleidomastoid

Deltoid

Pectoralis major

Brachialis

Biceps
brachii

Brachioradialis

Triceps
brachii

External oblique

Rectus abdominus

Iliopsoas

Pectineus

Sartorius

Adductor longus

Rectus femoris

Gracilis

Vastus lateralis

Vastus medialis

Gastrocnemius

Tibialis anterior

Soleus

B

Figure 11–6 *Continued.*

epimysium, perimysium, and endomysium converges at the end of the muscle to become continuous and indistinguishable from the periosteum. In some instances, this connective tissue penetrates the bone itself. When connective tissue fibers form a cord or strap, it is referred to as a **tendon**. This localizes a great deal of force in a small area of bone. Ligaments are composed of connective tissue and attach one bone to another. When the fibrous attachment spans a large area of a particular bone, the attachment is called an **aponeurosis**. Such attachments are found in the lumbar region of the back.

To become familiar with the names of major muscles, review Figure 11–6.

COMBINING FORMS

Skeletal System

Combining Form	Meaning	Example	Pronunciation
Bones of Upper Extremities			
brachi/o	arm	brachi/o/cephal/ic 　　　　head pertaining to	brăk-ē-ō-sĕ-FĂL-ĭk
carp/o	carpus (wrist bones)	carp/o/ptosis 　　　downward displacement, 　　　prolapse	kăr-pŏp-TŌ-sĭs
cephal/o	head	cephal/ad 　　　toward	SĔF-ă-lăd
cervic/o	neck	cervic/o/facial 　　　　face	sĕr-vĭ-kō-FĀ-shē-ăl
cost/o	ribs	cost/o/chondr/ itis 　　　cartilage inflammation	kŏs-tō-kŏn-DRĪ-tĭs
crani/o	cranium (skull)	crani/o/tomy 　　　incision	krā-nē-ŎT-ō-mē
dactyl/o	digit (a finger or toe)	syn/dactyl/　　　ism joined together condition	sĭn-DĂK-tĭl-ĭzm
humer/o	humerus	humer/al 　　　pertaining to	HŪ-mĕr-ăl
metacarp/o	metacarpus (bones of the hand)	metacarp/ectomy 　　　　excision	mĕt-ă-kăr-PĔK-tō-mē
phalang/o	phalanges (bones of fingers and toes)	phalang/eal 　　　pertaining to	fă-LĂN-jē-ăl
rachi/o	spine	rachi/o/plegia 　　　paralysis	rā-kē-ō-PLĒ-jē-ă
spondyl/o (used to make words about conditions of the structure) vertebr/o (used to make words that describe the structure)	vertebrae (backbone)	spondyl/itis 　　　inflammation cost/o/vertebr/al ribs　　　pertaining to	spŏn-dĭl-Ī-tĭs kŏs-tō-VĔR-tĕ-brăl
stern/o	sternum (breastbone)	stern/al 　　　pertaining to	STĔR-năl
thorac/o	chest	thorac/o/dynia 　　　pain	thō-răk-ō-DĬN-ē-ă
Bones of Lower Extremities			
calcane/o	calcaneum (heel bone)	calcane/o/dynia 　　　pain	kăl-kā-nē-ō-DĬN-ē-ă
femor/o	femur (thigh bone)	femor/al 　　　pertaining to	FĔM-or-ăl

Skeletal System (Continued)

Combining Form	Meaning	Example	Pronunciation
fibul/o	fibula (smaller, outer bone of lower leg)	fibul/ar pertaining to	FĬB-ū-lăr
ili/o	ilium (lateral flaring portion of hip bone)	ili/ac pertaining to	ĬL-ē-ăk
ischi/o	ischium (lower portion of hip bone)	ischi/al pertaining to	ĬS-kē-ăl
lumb/o	loins	lumb/o/dynia pain	lŭm-bō-DĬN-ē-ă
patell/o patell/a	patella (kneecap)	patell/a/pexy fixation	pă-TĔL-ă-pĕk-sē
ped/i	foot	ped/i/cure care	PĔD-ĭ-kūr
pod/o		pod/iatry treatment	pō-DĪ-ă-trē
pelv/i	pelvis	pelv/i/metry measuring	pĕl-VĬM-ĕt-rē
pub/o	pubis (part of hip bone)	pub/o/femor/al femur relating to	pū-bō-FĔM-or-ăl
tibi/o	tibia (larger, inner bone of lower leg)	tibi/o/femor/al femur pertaining to	tĭb-ē-ō-FĔM-or-ăl

Other Combining Forms

Combining Form	Meaning	Example	Pronunciation
acromi/o	acromion (projection of scapula)	acromi/o/humer/al humerus pertaining to	ăk-rō-mē-ō-HŪ-mĕr-ăl
ankyl/o	stiffness, bent, crooked	ankyl/osis abnormal condition	ăng-kĭ-LŌ-sĭs
arthr/o	joint	arthr/o/centesis puncture	ăr-thrō-sĕn-TĒ-sĭs
condyl/o	condyle (rounded protuberance at end of bone forming an articulation)	condyl/ectomy excision	kŏn-dĭl-ĔK-tō-mē
lamin/o	lamina (part of the vertebral arch)	lamin/ectomy excision	lăm-ĭ-NĔK-tō-mē
myel/o	bone marrow, spinal cord	myel/o/cele herniation	MĪ-ĕl-lō-sēl
orth/o	straight	orth/o/ped/ic child pertaining to	or-thō-PĒ-dĭk
oste/o	bone	oste/oma tumor	ŏs-tē-Ō-mă

Muscular System

Combining Form	Meaning	Example	Pronunciation
chondr/o	cartilage	chondr/itis inflammation	kŏn-DRĪ-tĭs
leiomy/o	smooth muscle (visceral)	leiomy/oma tumor	lī-ō-mī-Ō-mă
my/o	muscle	my/oma tumor	mī-Ō-mă
rhabd/o	rod-shaped (striated)	rhabd/oid resembling	RĂB-doyd
rhabdomy/o	rod-shaped (striated) muscle	rhabdomy/oma tumor	răb-dō-mī-Ō-mă
ten/o		ten/o/tomy incision	tĕn-ŎT-ō-mē
tend/o	tendon	tend/o/tome instrument to cut	TĔN-dō-tōm
tendin/o		tendin/itis inflammation	tĕn-dĭn-Ī-tĭs

SUFFIXES

Suffix	Meaning	Example	Pronunciation
-blast	embryonic cell	oste/o/blast bone	ŎS-tē-ō-blăst
-clasis	break, fracture, refracture	oste/o/clasis bone	ŏs-tē-ō-KLĂ-sĭs
-desis	binding, fixation (of a bone or joint)	arthr/o/desis joint	ăr-thrō-DĒ-sĭs
-malacia	softening	oste/o/malacia bone	ŏs-tē-ō-mă-LĀ-shē-ă
-physis	growth	dia/physis through	dī-ĂF-ĭ-sĭs
-plasty	surgical repair	arthr/o/plasty joint	ĂR-thrō-plăs-tē
-porosis	porous	oste/o/porosis bone	ŏs-tē-ō-pŏ-RŌ-sĭs
-schisis	a splitting	rachi/schisis spine	ră-KĬS-kĭ-sĭs
-scopy	visual examination	arthr/o/scopy joint	ăr-THRŎS-kō-pē

PATHOLOGY

Bones

Pus-forming (**pyogenic**) bacteria commonly cause **osteomyelitis**, an infection of bone and bone marrow. The disease usually begins with local trauma to the bone causing a blood clot (**hematoma**). Bacteria from an acute infection in another area of the body find their way to the injured bone and are frequently responsible for bone infection.

Most bone infections are more difficult to cure than soft-tissue infections. Eventually they may result in bone destruction (**necrosis**) and stiffening, or freezing, of the joints (**ankylosis**). Osteomyelitis may be acute or chronic. With early treatment, prognosis for acute osteomyelitis is good; prognosis for the chronic form of the disease is poor.

Paget's disease, also known as **osteitis deformans**, is a chronic inflammation of bones, resulting in thickening and softening of bones. It can occur in any bone but most often affects the long bones of the legs, the lower spine, the pelvis, and the skull. This disease is found in the population older than 40 years of age. Although a variety of causes have been proposed, a slow virus (not yet isolated) is currently thought to be the most likely cause.

Fractures

A fracture means that a bone has been broken. The different types of fractures are classified as to extent of damage (Fig. 11–7).

A (1) **closed** or **simple fracture** is one in which the bone is broken but no external wound exists. An (2) **open** or **compound fracture** involves a broken bone and an external wound that leads to the site of fracture. Fragments of bone often protrude through the skin. A (3) **complicated fracture** occurs when a broken bone has injured some internal organ, such as when a broken rib pierces a lung. In a (4) **comminuted fracture**, the bone has broken or splintered into pieces. An (5) **impacted fracture** occurs when the bone is broken and one end is wedged into the interior of the other. An (6) **incomplete fracture** is when the line of fracture does not include the whole bone. (7) A **greenstick fracture** occurs when the bone is partially bent and partially broken, as when a green stick breaks. It occurs in children because their bones contain more collagen than do adult bones and tend to splinter rather than break completely. A **hairline fracture** is a minor fracture in which all portions of the bone are in perfect alignment. The fracture is seen on radiographic examination as a very thin hairline between the two segments but not extending entirely through the bone. **Pathological** (spontaneous) **fractures** are usually caused by a disease process such as neoplasm or osteoporosis.

Unlike other repairs of the body, bones sometimes require months to heal. Several factors influence the rate at which fractures heal. Broken bones that lie close together heal faster than those that do not. Because of this, fractured bones are set in a cast (**immobilized**). Some bones have a natural tendency to heal more rapidly than others. For instance, the long bones of the arms have an inclination to mend twice as fast as those of the legs. Age also plays an important role in bone fracture healing rate. Older patients require more time for healing. Also, an adequate blood supply to the injured area and the nutritive state of the individual are crucial to the healing process.

Osteoporosis

Porous bone (**osteoporosis**) is a common bone disorder in older persons, especially women older than 60 years of age. A decrease of bone density occurs when the rate of bone reabsorption (loss of substance) exceeds that of bone formation. Among the many causes of osteoporosis are disturbances of protein metabolism, protein deficiency, disuse of bones because of prolonged periods of immobilization, estrogen deficiencies associated with menopause, a diet lacking vitamins or calcium, and long-term administration of high doses of corticosteroids.

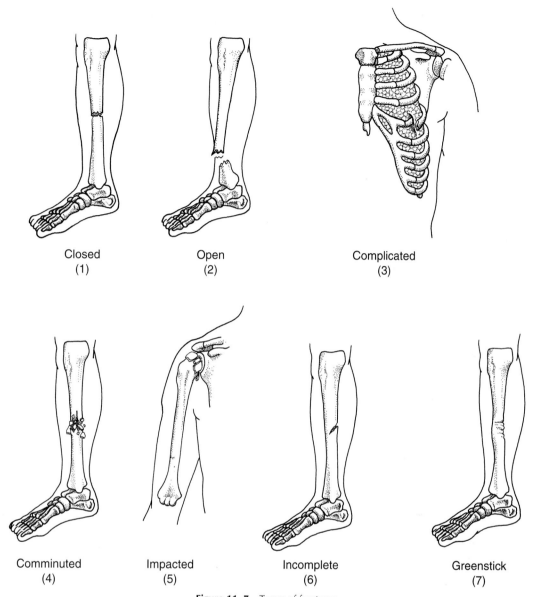

Closed
(1)

Open
(2)

Complicated
(3)

Comminuted
(4)

Impacted
(5)

Incomplete
(6)

Greenstick
(7)

Figure 11–7 Types of fractures.

Patients with osteoporosis frequently complain of bone pain, most commonly in the back, which may be caused by repeated microscopic fractures. Thin areas of porous bone are also evident. Deformity associated with osteoporosis is usually the result of pathological fractures.

Spinal Disorders

Because of various conditions, the normal curvature of the spine may become abnormally bent, causing **curvature** of the spine. A lateral curvature deviation of the spine to the right or left is called **scoliosis**. Scoliosis or C-shaped curvature of the spine may be congenital, caused by chronic poor posture during childhood while the vertebrae are still growing, or the result of one leg being longer than the other. Surgery, braces, casts, and corrective exercise may alleviate abnormal spine curvatures. Untreated scoliosis may result in pulmonary insufficiency (curvature may decrease lung capacity), back pain, sciatica, disk disease, or even degenerative arthritis.

Hunchback or humpback **(kyphosis)** is an exaggeration or angulation of the thoracic curve of the vertebral column. Rheumatoid arthritis, rickets, poor posture, or chronic respiratory diseases may cause kyphosis. Treatment for kyphosis caused by poor posture may consist of bedrest, therapeutic exercise, and a brace to straighten the kyphotic curve until growth is completed. Treatment for both adolescent and adult kyphosis includes appropriate measures for the underlying cause and, possibly, spinal arthrodesis for relief of symptoms. Surgery may be necessary when kyphosis causes neurological damage or intractable and disabling pain, but it is rarely necessary.

Swayback (**lordosis**), a forward curvature of the lumbar spine, may be caused by increased weight of the abdominal contents, resulting from obesity or excessive weight gain during pregnancy.

Spina bifida is a congenital defect characterized by defective closure of the spinal canal through which the spinal cord and meninges may or may not protrude. It usually occurs in the lumbosacral area and has several forms. **Spina bifida occulta** is the most common and least severe form. There is no protrusion of the spinal cord or meninges. **Spina bifida cystica** is a more severe type involving protrusion of the meninges (**meningocele**), spinal cord (**myelocele**), or both (**meningomyelocele**).

An inflammation of the vertebrae (**spondylitis**) is a serious chronic disorder. When it is associated with tuberculosis of the bones, it is called **Pott's disease**. Vertebrae become eroded and collapse, causing kyphosis. Spondylitis may also be associated with other infectious diseases. The intervertebral disks and the vertebrae are affected and sometimes destroyed, with resultant permanent stiffening or ankylosis of the back.

Joints

Because of their location and constant use, joints are prone to stress injuries and inflammation. The main diseases affecting the joints are rheumatoid arthritis, osteoarthritis, and gouty arthritis or gout.

Rheumatoid arthritis (**RA**), a systemic disease characterized by inflammatory changes in joints and their related structures, results in crippling deformities. This form of arthritis is believed to be caused by an autoimmune reaction of joint tissue. It begins most often in women between the ages of 23 and 35 years but can affect people of any age group. Intensified aggravations (**exacerbations**) of this disease are frequently associated with periods of increased physical or emotional stress. In addition to joint changes, muscles, bones, and skin adjacent to the affected joint atrophy. There is no specific cure, but nonsteroidal anti-inflammatory drugs (NSAIDs), physical therapy, and orthopedic measures are used in treatment of less severe cases.

Osteoarthritis, also called **degenerative joint disease (DJD)**, is the most common type of connective tissue disease. Cartilage destruction and new bone formation at the edges of joints (**spurs**) are the most common pathologies seen with osteoarthritis. Even though osteoarthritis is less crippling than rheumatoid arthritis, it may result in fusion of two bone surfaces, thereby completely immobilizing the joint. Small, hard nodules may form at the distal interphalangeal joints of the fingers (**Heberden's nodes**).

Gouty arthritis (gout) is a metabolic disease caused by accumulation of uric acid crystals in the blood. These crystals may become deposited in joints and soft tissue near joints, causing painful swelling and inflammation. Although the joint chiefly affected is the big toe, any joint may be involved. Often there is a formation of renal calculi (**nephrolithiasis**).

Muscles

Myasthenia gravis (MG), a neuromuscular disorder, causes fluctuating weakness of certain skeletal muscle groups (of the eyes, face, and, to a lesser degree, the limbs). It is characterized by destruction of the receptors in the synaptic region that respond to **acetylcholine**, a substance that transmits nerve impulses (**neurotransmitter**). As the disease progresses, the muscle becomes increasingly weaker and may eventually cease to function altogether. Women are affected slightly more often than men. Initial symptoms include a weakness of the eye muscles and difficulty in swallowing (**dysphagia**). Later, the individual has difficulty chewing and talking. Eventually, the muscles of the limbs may become involved.

Muscular dystrophy is a genetic disease characterized by gradual atrophy and weakening of muscle tissue. There are several kinds of muscular dystrophy. The most common type, Duchenne's dystrophy, affects children, boys more often than girls. It is transmitted as a sex-linked disease passed from mother to son. As muscular dystrophy progresses, the loss of muscle function affects not only skeletal muscle but also cardiac muscle. At present there is no cure for this disease, and most children with muscular dystrophy die before the age of 20 years.

Oncology

Some bone tumors present no problem. Others are exceedingly rare and rapidly become life threatening. Bone tumors (**osteomas**) can be either benign or malignant. Generally, benign tumors are slow growing and are usually treated by surgical excision. Malignant tumors that arise from bone (**sarcoma**) are rare. They usually develop rapidly and metastasize through lymph channels. Sarcomas are named for the specific tissue that they affect—for example, sarcoma in fibrous connective tissue (**fibrosarcoma**), sarcoma in lymphoid tissue (**lymphosarcoma**), or sarcoma in cartilage (**chondrosarcoma**). A sarcoma that often attacks the shafts rather than the ends of the long bones is called **Ewing's sarcoma**. This highly malignant tumor is found primarily in young men. Included in the treatment of malignant bone tumors are chemotherapy for management of metastasis and radiation when the tumor is radiosensitive.

DIAGNOSTIC, SYMPTOMATIC, AND THERAPEUTIC TERMS

Term	Meaning
carpal tunnel syndrome (CPT) KĂR-păl	painful condition resulting from compression of the median nerve within the carpal tunnel (wrist canal through which the flexor tendons and the median nerve pass)
claudication klăw-dĭ-KĀ-shŭn	lameness, limping
contracture kŏn-TRĂK-chŭr	fibrosis of connective tissue in skin, fascia, muscle, or joint capsule that prevents normal mobility of the related tissue or joint
crepitation krĕp-ĭ-TĀ-shŭn	dry, grating sound or sensation caused by bone ends rubbing together, indicating a fracture or joint destruction
electromyography ē-lĕk-trō-mī-ŎG-ră-fē	use of electrical stimulation to record the strength of muscle contraction
exacerbation ĕks-ăs-ĕr-BĀ-shŭn	increase in severity of a disease or of any of its symptoms
ganglion cyst GĂNG-lē-ŏn SĬST	tumor of tendon sheath or joint capsule, frequently found in the wrist. The cyst is aspirated and injected with an anti-inflammatory material
hypotonia hī-pō-TŌ-nē-ă	loss of muscular tonicity, in consequence of which the muscles may be stretched beyond their normal limits
hemarthrosis hĕm-ăr-THRŌ-sĭs	effusion of blood into a joint cavity
multiple myeloma MŬL-tĭ-pl mī-ĕ-LŌ-mă	primary malignant tumor that infiltrates the bone and red bone marrow. This progressive and often fatal disease causes multiple tumor masses that frequently cause bone fractures
osteophyte ŎS-tē-ō-fīt	a bony outgrowth that occasionally develops on the vertebra and may exert pressure on the spinal cord

DIAGNOSTIC, SYMPTOMATIC, AND THERAPEUTIC TERMS (Continued)

Term	Meaning
phantom limb	illusion, following amputation of a limb, that the limb still exists. The sensation that pain exists in the removed part is known as phantom limb pain
prosthesis PRŎS-thē-sĭs	replacement of a missing part by an artificial substitute, such as an artificial extremity
rickets, rachitis RĬK-ĕts, rā-KĪ-tĭs	form of osteomalacia in children, caused by vitamin D deficiency
sequestrum sē-KWĔS-trŭm	fragment of necrosed bone that has become separated from surrounding tissue
spondylolisthesis spŏn-dĭ-lō-lĭs-THĒ-sĭs	any forward slipping (subluxation) of a vertebra over the one below it
spondylosis spŏn-dĭ-LŌ-sĭs	degeneration of the cervical, thoracic, and lumbar vertebrae and related tissues; may cause pressure on nerve roots with subsequent pain or paresthesia in the extremities
sprain	tearing of ligament tissue that may be slight, moderate, or complete. A complete tear of a major ligament is especially painful and disabling. Ligamentous tissue does not heal well because of poor blood supply. Treatment consists of surgical reconstruction of the severed ligament
strain	excessive stretching of tissue composing the tendon or muscle, with no serious damage
subluxation sŭb-lŭk-SĀ-shŭn	partial or incomplete dislocation
talipes TĂL-ĭ-pēz	any number of foot deformities, especially those occurring congenitally; clubfoot

DIAGNOSTIC PROCEDURES

Imaging Procedure	Description
arthrography ăr-THRŎG-ră-fē	a series of radiographs taken after injection of a radiopaque substance into a joint cavity, especially the knee or shoulder, in order to outline the contour of the joint
CT scan (bone)	radiograph taken as a camera scans the entire body following injection of a radioactive substance; used to evaluate skeletal involvement related to connective tissue disease
CT scan (joint)	radiograph taken as a camera scan to determine joint damage throughout the entire body; one of the most sensitive studies for early detection of joint disease
diskography	radiological examination of the intervertebral disk structures in suspected cases of herniated disk
lumbosacral spinal radiography (LS spine) LŬM-bō-sā-krăl SPĪ-năl	radiography of the five lumbar vertebrae and the fused sacral vertebrae, including anteroposterior, lateral, and oblique views of the lower spine. The most common indication for this procedure is lower back pain, to identify or differentiate traumatic fractures, spondylosis, spondylolisthesis, and metastatic tumor
myelography, myelogram MĪ-ĕ-lŏg-ră-fē, MĪ-el-ō-gram	radiography of the spinal cord after injection of a contrast medium; used to identify and study spinal distortions caused by tumors, cysts, herniated intervertebral disks, or other lesions

SURGICAL AND THERAPEUTIC PROCEDURES

Procedure	Description
amputation ăm-pū-TĀ-shŭn	partial or complete removal of a limb
arthrocentesis ăr-thrō-sĕn-TĒ-sĭs	puncture of a joint space to remove accumulated fluid
arthroclasia ăr-thrō-KLĀ-zē-ă	surgical breaking of an ankylosed joint to provide movement
arthroscopy ăr-THRŎS-kŏ-pē	visual examination of a joint, especially the knee; used primarily to detect trauma or lesions and to obtain a biopsy of synovial tissue for microscopic examination. Synovial biopsy may also be obtained by needle or surgical incision
bone grafting bōn GRĂFT-ĭng	implanting or transplanting bone tissue from another part of the body or from another person to serve as replacement for damaged or missing bone tissue
bursectomy bĕr-SĔK-tō-mē	excision of bursa (a padlike sac or cavity found in connective tissue, usually in the vicinity of joints)
closed reduction of fractures	treatment of bone fractures by placing the bones in proper position (i.e., reducing the fragments without surgery); alignment is stabilized with the application of an external device to protect and hold the fracture while healing. Examples of closed reductions are listed here.
casting	immobilizing a limb or body part with a stiff, solid dressing during the healing process
splinting	an appliance made of bone, wood, metal, or plaster of Paris, used for the fixation, union, or protection of an injured part of the body. It may be movable or immovable
traction	the exertion of a pulling force that is applied to a fractured bone or dislocated joint to maintain proper position and facilitate healing
laminectomy lăm-ĭ-NĔK-tō-mē	excision of the posterior arch of a vertebra; most often performed to relieve the symptoms of a ruptured intervertebral (slipped) disk
open reduction of fractures	treatment of bone fractures by the use of surgery to place the bones in proper position (i.e., reducing the fragments)
sequestrectomy sē-kwĕs-TRĔK-tō-mē	excision of a sequestrum (segment of necrosed bone)
synovectomy sĭn-ō-VĔK-tō-mē	excision of a synovial membrane

PHARMACOLOGY

Medication	Action
anti-inflammatory drugs, antipyretics	non-narcotic analgesics used to relieve pain, fever, and swelling in musculoskeletal inflammatory diseases (e.g., rheumatoid arthritis, gout). The main antirheumatic is aspirin. Prescribed in much larger dosages for arthritis than those used to treat other types of pain. When used for arthritis and gout, these drugs are also called NSAIDs
corticosteroids	major anti-inflammatory drugs used for bone and joint disorders
gold therapy, aurotherapy, chrysotherapy	gold compounds used to treat rheumatoid arthritis
relaxants	drugs that reduce tension and produce relaxation (e.g., muscle relaxants provide therapeutic treatment that specifically relieves muscular tension)

ABBREVIATIONS

Abbreviation	Meaning
AE	above the elbow
AK	above the knee
AP	anteroposterior
BE	below the elbow
BK	below the knee
C1, C2, and so on	first cervical vertebra, second cervical vertebra, and so on
CDH	congenital dislocation of the hip
CPT	carpal tunnel syndrome
DJD	degenerative joint disease
Fx	fracture
HD	hip disarticulation
HNP	herniated nucleus pulposus (herniated disk)
HP	hemipelvectomy
IM	intramuscular
IS	intracostal space
KD	knee disarticulation
L1, L2, and so on	first lumbar vertebra, second lumbar vertebra, and so on
LAT, lat	lateral
MG	myasthenia gravis
NSAID	nonsteroidal anti-inflammatory drug
ORTH, ortho	orthopedics
RA	rheumatoid arthritis
SD	shoulder disarticulation
T1, T2, and so on	first thoracic vertebra, second thoracic vertebra, and so on
THA	total hip arthroplasty
THR	total hip replacement
TKA	total knee arthroplasty
TKR	total knee replacement

MEDICAL RECORD

Radiographic Consultation: Injury of Left Wrist and Hand

Left Wrist Images   were obtained with the patient's arm taped to an armboard. There are fractures through the distal shafts of the radius and ulna. The radial fracture fragments show approximately 8-mm overlap with dorsal displacement of the distal radial fracture fragment. The distal ulnar shaft fracture shows ventral-lateral angulation at the fracture apex. There is no overriding at this fracture. No additional fracture is seen. Soft-tissue deformity is present, correlating with the fracture sites.

Left Elbow and Left Humerus   Single view of the left elbow was obtained in the lateral projection. AP view of the humerus was obtained to include a portion of the elbow. A third radiograph was obtained but is not currently available for review. There is lucency through the distal humerus on the AP view along its medial aspect. It would be difficult to exclude fracture just above the medial epicondyle. On the lateral view, there is elevation of the anterior and posterior fat pad. These findings are of some concern. Repeat elbow study is recommended.

Worksheet 5 provides a dictionary and reading application and an analysis of this medical record.

WORKSHEET 1

■ ■ ■ ■ ■ ■ ■ ■ ■ ■ ■ ■ ■ ■

Use **oste/o** *(bone) to build a medical word meaning:*

1. bone cells _____

2. pain in the bones _____

3. disease of the bones and joints _____

4. beginning or formation of bones _____

Use **cervic/o** *(neck) to build a medical word meaning:*

5. pertaining to the neck _____

6. pertaining to the neck and arm _____

7. pertaining to the neck and face _____

Use **myel/o** *(bone marrow, spinal cord) to build a medical word meaning:*

8. herniation of the spinal cord _____

9. sarcoma of bone marrow (cells) _____

10. softening of the spinal cord _____

11. tumor containing myeloblasts _____

Use **stern/o** *(sternum, breastbone) to build a medical word meaning:*

12. pertaining to above the sternum _____

13. resembling the breastbone _____

Use **arthr/o** *(joint) or* **chondr/o** *(cartilage) to build a medical word meaning:*

14. embryonic cell that forms cartilage _____

15. inflammation of a joint _____

16. inflammation of bones and joints _____

Use **pelv/i** *(pelvis) to build a medical word meaning:*

17. instrument for measuring the pelvis _____

Use **my/o** *(muscle) to build a medical word meaning:*

18. tumor containing muscle (tissue) _____

19. hardening of a muscle _____

20. rupture of a muscle _____

WORKSHEET 2

Build a surgical term meaning:

1. excision of one or more of the phalanges (bones of a finger or toe) _____

2. incision of the thorax (chest wall) _____

3. excision of a vertebra _____

4. binding of a joint _____

5. repair of bones _____

6. repair of muscle (tissue) _____

7. excision of the lamina (part of the vertebral arch) _____

WORKSHEET 3

Match the following medical words with the definitions in the numbered list.

amputation   muscular dystrophy   sequestrum
claudication   myasthenia gravis   subluxation
ganglion cyst   prosthesis   spondylolisthesis
hypotonia   rickets   talipes

1. _____ incomplete or partial dislocation

2. _____ softening of the bones caused by a lack of vitamin D

3. _____ slipped vertebrae

4. _____ limping

5. _____ degeneration of the muscles

6. _____ congenital deformity of the foot, which is twisted out of shape or position

7. _____ part of dead or necrosed bone that has become separated from surrounding tissue

8. _____ chronic neuromuscular disorder characterized by weakness manifested in ocular muscles, resulting in bilateral ptosis of the eyelids

9. _____ replacement of a missing limb with an artificial part

10. _____ tendon sheath or joint capsule tumor, frequently found in the wrist

11. _____ diminution or loss of muscular tonicity; diminished resistance of muscles to passive stretching

ŋ

WORKSHEET 4

Select a term that best describes the statements that follow.

amputation	chrysotherapy	laminectomy
arthroclasia	corticosteroids	myelography
arthrodesis	HNP	open reduction
arthrography	L3	thermography

1. _____ radiograph of spinal cord after injection of a contrast medium

2. _____ treatment of bone fractures by use of surgery to place bones in proper position

3. _____ oral or injectable gold salts administered to treat rheumatoid arthritis

4. _____ major anti-inflammatory drugs used for bone and joint disorders

5. _____ excision of the posterior arch of a vertebra

6. _____ series of joint radiographs preceded by injection of a radiopaque substance or air into the joint cavity

7. _____ surgical immobilization of a joint

8. _____ partial or complete removal of a limb

9. _____ herniated nucleus pulposus

WORKSHEET 5

. . . .

MEDICAL RECORD RADIOGRAPHIC CONSULTATION: INJURY OF LEFT WRIST AND HAND

Underline the following terms in the medical record (see p. 209). Use a medical dictionary and other resources to define the terms and to determine their pronunciation; then practice reading the medical record aloud.

angulation _____

AP _____

apex _____

distal shafts _____

epicondyle _____

fracture _____

lucency _____

medial _____

mm _____

radiographic _____

radius _____

ulna _____

ventral-lateral _____

MEDICAL RECORD EVALUATION OF RADIOGRAPHIC CONSULTATION:
INJURY OF LEFT WRIST AND HAND

1. *What is the abbreviation for anteroposterior?*

2. *What caused the soft tissue deformity?*

3. *Why was an AP view of the humerus taken?*

4. *Where are the left wrist fractures located?*

5. *Did the radiologist take any side views of the left elbow?*

WORKSHEET 6

Label the parts of the bone on the following diagram. Check your answers by referring to Figure 11–1.

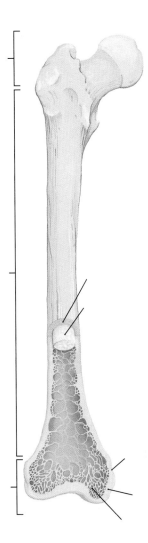

Compact bone   Medullary cavity   Proximal epiphysis
Diaphysis   Periosteum   Spongy bone
Distal epiphysis

WORSHEET 7

▪ ▪ ▪ ▪ ▪ ▪ ▪ ▪ ▪ ▪ ▪ ▪ ▪ ▪ ▪

Label the parts of the skeleton on the following diagram. Check your answers by referring to Figure 11–2.

Carpals
Cervical vertebrae
Clavicle
Coccyx
Femur
Fibula
Humerus
Ilium
Ischium
Lumbar vertebrae
Mandible
Maxilla
Metacarpals
Metatarsals
Patella
Phalanges
Pubis
Radius
Ribs
Sacrum
Scapula
Skull (cranium)
Sternum
Tarsals
Thoracic vertebrae
Tibia
Ulna
Zygomatic bone

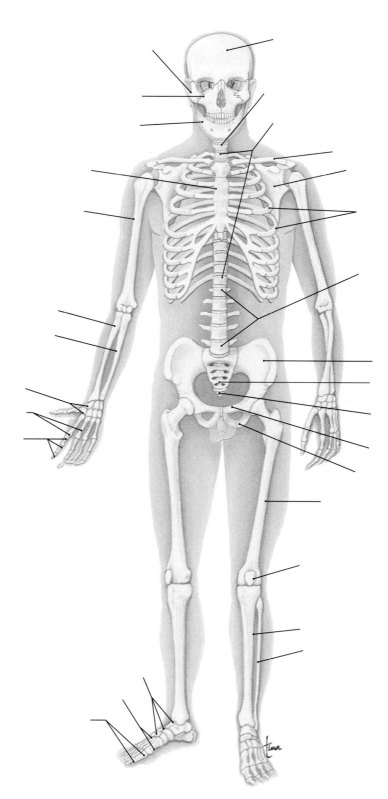

WORSHEET 8

Label the muscles and tendons on the following diagram. Check your answers by referring to Figure 11–6A.

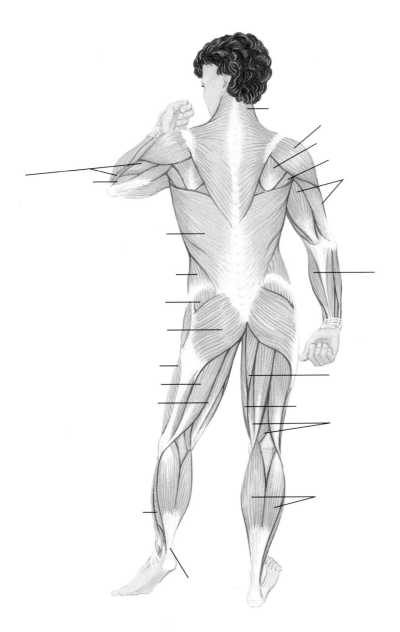

Achilles tendon	Deltoid	Gracilis	Soleus
Adductor magnus	External oblique	Infraspinatus	Teres major
Biceps brachii	Gastrocnemius	Latissimus dorsi	Trapezius
Biceps femoris	Gluteus maximus	Semimembranosus	Triceps brachii
Brachialis	Gluteus medius	Semitendinosus	Vastus lateralis
Brachioradialis			

WORKSHEET 9

▪ ▪ ▪ ▪ ▪ ▪ ▪ ▪ ▪ ▪ ▪ ▪ ▪ ▪ ▪

Label the muscles on the following diagram. Check your answers by referring to Figure 11–6B.

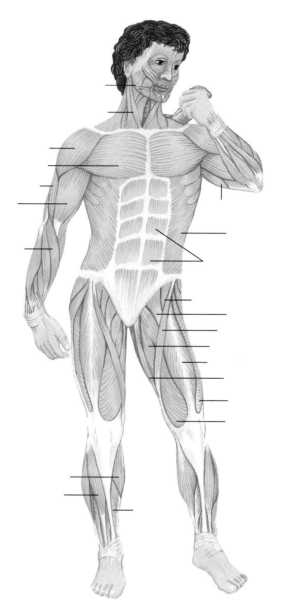

Adductor longus	Gastrocnemius	Pectoralis major	Sternocleidomastoid
Biceps brachii	Gracilis	Rectus abdominus	Tibialis anterior
Brachialis	Iliopsoas	Rectus femoris	Triceps brachii
Brachioradialis	Masseter	Sartorius	Vastus lateralis
Deltoid	Pectineus	Soleus	Vastus medialis
External oblique			

GENITOURINARY SYSTEM

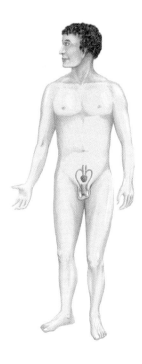

Chapter Outline

Student Objectives

Anatomy and Physiology
Urinary System
Macroscopic Structures
Microscopic Structures
Male Reproductive System

Combining Forms

Suffixes

Pathology
Pyelonephritis
Glomerulonephritis
Nephrolithiasis
Bladder Neck Obstruction
Benign Prostatic Hyperplasia
Cryptorchidism
Acute Tubular Necrosis

Oncology
Carcinoma of the Prostate

Diagnostic, Symptomatic, and Therapeutic Terms
Urinary System
Male Reproductive System

Diagnostic Procedures
Imaging Procedures
Endoscopic Procedures
Laboratory Procedures

Surgical and Therapeutic Procedures

Pharmacology

Abbreviations

Medical Record
Operative Report

Worksheets

Student Objectives

Upon completion of this chapter, you will be able to do the following:

1. List the macroscopic structures of the urinary system, and describe how they function.

2. Describe the structure and function of the nephron.

3. Explain physiological activities involved in the formation of urine.

4. Identify structures and functions associated with the reproductive process in the man.

5. Explain the function of the seminal vesicle, prostate, and Cowper's glands.

6. Name the reproductive structures that also function as part of the male urinary system.

7. Identify combining forms and suffixes related to the genitourinary system.

8. Identify and discuss pathology related to the genitourinary system.

9. Identify diagnostic, symptomatic, and therapeutic terms related to the genitourinary system.

10. Identify diagnostic procedures related to the genitourinary system.

Student Objectives (Continued)

11. Identify surgical and therapeutic procedures related to the genitourinary system.
12. Discuss pharmacology related to the treatment of genitourinary disorders.
13. Identify the abbreviations related to the genitourinary system.
14. Demonstrate your knowledge of the chapter by completing the worksheets.

ANATOMY AND PHYSIOLOGY

The male and female urinary systems consist of four major structures: two kidneys and ureters, a bladder, and a urethra (Fig. 12–1). This chapter presents information on these structures. In addition, it includes a discussion of the male reproductive system because some of the male reproductive organs also function as urinary structures.

Urinary System

The urinary system monitors and regulates the extracellular fluids (plasma, tissue fluid, and lymph) of the body. It filters a variety of substances from plasma. The harmful substances are excreted from the body as urine, and the useful products are returned to the blood.

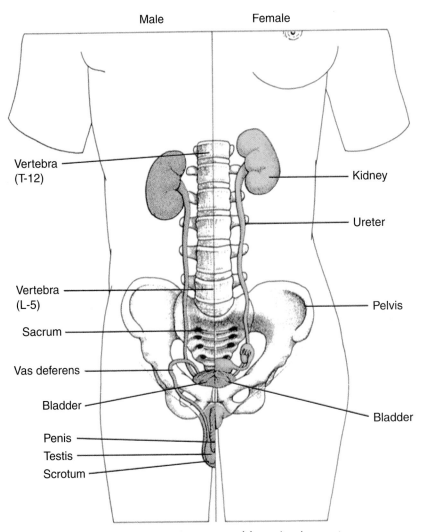

Figure 12–1 Macroscopic structures of the genitourinary system.

Some harmful products that must be filtered from blood are **nitrogenous wastes** and excess fluid **electrolytes** (sodium, potassium, and calcium). Nitrogenous wastes are products formed when the body metabolizes protein. Electrolytes are substances that have the ability to carry electrical charges. These are vital to the functioning of the musculoskeletal, cardiovascular, and nervous systems.

Macroscopic Structures

Refer to Figure 12–2 as you read the following material to identify the major structures of the kidneys.

Two kidneys, each about the size of a fist, are located in the abdominal cavity slightly above the waistline. Because they lie outside of the peritoneum, their location is said to be **retroperitoneal**. A concave medial border gives the kidney its beanlike shape. In a frontal section, two

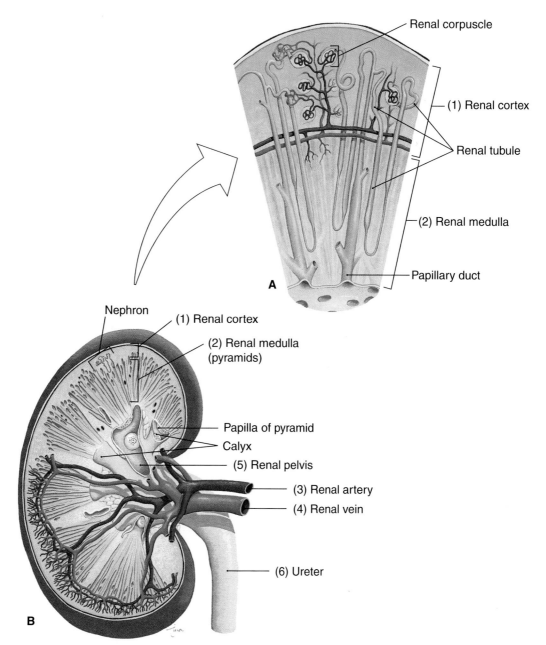

Figure 12–2   (*A*) Frontal section of the right kidney showing internal structure and blood vessels. (*B*) The magnified section of the kidney shows several nephrons. (From Scanlon, VC, and Sanders, T: Understanding Human Structure and Function. F.A. Davis, Philadelphia, 1997, p 326, with permission.)

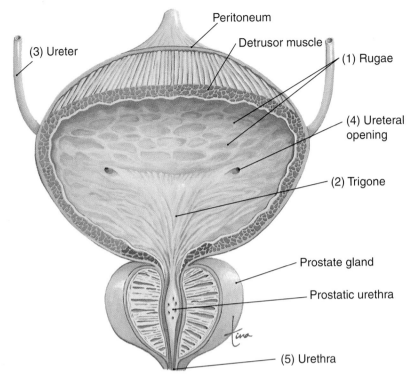

Figure 12–3 Urinary bladder and a portion of the urethra in the man. Anterior view of a frontal section. (From Scanlon, VC, and Sanders, T: Understanding Human Structure and Function. F.A. Davis, Philadelphia, 1997, p 333, with permission.)

distinct areas can be identified: an outer section, the (1) **renal cortex**, and a middle area, the (2) **renal medulla.** These two sections contain portions of the filtering units that compose the kidney. Near the medial border is an opening, the **hilum (hilus)**, where the (3) **renal artery** enters and the (4) **renal vein** exits the kidney. The renal artery carries blood, containing waste products, to the microscopic filtering structures located within the kidney for purification. After waste products are removed, blood leaves the kidney by way of the renal vein. Waste material, now in the form of urine, passes to a hollow chamber, the (5) **renal pelvis**. This cavity is an enlarged funnel-shaped extension of the (6) **ureter** located at the entrance to the kidney. Each ureter is a slender tube about 10 to 12 inches long that carries urine, in peristaltic waves, to the bladder.

As you read the following material, refer to Fig. 12–3 to identify the structures of the urinary bladder. The bladder, an expandable hollow organ, acts as a temporary reservoir for urine. When empty, the bladder has small folds called (1) **rugae** that allow expansion as the bladder fills. A triangular area at the base of the bladder is called the (2) **trigone**. The (3) **ureters** pass behind the bladder and enter its base at the (4) **ureteral opening** located at the trigone. The base of the trigone forms the (5) **urethra**, the tube that discharges urine from the bladder. The length of the urethra is approximately 1.5 inches in women and about 7 inches in men. In the male, the urethra passes through the prostate gland and the penis. During **voiding** or **micturition**, urine is expelled through the urethral opening, the **urinary meatus**.

Microscopic Structures

Microscopic examination of kidney tissue reveals the presence of approximately 1 million microscopic functional structures called **nephrons**. Nephrons are responsible for maintaining homeostasis by continually adjusting conditions that are necessary for survival. When the level of various products in the blood elevates beyond a normal range, nephrons selectively remove these products from the blood by producing a substance called urine. This helps to re-establish a level that can sustain life. Substances removed by nephrons are nitrogenous wastes, including urea, uric acid, and creatinine, the end products of metabolism. Nephrons also remove excess electrolytes and many other products that exceed the amount tolerated by the body.

Figure 12–4 is an illustration of a nephron. Locate each structure as you read the following material.

Each nephron includes a **renal corpuscle** and a **renal tubule**. The renal corpuscle is composed of a tuft of capillaries called the (1) **glomerulus** and a modified, funnel-shaped end of the

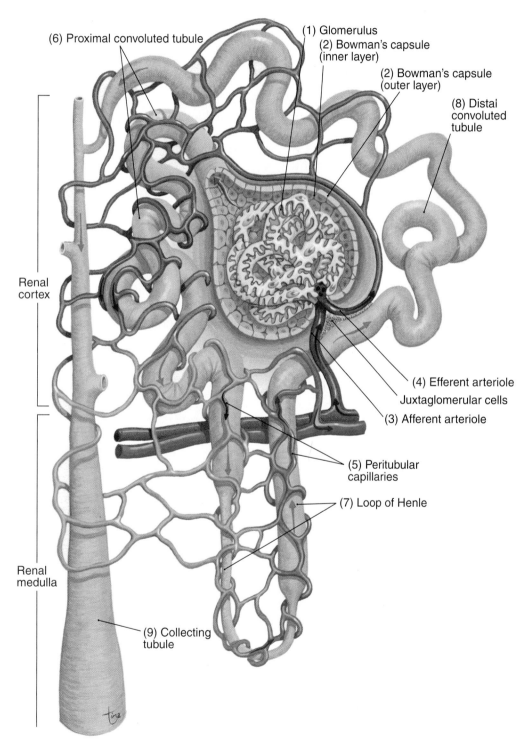

Figure 12–4   A nephron with its associated blood vessels. The arrows indicate the direction of blood flow and the flow of renal filtrate. (From Scanlon, VC, and Sanders, T: Understanding Human Structure and Function. F.A. Davis, Philadelphia, 1997, p 327, with permission.)

renal tubule known as (2) **Bowman's capsule**. This capsule encases the glomerulus. An (3) **afferent arteriole** carries blood to the glomerulus, and a smaller (4) **efferent arteriole** removes it from the glomerulus. As the efferent arteriole passes behind the renal corpuscle, it forms the (5) **peritubular capillaries**, which allow needed products that have been filtered from the blood to re-enter the vascular system.

Each renal tubule consists of four sections: the (6) **proximal convoluted tubule**; followed by the narrow (7) **loop of Henle**; then a larger portion, the (8) **distal tubule**; and finally, the (9) **collecting tubule**.

The nephron produces urine by three physiological activities:

- Filtration
- Reabsorption
- Secretion

Filtration takes place in the renal corpuscle. Here, water, electrolytes, sugar, amino acids, and other compounds pass from the blood in the glomerulus into Bowman's capsule. The fluid that is formed is called **filtrate**.

Reabsorption begins as filtrate passes through the four sections of the tubule. As filtrate travels the long and twisted pathway of the tubule, most of the water and some of the electrolytes and amino acids are absorbed by the peritubular capillaries, thus re-entering the circulating blood.

Secretion occurs when specialized cells of the collecting tubules secrete ammonia, uric acid, and other substances directly into the tubule. This process completes urine production.

Male Reproductive System

The male reproductive system serves two important functions. First, it produces sperm, the male sex cell, which contains one half of the genetic material necessary to produce a living being. Second, it provides structures necessary to transport and maintain viable sperm. As you read this section, identify the structures in Figure 12–5.

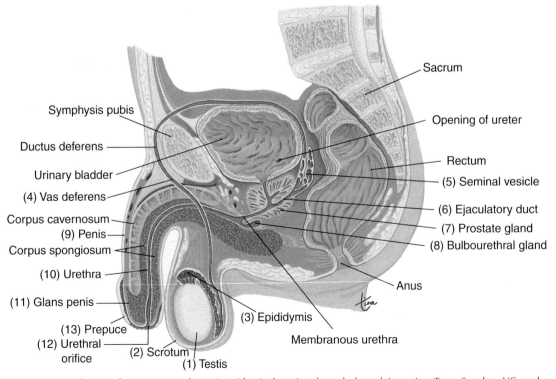

Figure 12–5 Male reproductive system shown in midsagittal section through the pelvic cavity. (From Scanlon, VC, and Sanders, T: Understanding Human Structure and Function. F.A. Davis, Philadelphia, 1997, p 357, with permission.)

The primary male reproductive organ consists of two (1) **testes** (singular, **testis**), located in an external sac called the (2) **scrotum**. Within the testes are numerous small tubes that twist and coil to form **seminiferous tubules**, which produce sperm, the male sex cell. The testes also secrete testosterone, which develops and maintains secondary sex characteristics. Lying over the superior surface of each testis is a single, tightly coiled tube, the (3) **epididymis**. This structure stores sperm after it leaves the seminiferous tubules. The epididymis is the first duct through which sperm passes after its production in the testes. Tracing the duct upward, the epididymis forms the (4) **vas deferens** (**seminal duct** or **ductus deferens**), a narrow tube that passes through the inguinal canal into the abdominal cavity. The vas deferens extends over the top and down the posterior surface of the bladder, where it joins the (5) **seminal vesicle**. The union of the vas deferens with the duct from the seminal vesicle forms the (6) **ejaculatory duct**.

The seminal vesicle secretes approximately 60 percent of the fluid that is ultimately ejaculated during sexual intercourse **(coitus)**. It contains nutrients that support sperm viability. The ejaculatory duct passes at an angle through the (7) **prostate gland**, a triple-lobed organ fused to the base of the bladder. The prostate secretes a thin, alkaline substance that accounts for about 30 percent of the seminal fluid. Its alkalinity helps protect sperm from the acidic environments of both the male urethra and the female vagina. The two pea-shaped (8) **bulbourethral (Cowper's) glands** are located below the prostate and are connected by a small duct to the urethra. Cowper's glands provide an alkaline fluid necessary for sperm viability. The (9) **penis** is the male organ of copulation. It is cylindrical and composed of erectile tissue that encloses the (10) **urethra**. The urethra expels both semen and urine from the body. During ejaculation, the sphincter at the base of the bladder closes. This not only stops the urine from being expelled with the semen but also prevents semen from entering the bladder.

The enlarged tip of the penis, the (11) **glans penis**, contains the (12) **urethral orifice (meatus)**. A movable hood of skin, called (13) **prepuce**, or **foreskin**, covers the glans penis.

COMBINING FORMS

Combining Form	Meaning	Example	Pronunciation
Urinary			
cyst/o	bladder	cyst/o/scopy visual examination	sĭs-TŎS-kō-pē
vesic/o		vesic/o/cele herniation	VĔS-ĭ-kō-sēl
glomerul/o	glomerulus	glomerul/o/pathy disease	glō-mĕr-ū-LŎP-ă-thē
nephr/o	kidney	nephr/o/pexy fixation	NĔF-rō-pĕks-ē
ren/o		ren/al pertaining to	RĒ-năl
ureter/o	ureter	ureter/ectasis dilation, expansion	ū-rē-tĕr-ĔK-tă-sĭs
urethr/o	urethra	urethr/o/plasty surgical repair	ū-RĒ-thrō-plăs-tē
ur/o	urine, urinary	ur/o/lith calculus, stone	Ū-rō-lĭth
Male Reproductive			
andr/o	male	andr/o/logy study	ăn-DRŎL-ō-jē

COMBINING FORMS (Continued)

Combining Form	Meaning	Example	Pronunciation
balan/o	glans penis	balan/o/rrhea flow, discharge	băl-ăn-ō-RĒ-ă
epididym/o	epididymis	epididym/itis inflammation	ĕp-ĭ-dĭd-ĭ-MĪ-tĭs
orch/i		orchi/algia pain	or-kē-ĂL-jē-ă
orchi/o	testes	orchi/o/rrhaphy suture	or-kē-OR-ră-fē
orchid/o		orchid/itis inflammation	or-kĭ-DĪ-tĭs
prostat/o	prostate	prostat/ectomy excision	prŏs-tă-TĔK-tō-mē
spermat/o	sperm	spermat/o/lysis destruction	spĕr-măt-ŎL-ĭ-sĭs
vas/o	vas deferens, duct, vessel	vas/ectomy excision	văs-ĔK-tō-mē
vesicul/o	seminal vesicle	vesicul/itis inflammation	vĕ-sĭk-ū-LĪ-tĭs
Other Combining Forms Related to the Genitourinary System			
albumin/o	albumin (protein)	albumin/oid resembling	ăl-BŪ-mĭ-noyd
bacteri/o	bacteria	bacteri/al pertaining to	băk-TĒ-rē-ăl
crypt/o	hidden	crypt/orchid/ism testes condition	krĭpt-OR-kĭd-ĭzm
noct/o	night	noct/uria urine	nŏk-TŪ-rē-ă
olig/o	scanty	olig/uria urine	ŏl-ĭg-Ū-rē-ă
py/o	pus	py/osis abnormal condition	pī-Ō-sĭs

SUFFIXES

Suffix	Meaning	Example	Pronunciation
-genesis	forming, producing, origin	spermat/o/genesis sperm	spĕr-măt-ō-JĔN-ĕ-sĭs
-iasis	abnormal condition (produced by something specified)	nephr/o/lith/iasis kidney stone	nĕf-rō-lĭth-Ī-ă-sĭs
-uria	urine	dys/uria painful, difficult	dĭs-Ū-rē-ă

PATHOLOGY

Pyelonephritis

One of the most common forms of kidney disease is **pyelonephritis**. In this disorder, bacteria invade the renal pelvis and kidney tissue, often as a consequence of a bladder infection that has ascended to the kidney via the ureters. When the infection is severe, lesions form in the renal pelvis, causing bleeding. The microscopic examination of urine reveals the following: large quantities of bacteria (**bacteriuria**), white blood cells (**pyuria**), and, when lesions are present, red blood cells (**hematuria**). The onset of the disease is usually acute, with symptoms including chills, fever, nausea, and vomiting.

Pyelonephritis is about eight times more common in women than in men, probably because of the shorter female urethra. Treatment includes the use of antibiotics.

Glomerulonephritis

Any condition that causes the glomerular walls to become inflamed is referred to as **glomerulonephritis**. One of the most common causes of glomerular inflammation is a reaction to the toxins given off by pathogenic streptococci that have recently infected another part of the body, especially the throat. Glomerulonephritis is also associated with autoimmune diseases such as systemic lupus erythematosus, polyarthritis, and scleroderma.

When the glomerular membrane is inflamed, it becomes highly permeable and permits blood cells and protein to enter the filtrate, causing hematuria and **proteinuria**. In some cases, protein solidifies in the nephron tubules and forms solid masses that take the shape of the tubules in which they develop. These masses are called **casts**. They often pass out of the kidney by way of the urine and may be visible when urine is examined microscopically. Most patients with acute glomerulonephritis associated with a streptococcal infection recover with no residual kidney damage.

Nephrolithiasis

Stones may form in any part of the urinary tract, but most arise in the kidney. They frequently form when dissolved urine salts begin to solidify. As these stones increase in size, they obstruct urinary structures. When they lodge in the ureters, they cause intense pulsating pain called **colic**. Because urine is hindered from flowing into the bladder, it refluxes into the renal pelvis and the tubules, causing them to dilate. This distension is called **hydronephrosis**. For calculi that cannot be dislodged or dissolved, ultrasound waves, directed through the skin (**percutaneous ultrasonic lithotripsy** or **extracorporeal shock-wave lithotripsy [ESWL]**), often prove effective.

Bladder Neck Obstruction

A blockage of the bladder outlet is referred to as **bladder neck obstruction (BNO)**. The obstruction may be caused by an enlarged prostate gland (**prostatic hypertrophy**) or by the presence of an obstructive mass such as a calculus, blood clot, or tumor. The resulting bladder distension may lead to hydronephrosis accompanied by bladder infection (**cystitis**). The patient experiences a need to void but can only void small quantities at a time. This is referred to as retention with overflow. Correction of BNO includes surgery that relieves or removes the obstruction.

Benign Prostatic Hyperplasia

Benign prostatic hyperplasia (BPH), sometimes called **nodular hyperplasia** or **benign prostatic hypertrophy**, is often associated with the aging process. The prostate enlarges and decreases the urethral lumen. Inability to empty the bladder completely may cause cystitis, which may then lead to nephritis. Surgical removal of the prostate may be necessary. The different operative procedures include the removal of the prostate through the perineum (**perineal prostatectomy**), excision through the urethra (**transurethral resection [TUR]**), or excision through an abdominal opening above the pubis and directly over the bladder (**suprapubic prostatectomy**).

Cryptorchidism

Failure of the testes to descend into the scrotal sac prior to birth is called **cryptorchidism**. In many infants born with this condition, the testes descend spontaneously by the end of the first year. If this does not occur, correction of the disorder involves surgical suspension of the testes (**orchiopexy**) in the scrotum. This procedure is usually done before the child reaches 2 years of age. Because an inguinal hernia often accompanies cryptorchidism, the hernia (**herniorrhaphy**) may be sutured at this time.

Acute Tubular Necrosis

Two major causes of **acute tubular necrosis (ATN)** are ischemia and nephrotoxic injury. In ATN, the tubular portion of the nephron is injured through either a decreased blood supply or the presence of toxic substances (usually after ingestion of toxic chemical agents). Ischemia may be the result of circulatory collapse, severe hypotension, hemorrhage, dehydration, or other disorders that affect blood supply.

Signs and symptoms of ATN include scanty urine production (**oliguria**) and increased blood levels of calcium (**hypercalcemia**). When tubular damage is not severe, the disorder is reversible.

Oncology

Carcinoma of the Prostate

The second most common form of cancer in men is carcinoma of the prostate. In the United States, the disease is rarely found in men younger than 50 years of age, but the incidence dramatically increases as the individual grows older. Susceptibility to the disease is influenced, to a large extent, by race, being extremely low in Asians, moderate in whites, and high in blacks.

Symptoms include difficulty in starting and stopping the urinary stream, dysuria, frequency, and hematuria. By the time these symptoms develop and the patient seeks treatment, the disease is quite advanced and long-term survival is not likely. Early presymptomatic tests include a blood test for **prostate-specific antigen (PSA)** and periodic **digital rectal examination (DRE)**.

Like other forms of cancer, prostatic carcinomas are staged and graded to determine metastatic potential, response to treatment, survival, and appropriate forms of therapy.

Surgical removal of the testes (**bilateral orchiectomy**) and administration of estrogens can usually arrest metastatic prostatic cancer.

DIAGNOSTIC, SYMPTOMATIC, AND THERAPEUTIC TERMS

Urinary System

Term	Meaning
anuria ăn-Ū-rē-ă	absence of urine production
azotemia, uremia ăz-ō-TĒ-mē-ă, ū-RĒ-mē-ă	metabolic wastes (urea, creatinine, and uric acid) in the blood

Urinary System (Continued)

Term	Meaning
chronic renal failure KRŎ-nĭk RĒ-năl	renal failure that occurs over a period of years, whereby the kidneys lose their ability to maintain volume and composition of body fluids with normal dietary intake; condition is due to deficiency in the total number of functioning nephrons in the kidneys
dysuria dĭs-Ū-rē-ă	painful or difficult urination, symptomatic of numerous conditions
enuresis, incontinence ĕn-ū-RĒ-sĭs, ĭn-KŎN-tĭ-nĕns	involuntary discharge of urine: during the night, nocturnal enuresis; during the day, diurnal enuresis
fistula FĬS-tū-lă	abnormal passage from a hollow organ to the surface, or from one organ to another
frequency FRĒ-kwĕn-sē	voiding at frequent intervals
hesitancy HĔZ-ĭ-tĕn-sē	involuntary delay in initiating urination
nephrotic syndrome nĕ-FRŎT-ĭk	loss of large amounts of plasma protein by way of urine, which results in systemic edema
nocturia, nycturia nŏk-TŪ-rē-ă, nĭk-TŪ-rē-ă	excessive urination during the night
oliguria ŏl-ĭg-Ū-rē-ă	scanty urine production
urgency ŬR-jĕn-sē	need to void immediately; commonly accompanies frequency in persons with urinary tract infections (UTIs)
urolithiasis ū-rō-lĭ-THĪ-ă-sĭs	presence of stones in any urinary structure; frequently treated by pulverizing the stones with an ultrasonic lithotriptor
Wilms' tumor	rapidly developing kidney tumor that usually occurs in children

Male Reproductive System

Term	Meaning
anorchism ăn-OR-kĭzm	congenital absence of one or both testes
aspermia ă-SPĔR-mē-ă	lack of or failure to ejaculate semen
balanitis băl-ă-NĪ-tĭs	inflammation of the skin covering the glans penis
epispadias ĕp-ĭ-SPĀ-dē-ăs	malformation in which the urethra opens on the dorsum of the penis
hydrocele HĪ-drō-sēl	accumulation of serous fluid in a saclike cavity, especially the testes and associated structures
hypospadias hī-pō-SPĀ-dē-ăs	developmental anomaly in the man in which the urethra opens on the underside of the penis or, in extreme cases, on the perineum
impotence ĬM-pō-tĕns	condition characterized by inability to achieve an erection
phimosis fī-MŌ-sĭs	stenosis or narrowing of preputial orifice so that the foreskin cannot be pushed back over the glans penis
sterility stĕr-ĬL-ĭ-tē	inability to fertilize the ovum; inability of reproducing an offspring
varicocele VĂR-ĭ-kō-sēl	swelling and distension of veins of the spermatic cord

DIAGNOSTIC PROCEDURES

Imaging Procedure	Description
cystography sĭs-TŎG-ră-fē	radiography of the urinary bladder using a contrast medium, used to diagnose tumors or defects in the bladder wall, vesicoureteral reflux, stones, or other pathological conditions of the bladder
cystometrography sĭs-tō-mĕ-TRŎG-ră-fē	a procedure that assesses volume and pressure in the bladder at varying stages of filling
cystourethrogram, cystourethrography sĭs-tō-ū-RĒ-thrō-grăm, sĭs-tō-ū-rē-THRŎG-ră-fē	radiological evaluation of the urinary bladder and urethra after the administration of a contrast medium
electromyogram, electromyography ē-lĕk-trō-MĪ-ō-grăm, ē-lĕk-trō-mī-ŎG-ră-fē	a graphic record of the contraction of a muscle as a result of electrical stimulation
sphincter SFĬNGK-tĕr	a test that assesses muscle function of the pelvic floor muscles during bladder filling and voiding
nephrotomography, CT scan (kidney) nĕf-rō-tō-MŎG-ră-fē	study visualizing several planes of the kidney, to differentiate solid renal and adrenal tumors from benign renal cysts; performed in conjunction with an IVP
pyelogram PĪ-ĕ-lō-grăm	radiography of the ureters and renal pelvis
intravenous ĭn-tră-VĒ-nŭs	radiography of the ureters and renal pelvis in which a radiopaque substance is injected intravenously
ultrasound ŬL-tră-sŏwnd	imaging procedure using ultra-high frequency sound waves
scrotal SKRŌ-tăl	assesses patency of vas deferens and other structures
urography ū-RŎG-ră-fē	radiography of the urinary tract after introduction of contrast medium
excretory ĔKS-krē-tō-rē	urography in which an injected dye is excreted by the kidney and studied by radiographic examination during excretion

Endoscopic Procedure	Description
cystoscopy sĭs-TŎS-kō-pē	visual examination of urinary bladder with a cystoscope inserted in the urethra; also used to obtain biopsies of tumors or other growths and to remove polyps
nephroscopy nĕ-FRŎS-kō-pē	visual examination of the kidney(s) using a specialized three-channel endoscope to provide for telescope, fiberoptic light input, and irrigation. The nephroscope is passed through a small incision made in the renal pelvis. Kidney pathology and congenital deformities may be observed
urethroscopy ū-rē-THRŎS-kō-pē	visualization of the urethra using a urethroscope; used for lithotripsy or for TUR

Laboratory Procedure	Description
blood urea nitrogen (BUN)	assesses kidney function by determining the nitrogen in blood in the form of urea (increased BUN usually indicates decreased renal function)
semen analysis	test that analyzes a semen sample for volume, sperm count, motility, and morphology; also used to verify sterilization after a vasectomy
urinalysis (UA)	a battery of physical observations, chemical tests, and microscopic evaluations performed on a urine specimen
urine culture and sensitivity (C&S)	used to determine the sensitivity of a urinary pathogen to the effects of various antibiotics

SURGICAL AND THERAPEUTIC PROCEDURES

Procedure	Description
circumcision sĕr-kŭm-SĬ-zhŭn	surgical removal of all or part of the foreskin, or prepuce, of the penis
dialysis dī-ĂL-ĭ-sĭs	the passage of a solution through a membrane
peritoneal pĕr-ĭ-tō-NĒ-ăl	removal of toxic substances from the body by perfusing the peritoneal cavity with warm sterile chemical solutions. The lining of the peritoneal cavity is used as the dialyzing membrane. Dialyzing fluid remains in the peritoneal cavity for 1 or 2 hours and then is removed. The procedure is repeated as often as necessary
hemodialysis hē-mō-dī-ĂL-ĭ-sĭs	dialysis of blood. Blood is shunted from the body and passed through a semipermeable membranous tube to remove liquid and chemicals that the kidneys would normally remove. At the completion of the process, the cleansed blood returns to the body
nephrolithotomy nĕf-rō-lĭth-ŎT-ō-mē	incision of a kidney to remove a stone
nephropexy NĔF-rō-pĕks-ē	fixation of a floating or mobile kidney
orchiectomy or-kē-ĔK-tō-mē	surgical removal of the testes
resection	partial excision of a structure
transurethral (TUR, TURP) trăns-ū-RĒ-thrăl rē-SĔK-shŭn	procedure to remove prostatic tissue by cauterization or cryosurgery, performed using an endoscope passed through the urethra
urethrorrhaphy ū-rē-THROR-ăf-ē	suture of the urethra, frequently employed to repair a fistula
urethrotomy ū-rē-THRŎT-ō-mē	incision of a urethral stricture
vasectomy văs-ĔK-tō-mē	excision of all or a segment of the vas deferens. Bilateral vasectomy is the most successful method of male contraception. Although the procedure is considered permanent, with advances in microsurgery vasectomy is sometimes reversible (Fig. 12–6)

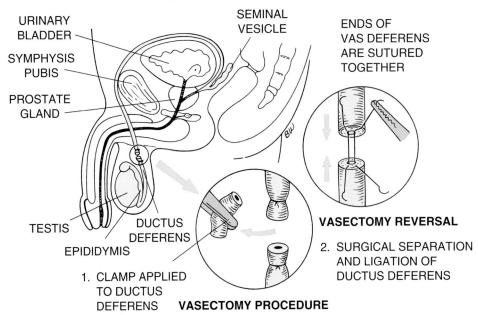

VASECTOMY AND ITS REVERSAL

Figure 12–6   Vasectomy and its reversal. (From Taber's Cyclopedic Medical Dictionary, ed 18. F.A. Davis, Philadelphia, 1997, p 2066, with permission.)

PHARMACOLOGY

Medication	Action
diuretics	agents that promote the secretion of urine
estrogen hormones	hormones used in men to suppress gonadotropic and testicular androgenic hormones; used to treat some prostatic cancers
gonadotropin	hormonal preparation used to raise sperm count in infertility cases
spermicidals	substances that destroy sperm; used within the woman's vagina for contraception
uricosurics	agents that increase the urinary excretion of uric acid; used to treat gout

ABBREVIATIONS

Abbreviation	Meaning
A/G	albumin-globulin ratio
AGN	acute glomerulonephritis
ARF	acute renal failure
ATN	acute tubular necrosis
BNO	bladder neck obstruction
BPH	benign prostatic hyperplasia; benign prostatic hypertrophy
BUN	blood urea nitrogen
C&S	culture and sensitivity
cath	catheterization, catheter
cysto	cystoscopy
DRE	digital rectal examination
ESL, ESWL	extracorporeal shock-wave lithotripsy

ABBREVIATIONS (Continued)

Abbreviation	Meaning
GU	genitourinary
HD	hemodialysis
IVP	intravenous pyelogram
K^+	potassium (an electrolyte)
KUB	kidney, ureter, and bladder
Na^+	sodium (an electrolyte)
pH	hydrogen ion concentration, degree of acidity
PSA	prostate-specific antigen
RP	retrograde pyelogram
TUR, TURP	transurethral resection of prostate
UA	urinalysis
UTI	urinary tract infection
VCU, VCUG	voiding cystourethrogram

MEDICAL RECORD

Operative Report

Preoperative and Postoperative Diagnosis   Hematuria with left ureterocele and ureterocele calculus.

Operation   Cystoscopy, transurethral incision of ureterocele, extraction of stone and cystolithotripsy

Anesthesia   General

Procedure   The patient was prepped and draped and placed in the lithotomy position. The urethra was calibrated with ease, using a #26 French Van Buren sound. A #24 resectoscope was inserted with ease. The prostate and bladder appeared normal, except for the presence of a left ureterocele; this was incised longitudinally and a large calculus was extracted from the ureterocele. There was minimal bleeding and no need for fulguration. The stone was crushed with the Storz stone-crushing instrument, and the fragments were evacuated. The bladder was emptied and the procedure terminated.

Worksheet 5 provides a dictionary and reading application and an analysis of this medical record.

WORKSHEET 1

■ ■ ■ ■ ■ ■ ■ ■ ■ ■ ■ ■ ■ ■ ■

*Use **nephr/o** (kidney) to build a medical word meaning:*

1. stone in the kidney _____

2. specialist in the study of the kidney _____

3. abnormal condition of pus in the kidney _____

4. abnormal condition of water in the kidney _____

*Use **pyel/o** (renal pelvis) to build a medical word meaning:*

5. dilation of the renal pelvis _____

6. disease of the renal pelvis _____

*Use **ureter/o** (ureter) to build a medical word meaning:*

7. dilation of the ureter _____

8. calculus in the ureter _____

9. enlargement of the ureter _____

*Use **cyst/o** (bladder) to build a medical word meaning:*

10. inflammation of the bladder _____

11. instrument to view the bladder _____

*Use **vesic/o** (bladder) to build a medical word meaning:*

12. herniation of the bladder _____

13. pertaining to the bladder and prostate _____

*Use **urethr/o** (urethra) to build a medical word meaning:*

14. narrowing or stricture of the urethra _____

15. an instrument to incise the urethra _____

*Use **ur/o** (urine, urinary) to build a medical word meaning:*

16. radiograph of urinary (structures) _____

17. disease of the urinary (tract) _____

*Use the suffix **-uria** (urine) to build a medical word meaning:*

18. blood in the urine _____

19. difficult or painful urination _____

20. scanty urination _____

Use orchid/o *or* orchi/o *(testes) to build a medical word meaning:*

21. disease of the testes _____

22. pain in the testes _____

Use vesicul/o *(seminal vesicle) to build a medical word meaning:*

23. disease of the seminal vesicle _____

Use prostat/o *(prostate) to build a medical word meaning:*

24. discharge from the prostate _____

Use balan/o *(glans penis) to build a medical word meaning:*

25. discharge from the glans penis _____

WORSHEET 2

■ ■ ■ ■ ■ ■ ■ ■ ■ ■ ■ ■ ■ ■

Build a surgical term meaning:

1. removal of the vas deferens _____

2. suturing of the urethra _____

3. surgical repair of ureter and renal pelvis _____

4. removal of the kidney and its ureter _____

5. excision of a stone from the bladder _____

6. surgical repair of the bladder _____

7. narrowing or stricture of the urethra _____

8. removal of the prostate _____

9. incision for removal of a stone in the prostate _____

10. removal of the testes _____

WORKSHEET 3

Match the following medical terms with the definitions in the numbered list:

anuria   hypertension   oliguria
aspermia   hypospadias   urgency
epispadias   impotence   urolithiasis
frequency   incontinence   varicocele

1. _____ involuntary discharge of urine

2. _____ scanty urine production

3. _____ malformation in which the urethra opens on the dorsum of the penis

4. _____ an inability to achieve an erection

5. _____ swelling and distension of the veins of the spermatic cord

6. _____ male developmental anomaly in which the urethra opens on the underside of the penis

7. _____ presence of stones in the urinary system

8. _____ voiding at frequent intervals either in small or large amounts

9. _____ lack of or failure to ejaculate semen

10. _____ the need to void immediately

WORKSHEET 4

■ ■ ■ ■ ■ ■ ■ ■ ■ ■ ■ ■ ■

Match the following medical terms with the definitions in the numbered list.

blood urea nitrogen (BUN)   gonadotropins   spermicidal preparations
circumcision   nephrotomography   urethroscopy
cystography   pH   uricosuric agents
cystoscopy   intravenous pyelogram (IVP) urinalysis (UA)
diuretics   retrograde pyelogram (RP) UTI
estrogenic hormones   semen analysis

1. _____ use of a radiopaque dye administered intravenously to visualize the urinary structures, especially the structures of the kidney

2. _____ one of the most widely used battery of tests performed on a urine specimen

3. _____ test that assesses kidney function by assessing the kidneys' ability to remove urea

4. _____ drugs that increase the excretion of uric acid by the kidney, used in the treatment of gout

5. _____ hormonal preparations used to raise sperm count in cases of infertility

6. _____ hydrogen ion concentration

7. _____ removal of all or part of the foreskin, or prepuce

8. _____ increase the production of urine

9. _____ substances that destroy sperm

10. _____ analysis of volume, sperm count, motility, and morphology, usually performed as part of an infertility work-up

11. _____ an infection found in any structure of the urinary tract

12. _____ study visualizing several planes of the kidney

13. _____ hormonal agents used to treat prostate cancer

14. _____ procedure that permits visualization of the urethra, often used for lithotripsy or TUR

15. _____ radiographic procedure that involves the introduction of a contrast medium into the bladder to visualize this structure

WORKSHEET 5

■ ■ ■ ■ ■ ■ ■ ■ ■ ■ ■ ■ ■ ■

MEDICAL RECORD: OPERATIVE REPORT

Underline the following terms in the medical record (see p. 233). Use a medical dictionary and other resources to define the terms and to determine their pronunciation; then practice reading the medical record aloud.

bladder _____

calculus _____

calibrated _____

cystolithotripsy _____

cystoscopy _____

evacuated _____

fulguration _____

hematuria _____

lithotomy position _____

prostate _____

resectoscope _____

sound _____

transurethral _____

ureterocele _____

urethra _____

MEDICAL RECORD EVALUATION: OPERATIVE REPORT

1. *Why did the doctor perform a cystoscopy?*

2. *What size of urethral sound was used?*

3. *Why is a sound used?*

4. *In what direction did the urologist cut the urethrocele?*

5. *Did the urologist need to use fulguration? If not, why?*

WORKSHEET 6

. . . .

Label the following diagram. Check your answers by referring to Figure 12–2.

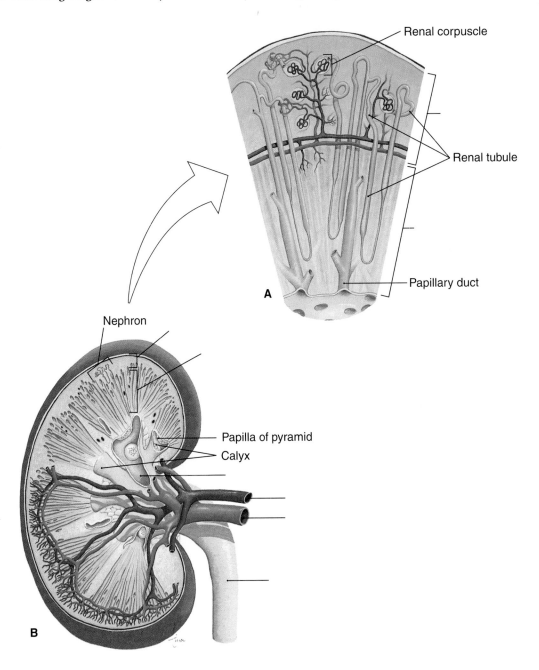

Renal corpuscle

Renal tubule

Papillary duct

A

Nephron

Papilla of pyramid

Calyx

B

Renal artery	Renal medulla	Renal vein
Renal cortex	Renal pelvis	Ureter

WORKSHEET 7

▪ ▪ ▪ ▪ ▪ ▪ ▪ ▪ ▪ ▪ ▪ ▪ ▪ ▪

Label the following diagram. Check your answers by referring to Figure 12–5.

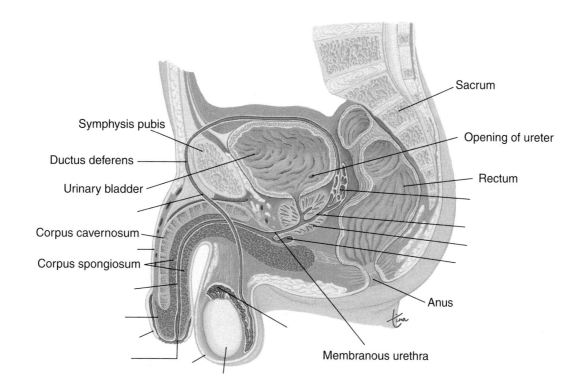

Sacrum

Symphysis pubis

Opening of ureter

Ductus deferens

Rectum

Urinary bladder

Corpus cavernosum

Corpus spongiosum

Anus

Membranous urethra

Bulbourethral gland	Ejaculatory duct	Epididymis
Glans penis	Penis	Prepuce
Prostate gland	Scrotum	Seminal vesicle
Testis	Urethra	Urethral orifice
Vas deferens		

Chapter 13

FEMALE REPRODUCTIVE SYSTEM

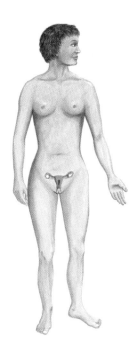

Chapter Outline
Student Objectives
Anatomy and Physiology
Internal Organs of Reproduction
  Ovaries
  Fallopian Tubes
  Uterus and Vagina
Menstrual Cycle
  Menstrual Phase
  Follicular Phase
  Luteal Phase
Pregnancy
Labor and Childbirth
Menopause
Combining Forms
Suffixes
Prefixes
Pathology
Menstrual Disturbances
Premenstrual Syndrome
Endometriosis
Pelvic Infections
Vaginal Infections

Sexually Transmitted Diseases
Uterine Tumors
Oncology
  Cervical Cancer
Diagnostic, Symptomatic, and Therapeutic Terms
Female Reproductive System
Obstetrics
Diagnostic Procedures
Imaging Procedures
Endoscopic Procedures
Laboratory Procedures
Surgical and Therapeutic Procedures
Pharmacology
Abbreviations
Maternal-Gynecological and Related
  Abbreviations
Fetal-Obstetric Abbreviations
Medical Record
Primary Herpes 1 Infection
Worksheets

Student Objectives

Upon completion of this chapter, you will be able to do the following:

1. List the organs of the female reproductive system.
2. Describe the position and function of each organ.
3. Explain the series of events associated with maturation of the ovum.
4. Describe the condition and stages of pregnancy.
5. Identify combining forms, prefixes, and suffixes related to the female reproductive system.

Student Objectives (Continued)

6. Identify and discuss pathology related to the female reproductive system.
7. Identify diagnostic, symptomatic, and therapeutic terms related to the female reproductive system.
8. Identify diagnostic procedures related to the female reproductive system.
9. Identify surgical and therapeutic procedures related to the female reproductive system.
10. Define the abbreviations related to the female reproductive system.
11. Discuss pharmacology related to treatment of female reproductive disorders.
12. Demonstrate your understanding of the chapter by completing the worksheets.

ANATOMY AND PHYSIOLOGY

The female reproductive system (Fig. 13–1) consists of internal and external organs of reproduction. The internal, or essential, organs of reproduction (Fig. 13–2) are the (1) **ovaries**, (2) **fal-**

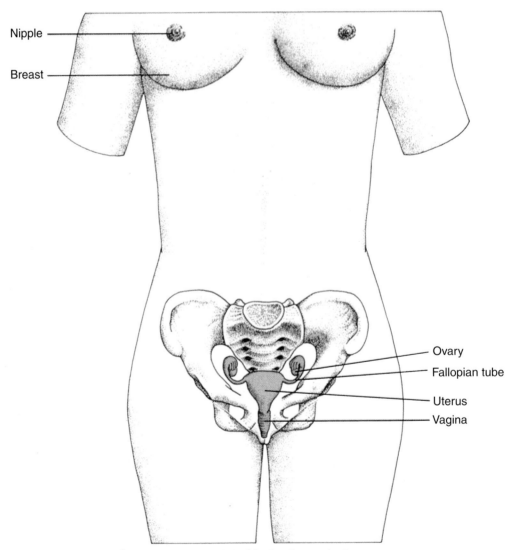

Figure 13–1   Anterior view of the female reproductive system.

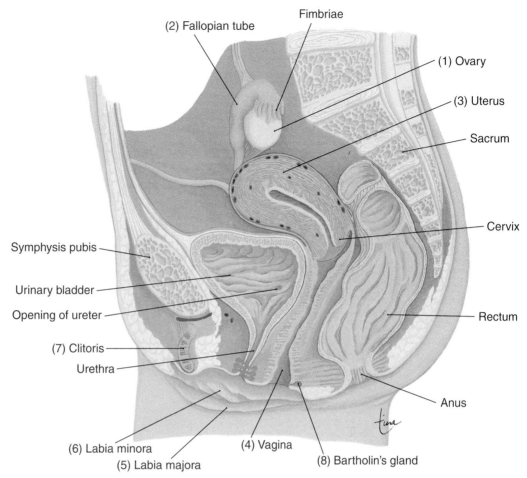

Figure 13–2 Structures of the female reproductive system. (From Scanlon, VC, and Sanders, T: Understanding Human Structure and Function. F.A. Davis, Philadelphia, 1997, p 361, with permission.)

lopian tubes (oviducts, uterine tubes), (3) **uterus**, and (4) **vagina**. The external genitalia include the (5) **labia majora**, (6) **labia minora**, (7) **clitoris**, and (8) **Bartholin's glands**. The combined structures of the external genitalia are known as the **vulva**.

Internal Organs of Reproduction

Ovaries

Refer to (Fig. 13–3) as you read the following material. The (1) **ovaries** are almond-shaped glands located in the pelvic cavity, one on each side of the uterus, which produce the ovum (egg), the female reproductive cell, and various hormones.

Two hormones secreted by the ovaries, estrogen and progesterone, are responsible for the menstrual cycle and menopause. In addition, both hormones prepare the uterus for implantation of the fertilized egg, help to maintain pregnancy, and promote growth of the placenta. Estrogen and progesterone also play an important role in development of secondary sex characteristics (see Chap. 14).

Fallopian Tubes

Two (2) **fallopian tubes (oviducts, uterine tubes)** extend laterally from superior angles of the uterus. Fingerlike projections, (3) **fimbriae**, create wavelike currents (peristalsis) in fluid sur-

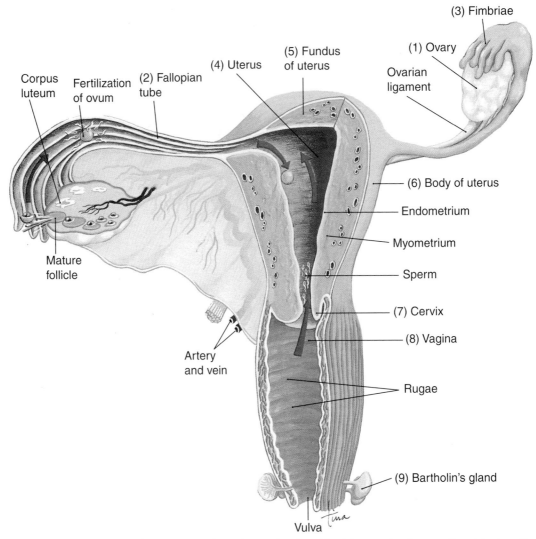

Figure 13–3 Female reproductive system shown in anterior view. The left ovary has been sectioned to show the developing follicles. The left fallopian tube has been sectioned to show fertilization. The uterus and vagina have been sectioned to show internal structures. Arrows indicate the movement of the ovum toward the uterus and the movement of sperm from the vagina toward the fallopian tube. (From Scanlon, VC, and Sanders, T: Essentials of Anatomy and Physiology, ed 2. F.A. Davis, Philadelphia, 1995, p 464, with permission.)

rounding the ovary to pull the ovum into the uterine tube. If the egg unites with a spermatozoon, the male reproductive cell, fertilization or conception takes place. If conception does not occur, the ovum disintegrates within 48 hours.

Uterus and Vagina

The (4) **uterus** contains and nourishes the embryo from the time the fertilized egg is implanted until the fetus is born. It is a muscular, hollow, pear-shaped structure located in the pelvic area between the bladder and rectum. The uterus is normally in a position of anteflexion (bent forward) and consists of three parts: the (5) **fundus**, which is the upper, rounded part; the (6) **body**, which is the central part; and the (7) **cervix**, also called the neck of the uterus or **cervix uteri**, which is the inferior constricted portion that opens into the vagina.

The (8) **vagina** is a muscular tube that extends from the cervix to the exterior of the body. Its lining consists of mucous membrane folds that give the organ an elastic quality. During sexual excitement, the vaginal orifice is lubricated by secretions from (9) **Bartholin's glands**. Besides serving as the organ of sexual intercourse and receptor of semen, the vagina discharges menstrual flow. The vagina also acts as a passageway for the delivery of the fetus.

Menstrual Cycle

Menarche, the initial menstrual period, occurs at puberty (about 13 years of age) and continues approximately 40 years, except during pregnancy. The menstrual cycle consists of approximately 28 days and can be described in terms of three phases: menstrual phase, follicular phase, and luteal phase.

Menstrual Phase

The loss of the functional layer of endometrium is known as menstruation. Menstruation may last 2 to 8 days, with an average of 3 to 6 days. Secretion of the follicle-stimulating hormone (FSH) increases, and several ovarian follicles begin to develop.

Follicular Phase

The FSH stimulates the ovarian follicles to develop and stimulates secretion of estrogen by the ovaries. Secretions of the luteinizing hormone (LH) work with FSH to bring about final maturation of the follicle and trigger its rupture a day or two later. This phase ends with ovulation, when a sharp increase in LH ruptures a mature ovarian follicle.

Luteal Phase

After ovulation, the empty graafian follicle is stimulated by LH to become a new structure, the corpus luteum. The corpus luteum secretes increasing quantities of estrogen and progesterone. If the ovum is not fertilized, another menstrual cycle is initiated by a decrease in secretions of progesterone and estrogen.

Pregnancy

During pregnancy, the uterus changes its shape, size, and consistency. The peritoneal covering becomes enlarged, and there is an enormous increase in muscle mass. The vaginal canal elongates as the uterus rises in the pelvis. The mucosa thickens, secretions increase, and the vascularity and elasticity of both the cervix and vagina become more pronounced.

The average pregnancy (**gestation**) lasts approximately 9 months and is followed by childbirth (**parturition**). Up to the third month of pregnancy, the product of conception is referred to as the embryo. From the third month to the time of birth, the unborn offspring is referred to as the fetus.

Pregnancy also causes enlargement of the breasts, sometimes to the point of painfulness. Many other changes occur throughout the body to accommodate the development and birth of the fetus.

Toward the end of gestation, the myometrium begins to contract weakly at irregular intervals. At this time the full-term fetus is usually positioned head down within the uterus.

Labor and Childbirth

Labor is the physiological process by which the fetus is expelled from the uterus. Labor occurs in three stages. The first is the **stage of dilation**, which begins with uterine contractions and terminates when there is complete dilation (10 cm) of the cervix. The second is the **stage of expulsion**. This is the time from complete cervical dilation to birth of the baby. The last is the **placental stage**, or afterbirth. It begins shortly after childbirth, when the uterine contractions discharge the placenta from the uterus (Fig. 13–4).

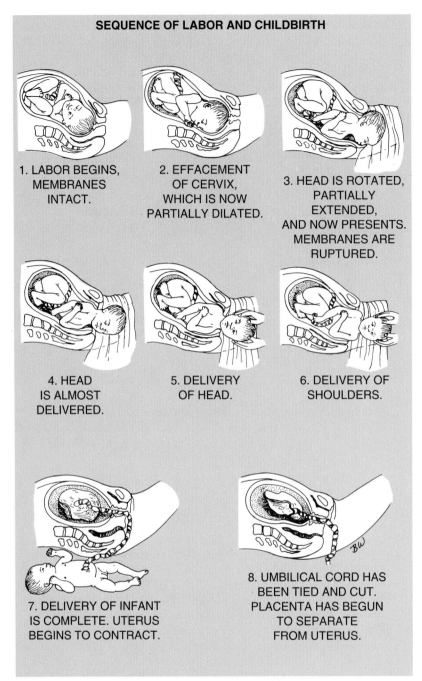

SEQUENCE OF LABOR AND CHILDBIRTH

1. LABOR BEGINS, MEMBRANES INTACT.

2. EFFACEMENT OF CERVIX, WHICH IS NOW PARTIALLY DILATED.

3. HEAD IS ROTATED, PARTIALLY EXTENDED, AND NOW PRESENTS. MEMBRANES ARE RUPTURED.

4. HEAD IS ALMOST DELIVERED.

5. DELIVERY OF HEAD.

6. DELIVERY OF SHOULDERS.

7. DELIVERY OF INFANT IS COMPLETE. UTERUS BEGINS TO CONTRACT.

8. UMBILICAL CORD HAS BEEN TIED AND CUT. PLACENTA HAS BEGUN TO SEPARATE FROM UTERUS.

Figure 13–4   Sequence of labor and childbirth. (From Taber's Cyclopedic Medical Dictionary, ed 18, F.A. Davis, Philadelphia, 1997, p 1063, with permission.)

Menopause

Menopause is the cessation of ovarian activity and diminished hormone production that occur at about 50 years of age. Menopause is usually diagnosed if absence of menses (**amenorrhea**) has persisted for 1 year. The period in which symptoms of approaching menopause occur is also known as **change of life** or **climacteric**.

Many women experience hot flashes and vaginal drying and thinning (**vaginal atrophy**) as estrogen levels fall. Although **estrogen replacement therapy (ERT)** is still controversial, it is used to treat vaginal atrophy and porous bones (**osteoporosis**), and is believed to play a role in prevention of heart attacks. Restraint in prescribing estrogens for long periods in all menopausal women arises from concern that there is an increased risk that long-term usage will induce neoplastic changes in estrogen-sensitive aging tissue.

COMBINING FORMS

Combining Form	Meaning	Example	Pronunciation
amni/o	amnion (amniotic sac)	amni/o/centesis puncture	ăm-nē-ō-sĕn-TĒ-sĭs
cervic/o	neck, cervix uteri (neck of uterus)	cervic/itis inflammation	sĕr-vĭ-SĪ-tĭs
colp/o	vagina	colp/o/rrhaphy suture	kŏl-POR-ă-fē
vagin/o		vagin/itis inflammation	văj-ĭn-Ī-tĭs
episi/o	vulva	episi/o/tomy incision	ĕ-pĭs-ē-ĕ-ŎT-ō-mē
vulv/o		vulv/ectomy excision	vŭl-VĚK-tō-mē
galact/o	milk	galact/o/rrhea flow	gă-lăk-tō-RĒ-ă
lact/o		lact/o/gen/ic production relating to	lăk-tō-JĚN-ĭk
gynec/o	woman, female	gynec/o/logy study of	gī-nĕ-KŎL-ō-jē
hyster/o	uterus, womb	hyster/ectomy excision	hĭs-tĕr-ĚK-tō-mē
metr/o		metr/o/rrhea discharge	mē-trō-RĒ-ă
uter/o		intra/uter/ine within pertaining to	ĭn-tră-Ū-tĕr-ĭn
labi/o	lip	labi/al pertaining to	LĀ-bē-ăl
lapar/o	abdomen	lapar/o/scopy visual examination	lăp-ăr-ŎS-kō-pē
mamm/o	breast	mamm/ary relating to	MĂM-ă-rē
mast/o		gynec/o/mast/ia female condition	gī-nĕ-kō-MĂS-tē-ă
men/o	menses, menstruation	men/o/rrhagia bursting forth	mĕn-ō-RĀ-jē-ă
nat/a	birth	post/nat/al after pertaining to	pōst-NĀ-tăl
oophor/o	ovary	oophor/itis inflammation	ō-ŏf-ō-RĪ-tĭs
ovari/o		ovari/o/cele herniation	ō-VĂ-rē-ō-sēl
perine/o	perineum	perine/al pertaining to	pĕr-ĭ-NĒ-ăl
salping/o	fallopian tubes, oviducts, uterine tubes	salping/o/rrhaphy suture	săl-pĭng-GOR-ă-fē

SUFFIXES

Suffix	Meaning	Example	Pronunciation
-arche	beginning	men/arche menses, menstruation	měn-ĂR-kē
-cyesis		pseud/o/cyesis false	soo-dō-sī-Ē-sĭs
-gravida	pregnancy	multi/gravida many	mŭl-tĭ-GRĂV-ĭ-dă
-para	to bear (offspring)	nulli/para none	nŭl-ĬP-ă-ră
-salpinx	fallopian tubes, oviducts, uterine tubes	hem/o/salpinx blood	hē-mō-SĂL-pĭnks
-tocia	childbirth, labor	dys/tocia difficult, painful	dĭs-TŌ-sē-ă
-version	act of turning	retr/o/version backward	rět-rō-VĔR-shŭn

PREFIXES

Prefix	Meaning	Example	Pronunciation
dys-	bad, painful, difficult	dys/men/o/rrhea menses, menstruation discharge, flow	dĭs-měn-ō-RĒ-ă
endo-	within	endo/metr/itis uterus, womb inflammation	ěn-dō-mē-TRĬ-tĭs
multi-	many	multi/gravida pregnant woman	mŭl-tĭ-GRĂV-ĭ-dă
primi-	first	primi/para to bear (offspring)	prī-MĬP-ă-ră

PATHOLOGY

Menstrual Disturbances

Menstrual disturbances are usually caused by hormonal dysfunctions or pathological conditions of the uterus and may produce a variety of symptoms.

Menstrual pain and tension (**dysmenorrhea**) may be the result of uterine contractions, a pathological growth, or general chronic disorders such as anemia, fatigue, diabetes, or tuberculosis. The female hormone estrogen is used to treat dysmenorrhea and also to regulate menstrual abnormalities.

Irregular uterine bleeding between menstrual periods (**metrorrhagia**) or after menopause is usually symptomatic of some disease, often benign or malignant uterine tumors. Consequently, early diagnosis and treatment are warranted. Metrorrhagia is probably the most significant form of menstrual dysfunction.

Profuse or prolonged bleeding during regular menstruation (**menorrhagia** or **hypermenorrhea**) may, during early life, be caused by endocrine disturbances. However, in later life, it is usually due to inflammatory diseases, tumors, or emotional disturbances, which also affect bleeding.

Premenstrual Syndrome

Premenstrual syndrome (PMS) occurs several days before the onset of menstruation and ends a short time after. A great number of symptoms involving almost every organ have been attributed to PMS. The direct cause of PMS is unknown, but the most common manifestations are irritability, emotional tension, anxiety, mood changes (especially depression), headaches, breast tenderness with or without swelling, and water retention, which may be sufficient enough to cause edema. The reason most individuals with PMS seek medical assistance is related to mood change.

Endometriosis

Endometriosis is the presence of functional endometrial tissue outside the uterus. Such **ectopic** (out-of-place) tissue or implants are usually confined to the pelvic area but may appear anywhere in the body. Like normal endometrial tissue, the ectopic endometrium responds to hormonal fluctuations of the menstrual cycle.

Pelvic Infections

Pelvic inflammatory disease (PID) is an acute, subacute, recurrent, or chronic condition of the oviducts and ovaries with adjacent tissue involvement. It includes inflammation of the cervix (**cervicitis**), uterus (**endometritis**), fallopian tubes (**salpingitis**), and ovaries (**oophoritis**). PID can extend to connective tissue lying between the broad ligaments (**parametritis**). If left untreated, PID may cause infertility and may lead to potentially fatal septicemia, pulmonary emboli, and shock.

Vaginal Infections

An inflammation of the vagina (**vaginitis**) is usually due to infection. The normal whitish vaginal discharge (**leukorrhea**), which usually occurs in slight amounts, becomes more profuse and yellowish in vaginitis. It is not uncommon for vaginitis to be accompanied by urethritis because of the proximity of the urethra to the vagina.

A curdy or cheeselike discharge and extreme itching (**pruritus**) characterize **candidiasis (moniliasis)**, a vaginal fungal infection caused by *Candida albicans*. Because the organism thrives in an environment rich in carbohydrates, it is commonly seen in patients with poorly controlled diabetes. Also, patients who have been receiving steroid therapy or antibiotics often develop a *Candida* infection. Antifungal agents (**mycostatics**) that suppress the growth of fungi are used to treat this disease.

Sexually Transmitted Diseases

Sexually transmitted diseases (STDs), also called venereal diseases (VDs), are contagious diseases acquired as a result of sexual activity with an infected individual. In the United States, the frequency of STDs is regarded as an epidemic. They include gonorrhea, syphilis, chlamydia, genital herpes, and a complex array of infections and clinical syndromes. All of these make up a new generation of STDs of which the newest and most serious is acquired immunodeficiency syndrome (AIDS) (see Chap. 10).

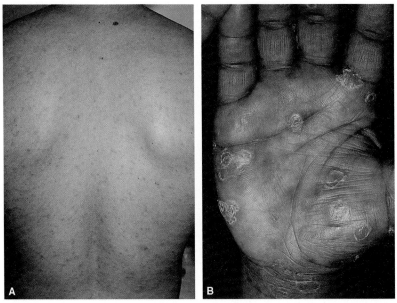

Figure 13–5   Syphilis: secondary syphilitic rash on (A) back and (B) palm. (From Reeves, JRT, and Maibach, HI. Clinical Dermatology Illustrated: A Regional Approach, ed 2. MacLennan & Petty, Rosebery, Australia, 1991 [distributed in America by F.A. Davis, Philadelphia], p 228, with permission.)

Gonorrhea is caused by infection with the bacterium *Neisseria gonorrhoeae* and involves the mucosal surface of the genitourinary tract, rectum, and possibly pharynx. This disease may be acquired through sexual intercourse and through orogenital and anogenital contacts between members of the opposite sex and between members of the same sex.

Some women do not experience pain or manifest overt clinical symptoms (**asymptomatic**) until the disease has spread to the ovaries (**oophoritis**) and uterine tubes (**salpingitis**), causing PID. The most common symptom of gonorrhea in women is a greenish-yellow cervical discharge. An untreated pregnant woman with gonorrhea may transmit the disease to the eyes of her newborn during vaginal delivery, which may result in blindness. Men with this disease suffer inflammation of the urethra (**urethritis**), which may cause painful urination (**dysuria**), along with a discharge of pus. If left untreated, the disease may infect the bladder (**cystitis**) and inflame the joints (**arthritis**). In addition, sterility may result from formation of scars that close the reproductive tubes of both sexes. Both sex partners must be treated because the infection can recur.

Syphilis, although less common than gonorrhea, is the more serious of the two diseases. It is caused by infection with the bacterium *Treponema pallidum*. Syphilis is a chronic infectious multisystemic disease acquired through sexual contact or at birth (**congenitally**). A primary sore (**chancre**) develops at the point where the bacteria entered the body. The chancre is an ulcerated sore with hard edges that contains contagious organisms for 10 days to 3 months. In pregnancy, the fetus is infected from the mother by way of the placenta. The vast majority of cases are contracted through sexual activity; the danger of transmission is greatest in the early stage of syphilis. If left untreated, the end result is blindness, insanity, and eventual death (Fig. 13–5).

Genital herpes, which causes red blisterlike sores, is the most common infectious genital ulceration in the United States. The fluid in the blisters is highly infectious. Most genital herpes infections are caused by the herpes simplex virus 2 (HSV-2) and are transmitted primarily through direct sexual contact. Individuals with herpes infection may have only one episode or may have repeated attacks. There is a much a greater incidence of cervical cancer and miscarriages in individuals with this disease. Genital herpes is also associated with the danger of seriously infecting children during childbirth. In men, lesions appear on the glans, foreskin, or penile shaft (Fig. 13–6).

Chlamydia, caused by infection with the bacterium *Chlamydia trachomatis,* is the most prevalent and among the most damaging of all STDs seen in the United States. In men, chlamydial infections cause urethritis with a whitish discharge from the penis. In women, chlamydial infec-

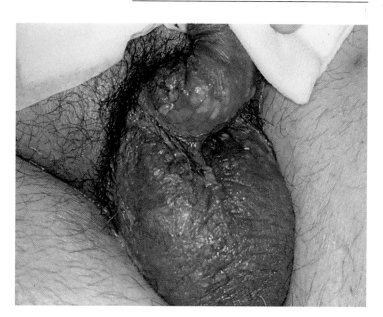

Figure 13–6 Genital herpes. (From Reeves, JRT, and Maibach, HI: Clinical Dermatology Illustrated: A Regional Approach, ed 2. MacLennan & Petty, Rosebery, Australia, 1991 [distributed in America by F.A. Davis, Philadelphia], p 78, with permission.)

tions cause an inflammation of the cervix uteri (**cervicitis**) with a mucopurulent discharge and an alarming increase in pelvic infections. These complications contribute significantly to the increase in the number of women who experience ectopic pregnancies. In pregnant women, transmission of chlamydia to the fetus can result in substantial newborn morbidity. In both sexes, chlamydia has been associated with many other health problems.

Trichomoniasis, caused by the protozoan *Trichomonas vaginalis*, is now known to be one of the most common causes of sexually transmitted lower genital tract infections. It is more commonly found in women and causes **vaginitis**, **urethritis**, and **cystitis**.

Uterine Tumors

About 30 to 40 percent of all women develop myomatous or fibroid tumors of the uterus (**leiomyomas**) that are benign. These benign tumors develop slowly between the ages of 25 and 40, and often enlarge in response to fluctuating endocrine stimulation after this period. Some persons with this type of tumor experience no symptoms. When symptoms are present, the most common is menorrhagia. Other symptoms are due to pressure on surrounding organs: pain, backache, constipation, and urinary symptoms. In addition, such tumors often cause metrorrhagia and even sterility.

Treatment of uterine fibroid tumors frequently depends on their size and location. If the patient plans to have children, treatment is as conservative as possible. As a rule, large tumors that produce pressure symptoms should be removed. Usually, the uterus is removed (**hysterectomy**), but the ovaries are preserved. If the tumor is small, a myomectomy may be performed to remove it. However, when the tumor is producing excessive bleeding, both the uterus and the tumor are excised.

Oncology

Cervical Cancer

Cancer of the cervix, a malignancy of the female reproductive system, most often affects women who are 40 to 49 years of age. Statistics indicate that infection owing to sexual activity has some relationship to the incidence of cervical cancer. First coitus at a young age, large number of sex partners, infection with certain sexually transmitted viruses, and frequent intercourse with men whose previous partners had cervical cancer are all associated with increased risk of developing cervical cancer.

A cytological examination known as a Papanicolaou test (Pap smear) can detect cervical cancer before the disease becomes clinically evident. Abnormal cervical cytology routinely calls for colposcopy, which can detect the presence and extent of preclinical lesions requiring biopsy and histological examination. Treatment of cervical cancer consists of surgery, radiation, and/or chemotherapy. If left untreated, the cancer will eventually metastasize and lead to death.

DIAGNOSTIC, SYMPTOMATIC, AND RELATED TERMS

Female Reproductive System

Term	Meaning
adnexa ăd-NĔK-să	accessory parts of a structure (adnexa uteri are the ovaries and fallopian tubes)
atresia ă-TRĒ-zē-ă	congenital absence or closure of a normal body opening (e.g., vagina)
choriocarcinoma kō-rē-ō-kăr-sĭ-NŌ-mă	malignant neoplasm of the uterus or at the site of an ectopic pregnancy. Although its actual cause is unknown, this rare tumor may occur after pregnancy or abortion
corpus luteum KOR-pŭs LŪ-tē-ŭm	ovarian scar tissue that results from rupturing of a follicle during ovulation. This small yellow body produces progesterone after ovulation
dyspareunia dĭs-pă-RŪ-nē-ă	occurrence of pain during sexual intercourse
endocervicitis ĕn-dō-sĕr-vĭ-SĪ-tĭs	inflammation of mucous lining of the cervix uteri; usually chronic, often due to infection, and accompanied by cervical erosion
fibroids, fibromyoma uteri FĪ-broyds, fĭ-brō-mī-Ō-mă	benign uterine tumors composed of muscle and fibrous tissue; leiomyomas. Myomectomy or hysterectomy may be indicated if the fibroids grow too large, causing symptoms such as metrorrhagia, pelvic pain, or menorrhagia
gynecology gī-nĕ-KŎL-ō-jē	study of the female reproductive system, including the breasts
infertility ĭn-fĕr-TĬL-ĭ-tē	inability or diminished ability to produce offspring
menarche mĕn-ĂR-kē	beginning of the menstrual function
oligomenorrhea ŏl-ĭ-gō-mĕn-ō-RĒ-ă	scanty or infrequent menstrual flow
perineum pĕr-ĭ-NĒ-ŭm	region between the vulva and anus that constitutes the pelvic floor
puberty PŪ-bĕr-tē	period during which secondary sex characteristics begin to develop and the capability of sexual reproduction is attained
pyosalpinx pī-ō-SĂL-pĭnks	pus in the fallopian tube
retroversion rĕt-rō-VĔR-shŭn	turning, or state of being turned back, especially an entire organ being tipped from its normal position (e.g., the uterus)
sterility stĕr-ĬL-ĭ-tē	inability of the female to become pregnant or for the male to impregnate female
vaginismus văj-ĭn-ĬZ-mŭs	painful spasm of the vagina from contraction of the muscles surrounding the vagina

Obstetrics

Term	Meaning
abruptio placentae ă-BRŬP-shē-ō plă-SĔN-tă	premature separation of a normally situated placenta
abortion ă-BOR-shŭn	termination of pregnancy before the embryo or fetus is capable of surviving outside the uterus
amnion ĂM-nē-ŏn	innermost membrane enclosing the developing fetus; the transparent sac that holds the fetus suspended in amniotic fluid
breech presentation	common abnormality of delivery in which the fetal buttocks or feet present rather than the head
Down syndrome, trisomy 21 dŏwn SĬN-drōm	congenital condition characterized by physical malformations and some degree of mental retardation. Trisomy of chromosome 21 usually occurs in 1 of 700 live births; preferred terms for mongolism
dystocia dĭs-TŌ-sē-ă	difficult labor; may be produced by either the large size of the fetus or the small size of the pelvic outlet
eclampsia ĕ-KLĂMP-sē-ă	most serious form of toxemia of pregnancy, manifested by high blood pressure, edema, convulsions, renal dysfunction, proteinuria, and, in severe cases, coma
ectopic pregnancy ĕk-TŎP-ĭk PRĔG-năn-sē	pregnancy in which the fertilized ovum does not reach the uterine cavity but instead becomes implanted on any tissue other than the lining of the uterine cavity (e.g., fallopian tube, ovary, abdomen, or even the cervix uteri). In a tubal pregnancy, as the fertilized ovum increases in size, the tube becomes more and more distended until, about 4 to 6 weeks after conception, it ruptures and the fertilized ovum is discharged into the abdominal cavity
gestation jĕs-TĀ-shŭn	pregnancy; the 9-month period from conception to birth
gravida GRĂV-ĭ-dă	pregnant woman; may be followed by numbers, indicating number of pregnancies (i.e., gravida 1, 2, 3, 4 or I, II, III, IV, and so on)
multigravida mŭl-tĭ-GRĂV-ĭ-dă	a woman who is experiencing her second pregnancy or who has been pregnant more than once
multipara mŭl-TĬP-ă-ră	woman who has borne more than one viable fetus, whether or not the offspring were alive at birth.
obstetrician ŏb-stĕ-TRĬSH-ăn	physician who specializes in the branch of medicine dealing with pregnancy, labor, and the puerperium
obstetrics ŏb-STĔT-rĭks	specialty concerned with pregnancy and delivery of the fetus
para PĂR-ă	woman who has borne one viable offspring; para may be followed by numbers, indicating number of deliveries (i.e., para 1, 2, 3, 4 or I, II, III, IV, and so on)
parturition păr-tū-RĬSH-ŭn	act or process of giving birth to a child
pelvimetry pĕl-VĬM-ĕ-trē	measurement of the pelvic dimensions or proportions; helps to determine whether the fetus can be delivered by the normal route
placenta previa plă-SĔN-tă PRĒ-vē-ă	condition in which the placenta is attached near the cervix and ruptures prematurely, with spotting as the early symptom. Prevention of hemorrhage may necessitate a cesarean section
primigravida prī-mĭ-GRĂV-ĭ-dă	woman during her first pregnancy
primipara prī-MĬP-ă-ră	woman who has delivered one viable offspring
puerperium pū-ĕr-PĒ-rē-ŭm	period of 42 days after childbirth and expulsion of the placenta and membranes, during which the reproductive organs usually return to normal
viable	capable of living outside of the uterus

DIAGNOSTIC PROCEDURES

Imaging Procedure	Description
endovaginal ultrasound ĕn-dō-VĂJ-ĭn-ăl	ultrasound procedure that provides a sharper look at pathological and normal structures within the pelvis. Instead of placing the sound probe across the pelvis, it is placed in the vagina
hysterosalpingography, hysterosalpingogram hĭs-tĕr-ō-săl-pĭn-GŎG-ră-fē, hĭs-tĕr-ō-săl-PĬNG-gō-grăm	radiography of the uterus and oviducts after a contrast medium is injected into those organs; used to determine pathology in the uterine cavity, evaluate tubal patency, and determine the cause of infertility
ultrasonography, ultrasonogram ŭl-tră-sŏn-ŎG-ră-fē, ŭl-tră-SŎN-ō-grăm	noninvasive technique in which ultrasonic echoes are recorded as they strike organs or tissues of different densities, producing an image of a structure; used to evaluate the female reproductive system as well as the fetus in the obstetric patient

Endoscopic Procedure	Description
colposcopy kŏl-PŎS-kō-pē	visual examination of the vagina and cervix using a colposcope. Colposcopy is used to select sites of abnormal epithelium for biopsy in patients with abnormal Pap smears
laparoscopy, peritoneoscopy lăp-ăr-ŎS-kō-pē, pĕr-ĭ-tō-nē-ŎS-kō-pē	visual examination of the abdominal cavity after a small incision of the abdominal wall to admit a laparoscope; used to examine the ovaries or fallopian tubes and to perform gynecological sterilization

Laboratory Procedure	Description
chorionic villus sampling (CVS)	a sample of chorionic villi is obtained using a catheter inserted into the cervix and into the outer portion of the membranes surrounding the fetus; used to detect chromosomal abnormalities and fetal biochemical disorders
endometrial biopsy, endometrial smear	used in screening high-risk patients for endometrial cancer; performed during the gynecological examination. After the administration of a small amount of anesthetic, a thin, hollow curette is used to remove endometrial tissue for laboratory analysis
exfoliative cytology	microscopic examination of cells sloughed from a body surface or lesion to detect malignancy and microbiological changes
Papanicolaou test, Pap smear	simple smear method of examining exfoliative cells; used most commonly to detect cervical cancer but may be used for tissue specimens from any organ; usually obtained during a routine pelvic examination

SURGICAL AND THERAPEUTIC PROCEDURES

Term	Description
amniocentesis ăm-nē-ō-sĕn-TĒ-sĭs	transabdominal puncture of the amniotic sac to remove amniotic fluid. The material obtained is cultured for biochemical and cytological studies
barrier contraceptive condom, diaphragm, and cervical cap	products that provide a physical barrier to prevent sperm from reaching the uterus and fallopian tubes
cerclage sār-KLŌZH	applying a nonabsorbable ligature around the cervix uteri to treat for an incompetent uterus, thus decreasing the chance of a spontaneous abortion
cesarean birth, C-section sē-SĀR-ē-ăn	incision of the abdomen and uterus to remove the fetus; most commonly used in the event of cephalopelvic disproportion, presence of sexually transmitted disease organisms in the birth canal, fetal distress, and breech presentation
colpectomy, vaginectomy kŏl-PĔK-tō-mē, văj-ĭn-ĔK-tō-mē	surgical excision of the vagina
colpocleisis kŏl-pō-KLĪ-sĭs	surgical closure of the vaginal canal
colpoperineoplasty, colpoperineorrhaphy kŏl-pō-pĕr-ĭn-Ē-ō-plăs-tē, kŏl-pō-pĕr-ĭn-ē-OR-ră-fē	plastic surgery of the vagina and perineum
conization kŏn-ĭ-ZĀ-shŭn	excision of a cone of tissue (e.g., mucosa of the cervix) for histological examination; uses cold knife blade or laser so as to preserve histological characteristics
contraception	any process, device, or method that prevents conception. See Pharmacology, p. 258.
cordocentesis kŏr-dō-sĕn-TĒ-sĭs	the sampling of fetal blood drawn from the umbilical vein. This may assist in managing hemolytic diseases or genetic abnormalities
cryosurgery, cryocautery krī-ō-SĔR-jĕr-ē, krī-ō-KAW-tĕr-ē	process of freezing tissue to destroy cells; used for chronic cervical infections and erosions because offending organisms may be entrenched in cervical cells and glands. Process destroys these infected areas, and in the healing process, normal cells are replenished. May also be used when a patient shows atypical or possible malignancy, as seen on a Pap smear
dilatation and curettage (D&C) dĭl-ă-TĀ-shŭn, kū-rĕ-TĀZH	widening of the cervical canal with a dilator and the scraping of the uterine endometrium with a curette; used for cytological examination of tissue, to control abnormal uterine bleeding, and as a therapeutic measure for incomplete abortion. Because this procedure usually is performed under anesthesia and requires surgical asepsis, it is done in the operating room
episiotomy ĕ-pĭs-ē-ŎT-ō-mē	incision of perineum from the vaginal orifice; usually done to facilitate childbirth
episiorrhaphy ĕ-pĭs-ē-OR-ă-fē	suturing of a lacerated perineum
hormonal contraception	use of hormones to suppress ovulation and to prevent conception
oral contraceptive pills (OCP)	birth control pills containing estrogen and progesterone in varying proportions. When taken according to schedule, they are about 98 percent effective
contraceptive implant	hormone injection and implant under the skin, such as Norplant. The implant procedure takes approximately 15 minutes and is performed in a physician's office under a local anesthetic. When the implant is removed, fertility is restored

SURGICAL AND THERAPEUTIC PROCEDURES (Continued)

Term	Description
hymenotomy hī-měn-ŎT-ō-mē	incision of the hymen
hysterectomy hǐs-těr-ĔK-tō-mē	excision of the uterus. Abdominal: excision of the uterus through an abdominal incision. Vaginal: excision of the uterus through the vagina. Total abdominal hysterectomy (TAH): excision of the uterus, including the cervix, through an abdominal incision
insufflation ǐn-sǔ-FLĀ-shǔn	the act of blowing a powder, vapor, gas, or air into a body cavity
tubal TŪ-băl	see Rubin's test
intrauterine devices (IUDs)	plastic or metal objects placed inside the uterus; prevents implantation of fertilized egg in the uterine lining
myomectomy mī-ō-MĔK-tō-mē	excision of a myomatous tumor, generally uterine
Rubin's test ROO-bǐns těst	a test for patency of the uterine tubes made by transuterine insufflation with carbon dioxide
salpingo-oophorectomy săl-pǐng-gō-ō-ŏf-ō-RĔK-tō-mē	excision of an ovary and fallopian tube, usually identified as right (R), left (L), or bilateral
tubal ligation TŪ-băl lǐ-GĀ-shǔn	ligating (tying) the uterine tubes to prevent pregnancy; sterilization surgery

PHARMACOLOGY

Medication	Action
contraceptives	used to prevent pregnancy by suppressing ovulation
steroids	oral contraceptive pills (OCPs): birth control pills containing estrogen and progesterone in varying proportions. When taken according to schedule, they are 98 percent effective
chemical	spermicidals, foam, cream, jelly, spermicide-impregnated sponge, or suppositories that are placed in the vagina before intercourse. Used alone or in combination with a barrier contraceptive. They act by killing the sperm
estrogen hormones	used in oral contraceptives and as a replacement hormone in the treatment of menopause and prevents postmenopausal osteoporosis. Its long-term, continued use increases the risk of endometrial carcinoma
oxytocins	stimulate the uterus to contract, thus inducing labor; also used to rid the uterus of an unexpelled placenta or a fetus that has died

ABBREVIATIONS

Maternal-Gynecological and Related Abbreviations

Abbreviation	Meaning
AB, ab	abortion
AI	artificial insemination
CPD	cephalopelvic disproportion
D&C	dilatation and curettage
DC	discharge
DUB	dysfunctional uterine bleeding
Dx	diagnosis
EDC	estimated date of confinement
ERT	estrogen replacement therapy
FH	family history
FSH	follicle-stimulating hormone
GC	gonorrhea
GYN	gynecology
HSV	herpes simplex virus
IUD	intrauterine device
IVF	in vitro fertilization
LH	luteinizing hormone
LMP	last menstrual period
Ⓛ, lt	left
MH	marital history
OCPs	oral contraceptive pills
Pap	Papanicolaou's smear (test for cervical or vaginal cancer)
PID	pelvic inflammatory disease
PMP	previous menstrual period
PMS	premenstrual syndrome
R/O	rule out
Ⓡ, rt	right
STDs	sexually transmitted diseases
TSS	toxic shock syndrome
VD	venereal disease

Fetal-Obstetric Abbreviations

Abbreviation	Meaning
CS, C-section	cesarean section
CVS	chorionic villus sampling
CWP	childbirth without pain
DOB	date of birth
FEKG	fetal electrocardiogram
FHR	fetal heart rate
FHT	fetal heart tone
FTND	full-term normal delivery
HSG	hysterosalpingography
HCG	human chorionic gonadotropin
IUGR	intrauterine growth rate, intrauterine growth retardation
NB	newborn
OB	obstetrics
TAH	total abdominal hysterectomy
UC	uterine contractions
XX	female sex chromosomes
XY	male sex chromosomes

MEDICAL RECORD

Primary Herpes 1 Infection

A family practice resident, aged 24 years, started having some sore areas around the labia, both rt and lt side. She stated that the last few days she started having a brownish DC. She has pruritus and pain of her vulvar area with adenopathy and fever at pm, and blisters. Apparently her partner had a cold sore and they had oral genital sex.

Has been using condoms since last seen in April. LMP 5/15/xx. She has not missed any OCPs. Patient has what looks like herpes lesions and ulcers all over vulva and introitus area. Rt labia appears as an ulcerlike lesion; it appears to be almost like an infected follicle. Speculum inserted, a brown DC noted. GC screen, chlamydia screen, and general culture obtained from that. Wet prep revealed monilial forms. Viral culture obtained from the ulcerlike lesion on the right.

Dx   Primary herpes 1 infection; will R/O other infectious etiologies.

Worksheet 5 provides a dictionary exercise and an analysis of this medical record.

WORKSHEET 1

∎ ∎ ∎ ∎ ∎ ∎ ∎ ∎ ∎ ∎ ∎ ∎ ∎ ∎

Use **gynec/o** *(woman, female) to build a medical word meaning:*

1. disease (specific to) women _____

2. study (of diseases) of the female _____

3. physician who specializes in diseases of the female _____

Use **cervic/o** *(neck, cervix uteri) to build a medical word meaning:*

4. inflammation of the cervix uteri and vagina _____

5. pertaining to the cervix uteri and bladder _____

Use **colp/o** *(vagina) to build a medical word meaning:*

6. instrument used to examine the vagina _____

7. visual examination of the vagina _____

Use **vagin/o** *(vagina) to build a medical word meaning:*

8. inflammation of the vagina _____

9. relating to the vagina _____

10. abnormal condition of a vaginal fungus _____

11. related to the vagina and the labia _____

Use **hyster/o** *(uterus) to build a medical word meaning:*

12. myoma of the uterus _____

13. disease of the uterus _____

14. radiography of the uterus and oviducts _____

Use **metr/o** *(uterus) to build a medical word meaning:*

15. hemorrhage from the uterus _____

16. inflammation around the uterus _____

Use **uter/o** *(uterus) to build a medical word meaning:*

17. herniation of the uterus _____

18. relating to the uterus and cervix _____

19. pertaining to the uterus and rectum _____

20. pertaining to the uterus and bladder _____

Use oophor/o (ovary) to build a medical word meaning:

21. inflammation of an ovary ——————————————————————

22. pain in an ovary ——————————————————————————

23. inflammation of an ovary and oviduct ——————————————

Use salping/o (fallopian tube) to build a medical word meaning:

24. herniation of a fallopian tube ————————————————————

25. radiography of the uterine tubes —————————————————

WORKSHEET 2

∎ ∎ ∎ ∎ ∎ ∎ ∎ ∎ ∎ ∎ ∎ ∎ ∎ ∎ ∎ ∎

Build a surgical term meaning:

1. fixation of (a displaced) ovary _____

2. suture of a displaced ovary (to the pelvic wall) _____

3. surgical repair of the vagina _____

4. excision of the uterus and ovaries _____

5. surgical repair of the vagina and perineum _____

6. suturing the perineum _____

7. excision of the uterus, oviducts, and ovaries _____

8. puncture of the amnion (amniotic sac) _____

WORKSHEET 3

∎ ∎ ∎ ∎ ∎ ∎ ∎ ∎ ∎ ∎ ∎ ∎

Match the following medical terms with the definitions in the numbered list.

atresia	dyspareunia	primipara
corpus luteum	dystocia	pruritus vulvae
cerclage	gestation	pyosalpinx
Down syndrome	laparomyitis	retroversion

1. _____ accumulation of pus in a uterine tube

2. _____ woman who has had one pregnancy that has resulted in a viable offspring

3. _____ pregnancy; 40 weeks in human beings

4. _____ procedure used to decrease the chance of a spontaneous abortion

5. _____ an entire organ being tipped from its normal position (e.g., uterus)

6. _____ yellow glandular mass in the ovary formed by an ovarian follicle that has matured and discharged its ovum

7. _____ difficult labor or childbirth

8. _____ congenital absence or closure of a normal body opening

9. _____ trisomy 21

10. _____ intense itching of the external female genitalia

WORSHEET 4

■ ■ ■ ■ ■ ■ ■ ■ ■ ■ ■ ■ ■ ■ ■

Select the word that best describes statements that follow.

amniocentesis	D&C	spermicidals
chorionic villus sampling	estrogens	tubal ligation
colpocleisis	hysterosalpingography	total abdominal hysterectomy (TAH)
contraceptives	laparoscopy	ultrasonography
CPD	oxytocin	
cryosurgery	Pap smear	

1. _____ cervical scrapings to detect cancerous cells in the mucus of the uterus and cervix

2. _____ radiography of the uterus and oviducts after a contrast medium is injected into those organs

3. _____ transabdominal puncture of the amniotic sac to remove amniotic fluid for biochemical and cytological studies

4. _____ destroying cells by the process of freezing tissue

5. _____ surgical closure of the vaginal canal

6. _____ widening of the cervical canal with a dilator and scraping the uterine endometrium with a curette

7. _____ excision of the entire uterus, including the cervix, through an abdominal incision

8. _____ tying the uterine tubes to prevent pregnancy; sterilization surgery

9. _____ cephalopelvic disproportion

10. _____ small incision in the abdominal wall that permits examination of the abdominal cavity to determine abnormalities

11. _____ agents that destroy sperm, used within the vagina for contraceptive purposes

12. _____ noninvasive ultrasound technique used to evaluate the female genital tract and fetus in the obstetric patient

13. _____ test to detect chromosomal abnormalities that can be done earlier than amniocentesis

14. _____ replacement hormones used during menopause to ease discomforts as the production of natural hormones decreases

15. _____ agent used to induce labor and to rid uterus of unexpelled placenta or fetus that has died

WORKSHEET 5

■ ■ ■ ■ ■ ■ ■ ■ ■ ■ ■ ■ ■

MEDICAL RECORD: PRIMARY HERPES 1 INFECTION

Underline the following terms in the medical record (see p. 260). Use a medical dictionary and other resources to define the terms and to determine their pronunciation; then practice reading the medical record aloud.

chlamydia _____

DC _____

Dx _____

GC _____

genital _____

herpes _____

introitus _____

labia _____

LMP _____

monilial _____

OCPs _____

primary herpes 1 _____

pruritus _____

speculum _____

vulvar _____

MEDICAL RECORD EVALUATION: PRIMARY HERPES I INFECTION

1. *Did the patient have any discharge? If so, describe it.*

2. *What type of discomfort was she experiencing around the vulvar area?*

3. *Has she been taking her oral contraceptive pills regularly?*

4. *Where was the viral culture obtained from?*

5. *Even though her partner used a condom, how do you think she became infected with herpes?*

WORKSHEET 6

Label the following diagram. Check your answers by referring to Figure 13–2.

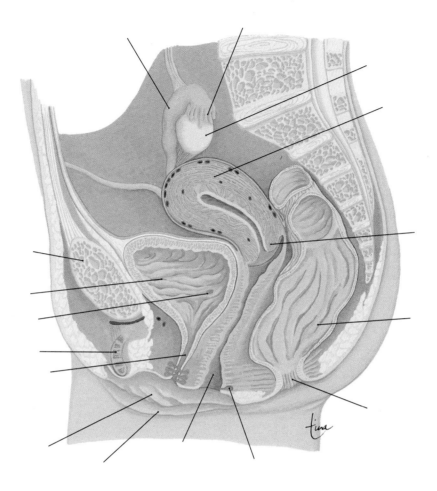

Anus	Labia majora	Symphysis pubis
Bartholin's gland	Labia minora	Urethra
Cervix	Opening of ureter	Urinary bladder
Clitoris	Ovary	Uterus
Fallopian tube	Rectum	Vagina
Fimbriae		

WORKSHEET 7

■ ■ ■ ■ ■ ■ ■ ■ ■ ■ ■ ■ ■

Label the following diagram. Check your answers by referring to Figure 13–3.

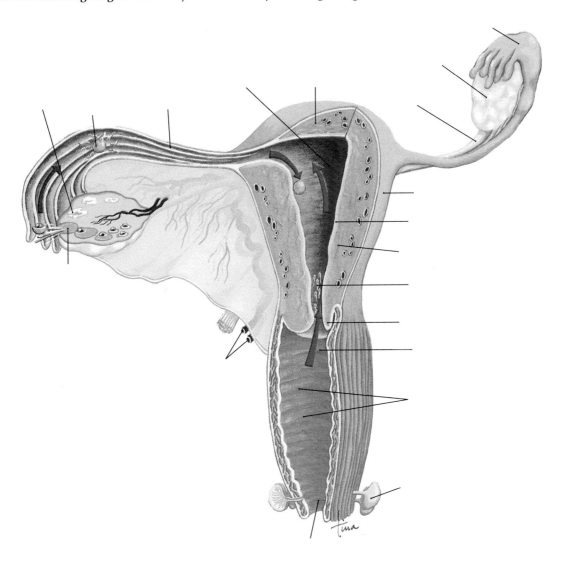

Artery and vein	Fertilization of ovum	Ovary
Bartholin's gland	Fimbriae	Rugae
Body of uterus	Fundus of uterus	Sperm
Cervix	Mature follicle	Uterus
Corpus luteum	Myometrium	Vagina
Endometrium	Ovarian ligament	Vulva
Fallopian tube		

ENDOCRINE SYSTEM

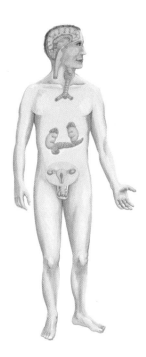

Chapter Outline

Student Objectives

Anatomy and Physiology
Pituitary Gland
Thyroid Gland
Parathyroid Glands
Adrenal Glands
  Adrenal Cortex
  Adrenal Medulla
Pancreas (Islets of Langerhans)
Pineal Gland

Combining Forms

Suffixes

Pathology
Pituitary Disorders
Thyroid Disorders
Parathyroid Disorders
Disorders of the Adrenal Glands
  Adrenal Medulla

  Adrenal Cortex
Pancreatic Disorders
Oncology
  Pancreatic Cancer
  Pituitary Tumors
  Thyroid Cancer

Diagnostic, Symptomatic, and Therapeutic Terms

Diagnostic Procedures
Imaging Procedures
Laboratory Procedures

Surgical and Therapeutic Procedures

Pharmacology

Abbreviations

Medical Record
Hyperparathyroidism and Diabetes Mellitus

Worksheets

Student Objectives

Upon completion of this chapter, you will be able to do the following:

1. List the glands of the endocrine system.

2. Describe the function of each endocrine gland.

3. Differentiate between endocrine and exocrine glands.

4. Identify the principal hormones secreted by the endocrine glands, and briefly explain their function.

5. Identify the combining forms and suffixes related to the endocrine system.

6. Identify and discuss pathology related to the endocrine system.

7. Identify diagnostic, symptomatic, and therapeutic terms related to the endocrine system.

8. Identify diagnostic procedures related to the endocrine system.

9. Identify surgical and therapeutic procedures related to the endocrine system.

Student Objectives (Continued)

10. Define the abbreviations related to the endocrine system.
11. Discuss pharmacology related to the treatment of endocrine disorders.
12. Demonstrate your knowledge of the chapter by completing the worksheets.

ANATOMY AND PHYSIOLOGY

The endocrine and the nervous systems work together like an interlocking supersystem to control many intricate activities of the body. Their functions are closely related because they strive to maintain **homeostasis** (the state of equilibrium in the internal environment of the body).

The ductless glands of the endocrine system produce specific effects on body functions by slowly discharging hormones into the bloodstream (Table 14–1). The general effects of most hormones are well known. However, the manner in which specific hormones affect different organs or tissues of the body is just starting to become clear. The tissues or organs that respond to the effects of a hormone are called **target tissues** or **target organs** (Figure 14–1). Hormones released by an endocrine gland to a target organ is determined by the body's need for the hormone at any given time and is regulated so that there is no overproduction (hypersecretion) or underproduction (hyposecretion) of a particular hormone. Unfortunately, there are times when the regulating mechanism does not operate properly and hormonal levels are excessive or deficient. When this happens, disorders result from or are associated with endocrine dysfunction. In contrast, the nervous system is designed to act instantaneously through the transmission of electrical impulses to specific body locations. The nervous system is covered in Chapter 15.

Included in the endocrine system are a number of ductless glands located in various parts of the body (Fig. 14–2), which release their secretions directly into blood vessels. These glands are not to be confused with exocrine glands such as the sweat and oil glands of the skin, which release their secretions externally through ducts.

This chapter discusses the function of the **pituitary**, **thyroid**, **parathyroid**, **adrenal**, **pancreatic**, and **pineal glands**. The functions of the other endocrine glands are discussed in the following chapters: Chapter 10, Blood, Lymph, and Immune Systems (thymus); Chapter 12, Genitourinary (testes); and Chapter 13, Female Reproductive System (ovaries).

Pituitary Gland

Refer to Figure 14–2 as you read the following material. The (1) **pituitary gland**, or **hypophysis**, is no larger than a pea and is located at the base of the brain. It is known as the "master gland" because it regulates many body activities and stimulates other glands to secrete their own specific hormones.

The gland consists of two distinct portions: an anterior lobe (adenohypophysis) that secretes adenohypophyseal hormones and a posterior lobe (neurohypophysis) that secretes neurohypophyseal hormones. The hormones of the anterior and posterior lobes are summarized in Table 14–2.

Table 14–1   DEFINITION AND CHARACTERISTICS OF HORMONES

Hormones are chemical substances produced by specialized cells of the body.
Hormones are released slowly in minute amounts directly into the bloodstream.
Hormones are produced primarily by the endocrine glands.
Most hormones are inactivated or excreted by the liver and kidneys.

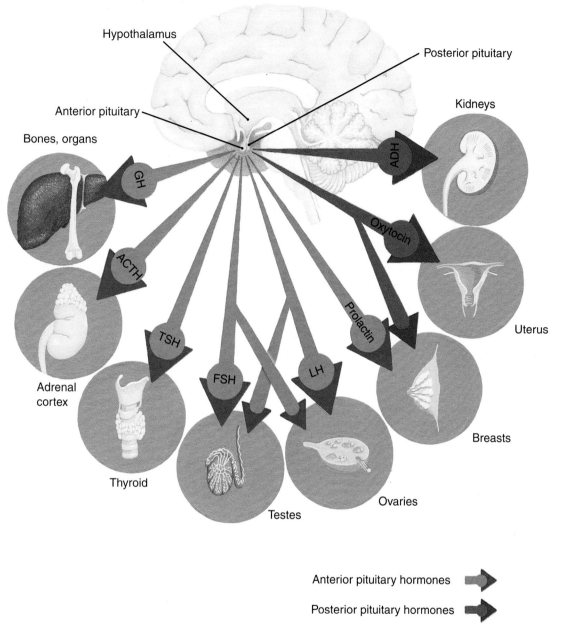

Figure 14–1 Hormones of the pituitary gland and their target organs. (From Scanlon, VC, and Sanders, T: Understanding Human Structure and Function. F.A. Davis, Philadelphia, 1997, p 183, with permission.)

Thyroid Gland

The (2) **thyroid gland** is the largest gland of the endocrine system. An H-shaped organ located in the neck just below the larynx, this gland is composed of two large lobes that are separated by a strip of tissue called an **isthmus**.

The function of the thyroid gland is to produce, store, and release **thyroxine (T_4)** and **triiodothyronine (T_3)**, the major thyroid hormones. Both T_3 and T_4 regulate metabolism and are responsible for energy level. They increase the rate of oxygen consumption and thus the rate at which carbohydrates, proteins, and fats are metabolized. In addition, both hormones work with the growth hormone (GH) and stimulate activity in the nervous system. Refer to Table 14–3 for a summary of hormones of the thyroid gland.

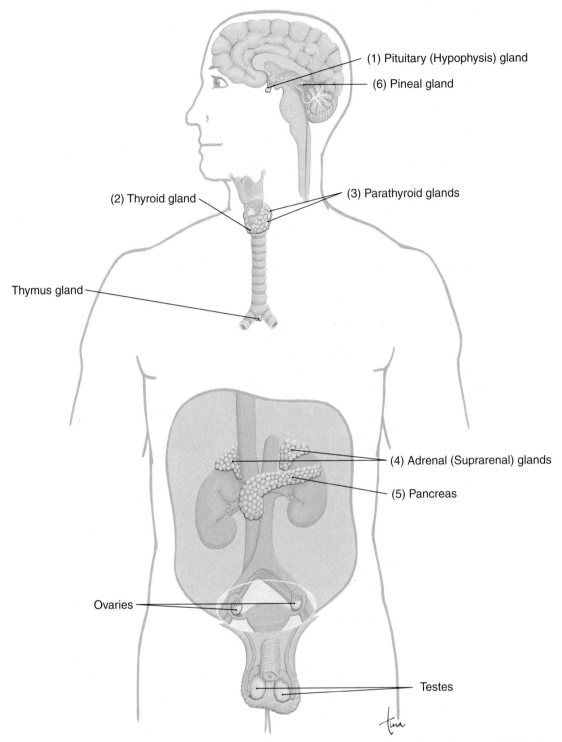

Figure 14–2   The glands of the endocrine system (ductless, internally secreting) are located in various parts of the body. (From Scanlon, VC, and Sanders, T: Understanding Human Structure and Function. F.A. Davis, Philadelphia, 1997, p 178, with permission.)

Table 14–2 ANTERIOR AND POSTERIOR PITUITARY GLAND HORMONES, FUNCTIONS, AND DISORDERS

Hormone	Function(s)	Disorders
Adenohypophyseal (Anterior Lobe) Hormones		
Growth hormone (GH)	Stimulates bone and body growth	Hyposecretion of GH during the growth years results in pituitary dwarfism.
		Possible cause: A congenital deficiency or destruction of GH-producing cells.
		Effects: Small but well-proportioned body; sexual immaturity.
		Hypersecretion of GH during the growth years results in giantism.
		Possible cause: Pituitary tumor before puberty.
		Effects: Abnormal overgrowth of body.
		Hypersecretion of GH during adulthood results in acromegaly.
		Possible cause: Primary tumor after puberty.
		Effects: Disproportionate increase in size of bones of face, hands, and feet.
Thyroid-stimulating hormone (TSH), or thyrotropin	Controls secretion of hormones by thyroid gland	
Prolactin	In conjunction with other hormones, initiates and maintains milk secretion by the mammary glands	
Adrenocorticotropic hormone (ACTH)	Controls secretions of some hormones by adrenal cortex, especially cortisol	
Follicle-stimulating hormone (FSH)	In Women:	
	Initiates development of ova in ovarian follicles	
	Induces secretion of estrogen by follicle cells	
	In Men:	
	Initiates sperm production in the testes	
Luteinizing hormone (LH), or interstitial cell-stimulating hormone (ICSH) in men	In Women:	
	Together with estrogens, stimulates ovulation	
	Together with estrogens, stimulates formation of progesterone-producing corpus luteum	
	Together with estrogens, prepares uterus for implantation, and readies mammary glands to secrete milk	
	In Men:	
	Stimulates interstitial cells in testes to develop and produce semen	

Table 14–2 ANTERIOR AND POSTERIOR PITUITARY GLAND HORMONES, FUNCTIONS, AND DISORDERS (Continued)

Hormone	Function(s)	Disorders
Neurohypophyseal (Posterior Lobe) Hormones		
Antidiuretic hormone (ADH)	Decreases volume of urine excreted Increases water reabsorption by the kidney (water returns to the blood)	Hyposecretion of ADH results in diabetes insipidus. Possible cause: Damage to the hypothalamus. Effects: Failure of kidneys to reabsorb needed salts and water. Hypersecretion of ADH results in high levels of ADH in blood. Possible cause: Pituitary tumor, head injury. Effects: Excessive sodium, water retention in the body.
Oxytocin	Stimulates contraction of pregnant uterus, labor, and childbirth Stimulates milk secretion from the mammary glands	

Parathyroid Glands

The (3) **parathyroid glands** consist of at least four separate glands located on the posterior surface of the lobes of the thyroid gland. The only hormone known to be secreted by the parathyroid glands is parathyroid hormone (PTH). PTH helps to regulate homeostasis of calcium by stimulating three target organs: bones, intestines, and kidneys. Refer to Table 14–4 for a summary of the hormone of the parathyroid gland.

Because of PTH stimulation, calcium, and phosphates are released from bones, increasing concentration of these substances in blood. Thus, calcium that is necessary for the proper functioning of body tissues is available in the bloodstream. At the same time, PTH enhances the absorption of calcium and phosphates from foods in the intestine, and this action also produces a rise in the blood levels of calcium and phosphates. PTH causes the kidneys to conserve blood calcium and to increase the excretion of phosphates in the urine.

Adrenal Glands

The (4) **adrenal glands** are paired organs covering the superior surface of the kidneys. Because of their location, the adrenal glands are also known as **suprarenal glands**. Each adrenal gland is

Table 14–3 HORMONES OF THE THYROID GLAND

Hormone	Function(s)	Disorders
Thyroxine (T_4) and triiodothyronine (T_3)	Regulates metabolism Increases energy production from all food types Increases rate of protein synthesis	Hyposecretion of thyroid hormones during the growth years results in cretinism. Hypothyroidism during adulthood produces myxedema. Hypersecretion of thyroid hormones produces exophthalmic goiter.
Calcitonin	Lowers blood calcium levels by accelerating calcium absorption by bones	

Table 14–4 HORMONE OF THE PARATHYROID GLANDS

Hormone	Function(s)	Disorders
Parathyroid hormone (PTH)	Increases blood calcium level and decreases blood phosphate level by increasing rate of calcium absorption from gastrointestinal tract into blood Increases calcium absorption and phosphate excretion by kidneys Increases number and activity of osteoclasts	Hypoparathyroidism results in tetany. Hyperparathyroidism produces osteitis fibrosa cystica.

structurally and functionally differentiated into two sections: the outer **adrenal cortex**, which makes up the bulk of the gland, and the inner **adrenal medulla**. Although these regions are not sharply divided, they represent distinct glands that secrete different hormones. Steroids are secreted by the adrenal cortex. Cells of the adrenal medulla secrete two closely related hormones, epinephrine (adrenaline), and norepinephrine (noradrenaline).

Adrenal Cortex

The adrenal cortex secretes three types of steroid hormones: mineralocorticoids, glucocorticoids, and gonadocorticoids (sex hormones). The sex hormones are produced in very small amounts, and their importance is not known with certainty. The functions of the other two cortical hormones, **mineralocorticoids** and **glucocorticoids**, are considered vital and are summarized here.

Mineralocorticoids help to regulate water and mineral salts (also called electrolytes) that are retained in the body. One of the major mineralocorticoids is **aldosterone**. Like all hormones of the adrenal cortex, aldosterone is a steroid. This hormone acts mainly through the kidneys to maintain homeostasis of sodium and potassium. More specifically, aldosterone causes the kidneys to conserve sodium and to excrete potassium. At the same time, it promotes water conservation and reduces urine output.

Glucocorticoids influence the metabolism of carbohydrates, fats, and proteins. The glucocorticoid with the greatest activity is **cortisol**. It helps to regulate the concentration of glucose in the blood, protecting against low blood sugar levels between meals. Cortisol also stimulates the breakdown of fats in adipose tissue and releases fatty acids into the blood. The increase in fatty acids causes many cells to use relatively less glucose. Refer to Table 14–5 for a summary of adrenal cortical hormones.

Adrenal Medulla

Epinephrine (adrenaline) and norepinephrine (noradrenaline) are two closely related hormones secreted by the adrenal medulla. The effects of the medullary hormones resemble those of the sympathetic nervous system. The adrenal medulla, like the rest of the sympathetic nervous system, is not essential to life, but it is important because it stimulates the responses necessary to meet emergencies. Refer to Table 14–5 for a summary of adrenal medullary hormones.

Pancreas (Islets of Langerhans)

Continue to refer to Figure 14–2 as you read the following material.

The (5) **pancreas** lies inferior to the stomach in a bend of the duodenum. It functions both as an exocrine and endocrine gland. A large pancreatic duct runs through the gland, carrying enzymes and other exocrine digestive secretions from the pancreas to the small intestine (see Chap. 7). The pancreas has groups of cells called islets of Langerhans, which produce endocrine secretions. There are two kinds of cells in the islets: A cells (alpha cells), which produce glucagon and constitute about 25 percent of the islet cells; and B cells (beta cells), which produce insulin

Table 14-5   HORMONES OF THE ADRENAL GLANDS, FUNCTIONS, AND DISORDERS

Hormone	Function(s)	Disorders
Adrenal Cortical Hormones		
Mineralocorticoids (mainly aldosterone)	Increases reabsorption of sodium by the kidneys to the blood	Hypersecretion of aldosterone results in aldosteronism.
	Increases excretion of potassium by the kidneys in urine. Decreases blood levels of potassium	
Glucocorticoids (mainly cortisol)	Regulates the metabolism of carbohydrates, proteins, and fats	Hyposecretion of glucocorticoids produces Addison's disease.
		Hypersecretion of glucocorticoids results in Cushing's syndrome.
Adrenal Medullary Hormones		
Epinephrine (adrenaline)	Increases cardiac activity	Hypersecretion of medullary hormones results in a prolonged "fight-or-flight" reaction.
	Dilates bronchial tubes	
	Increases conversion of glycogen to glucose in the liver	
	Increases use of fats for energy	
	Increases the rate of cell respiration	
	Causes vasoconstriction in skeletal muscle	
	Decreases peristalsis	
Norepinephrine (noradrenaline)	Raises blood pressure and constricts vessels	

and constitute about 75 percent of the islet cells. Both of these hormones, glucagon and insulin, play important roles in the proper metabolism of sugars and starches in the body. Refer to Table 14–6 for a summary of pancreatic hormones.

Pineal Gland

The (6) **pineal gland**, which is shaped like a pinecone, is attached to the posterior part of the third ventricle of the brain. Although the exact functions of this gland have not been established, there is evidence that it secretes melatonin hormone. It is believed that melatonin may inhibit the activities of the ovaries. When melatonin production is high, ovulation is blocked, and there may be a delay in puberty development. The pineal gland starts to degenerate at about 7 years of age; in the adult, it consists mostly of fibrous tissue.

Table 14-6   HORMONES OF THE PANCREAS

Hormone	Function(s)	Disorders
Insulin	Lowers blood sugar by accelerating glucose transport into cells	Hyposecretion of insulin produces diabetes mellitus.
		Hypersecretion of insulin results in hyperinsulinism.
Glucagon	Raises blood sugar level by accelerating conversion of glycogen into glucose in liver (glycogenolysis) and conversion of other nutrients into glucose in the liver (gluconeogenesis) and releasing glucose into blood	

COMBINING FORMS

Combining Form	Meaning	Example	Pronunciation
acr/o	extremity	acr/o/megaly enlargement	ăk-rō-MĔG-ă-lē
adren/o adrenal/o	adrenal glands	adren/al relating to adrenal/ism condition	ăd-RĒ-năl ă-DRĔN-ăl-ĭzm
andr/o	male	andr/o/gen forming, producing, origin	ĂN-drō-jĕn
calc/o	calcium	hypo/calc/emia under, blood below	hī-pō-kăl-SĒ-mē-ă
gluc/o	sugar, sweetness	gluc/o/genesis producing	gloo-kō-JĔN-ĕ-sĭs
glyc/o		hyper/glyc/emia excessive blood	hī-pĕr-glī-SĒ-mē-ă
gonad/o	gonads, sex glands	hypo/gonad/ism below condition	hī-pō-GŌ-năd-ĭzm
home/o	same, alike	home/o/stasis standing still	hō-mē-ō-STĀ-sĭs
pancreat/o	pancreas	pancreat/itis inflammation	păn-krē-ă-TĪ-tĭs
parathyroid/o	parathyroid glands	parathyroid/ectomy excision	păr-ă-thī-royd-ĔK-tō-mē
somat/o	body	somat/ic pertaining to	sō-MĂT-ĭc
thym/o	thymus	thym/o/lysis destruction	thī-MŎL-ĭ-sĭs
thyr/o thyroid/o	thyroid	thyr/o/toxic/ osis poison abnormal condition thyroid/ectomy excision	thī-rō-tŏks-ĭ-KŌ-sĭs thī-royd-ĔK-tō-mē

SUFFIXES

Suffix	Meaning	Example	Pronunciation
-crine	secrete	endo/crine within	ĔN-dō-krīn (or) krĭn
-dipsia	thirst	poly/dipsia many, much	pŏl-ē-DĬP-sē-ă
-phagia	eating, swallowing	poly/phagia many, much	pŏl-ē-FĀ-jē-ă

SUFFIXES (Continued)

Suffix	Meaning	Example	Pronunciation
-physis	growth	adeno/hypo/physis gland under	ăd-ĕ-nō-hī-PŎF-ĭ-sĭs
-toxic	poison	thyr/o/toxic thyroid	thī-rō-TŎKS-ĭk
-tropin	stimulate	somat/o/tropin body	sō-măt-ō-TRŌ-pĭn
-trophy	nourishment, development	a/trophy without	ĂT-rō-fē
-uria	urine	poly/uria much	pŏl-ē-Ū-rē-ă

PATHOLOGY

Disorders of the endocrine system are caused by underproduction (**hyposecretion**) or overproduction (**hypersecretion**) of hormones. In general, hyposecretion is treated by the use of hormones in drug therapy replacement. Hypersecretion is generally treated by surgery. Most hormone deficiencies result from genetic defects in the glands, surgical removal of the glands, or production of poor-quality hormones.

Pituitary Disorders

Hypersecretion or hyposecretion of GH leads to body-size abnormalities. Abnormal variations of antidiuretic hormone (ADH) secretions lead to disorders in the composition of the blood and marked electrolyte imbalance. Some pituitary disorders are summarized in Table 14–2.

Thyroid Disorders

Thyroid gland disorders are common and may develop at any time during life. They may be the result of a developmental problem, injury, disease, or dietary deficiency. One form of hypothyroidism that develops in infants is called **cretinism**. If not treated, this disorder leads to mental retardation, impaired growth, low body temperatures, and abnormal bone formation. Usually these symptoms do not appear at birth because the infant has received thyroid hormones from the mother's blood during fetal development.

When hypothyroidism develops during adulthood, it is known as **myxedema**. The characteristics of this disease are edema, low blood levels of T_3 and T_4, mental retardation, weight gain, and sluggishness.

Hyperthyroidism results from excessive secretions of T_3, T_4, or both. Two of the most common disorders of hyperthyroidism are **Graves' disease** and **toxic goiter**. Graves' disease is considerably more prevalent and is characterized by an elevated metabolic rate, abnormal weight loss, excessive perspiration, muscular weakness, and emotional instability. Also, the eyes are likely to protrude (**exophthalmos**) because of edematous swelling in the tissues behind them. At the same time, the thyroid gland is likely to enlarge, producing goiter.

It is believed that toxic goiter may occur because of excessive release of thyroid-stimulating hormone (TSH) from the anterior lobe of the pituitary gland. Overstimulation by TSH causes thyroid cells to enlarge and secrete extra amounts of hormones. Treatment for this condition may involve drug therapy to block the production of thyroid hormones or surgical removal of all or part of the thyroid gland. Another method for treating this disorder is to administer a sufficient amount of radioactive iodine to destroy the thyroid secretory cells. Some thyroid disorders are summarized in Table 14–3.

Parathyroid Disorders

As with the thyroid gland, dysfunction of the parathyroids is usually characterized by excessive hormone secretion (**hyperparathyroidism**) or inadequate hormone secretion (**hypoparathyroidism**).

Hypoparathyroidism can result from an injury or from surgical removal of the glands, sometimes in conjunction with thyroid surgery. The primary effect of hypoparathyroidism is the lowering of the blood calcium level. The decreased calcium (**hypocalcemia**) lowers the electrical threshold and causes neurons to depolarize more easily and the number of nerve impulses to increase. This results in muscle twitches and spasms, causing a condition called **tetany**.

Hyperparathyroidism is most often caused by a benign tumor. The resulting increase in PTH secretion leads to demineralization of bones (**osteitis fibrosa cystica**), making them porous (**osteoporosis**) and highly susceptible to fracture and deformity. When this condition is the result of a benign glandular tumor (**adenoma**) of the parathyroid, the tumor is removed. Treatment may also include orthopedic surgery to correct severe bone deformities. An excess of PTH also causes calcium to be deposited in the kidneys. When the disease is generalized and all bones are affected, this disorder is known as **von Recklinghausen's disease**. Renal symptoms and kidney stones (**nephrolithiasis**) may also develop. Some parathyroid disorders are summarized in Table 14–4.

Disorders of the Adrenal Glands

Adrenal Medulla

No specific diseases can be traced directly to a deficiency of hormones from the medulla. However, medullary tumors sometimes cause excess secretions. The most common disorder is in the form of a neoplasm known as **pheochromocytoma**, which produces excessive amounts of epinephrine and norepinephrine. Most of these tumors are encapsulated and benign. These hypersecretions produce stress, fear, palpitations, headaches, visual blurring, muscle spasms, and sweating. The usual form of treatment consists of administration of antihypertensive drugs and surgery.

Adrenal Cortex

Addison's disease, a relatively uncommon chronic disorder caused by a deficiency of cortical hormones, results when the adrenal cortex is destroyed. It is caused by atrophy of the adrenals, probably the result of some autoimmune process in which circulating adrenal antibodies slowly destroy the gland. Ninety percent of the gland is usually destroyed before clinical signs of adrenal insufficiency appear. Hypofunction of the adrenal cortex interferes with the body's ability to handle internal and external stress. In severe cases, the disturbance of sodium and potassium metabolism may be marked by depletion of sodium and water through urination, resulting in severe chronic dehydration. Other clinical manifestations include muscular weakness, anorexia, gastrointestinal symptoms, fatigue, hypoglycemia, hypotension, low blood sodium (**hyponatremia**), and high serum potassium (**hyperkalemia**). If treatment for this condition begins early, usually with adrenocortical hormone therapy, the prognosis is excellent. If untreated, the disease will continue a chronic course with progressive but relatively slow deterioration. In some patients, the deterioration may be rapid.

Cushing's syndrome, caused by hypersecretion of the adrenal cortex, results in excessive production of glucocorticoids. This overactivity is commonly due to an abnormal growth of the adrenal cortices. It may also be caused by a tumor arising in the cortex of one of the adrenal glands, a pituitary tumor, or excessive administration of cortisone. Symptoms include rapidly developing adiposity of the face ("moon face") and neck, purple striae on the skin, fatigue, high blood pressure, and excessive hair growth in unusual places (**hirsutism**), especially in women. Treatment is partial removal of the adrenal gland (**adrenalectomy**) or removal of the tumor. Some adrenal gland disorders are summarized in Table 14–5.

Pancreatic Disorders

Diabetes mellitus (DM), in its two forms, is by far the most common pancreatic disorder. **Type 1 diabetes**, also known as **insulin-dependent diabetes mellitus (IDDM)**, occurs mostly in children and adolescents (juvenile onset) and may be associated with a genetic predisposition for the disorder. It is characterized by destruction of beta cells of the islets of Langerhans with complete insulin deficiency in the body. Treatment includes injection of insulin in order to maintain a normal level of glucose in the blood.

Type 2 diabetes, also known as **non-insulin-dependent diabetes mellitus (NIDDM)**, is distinctively different from type 1. Its onset is usually later in life (maturity onset), and risk factors include a family history of diabetes and obesity. Even though insulin is produced, the insulin cannot exert its effects on cells because of the body's insensitivity to insulin. Treatment includes medications that stimulate the release of pancreatic insulin and improve the body's sensitivity to insulin (**oral hypoglycemic agents**), weight reduction, and diet. Clinical manifestations of both forms are summarized in Tables 14–7 and 14–8.

Diabetes is characterized by numerous complications, such as upsets in carbohydrate metabolism as well as disturbances in protein and fat metabolism. There is a rise in the concentration of blood sugar (**hyperglycemia**). Some of the glucose, along with electrolytes (particularly sodium), is excreted in the urine (**glycosuria**), causing excessive urination (**diuresis**), dehydration, and thirst (**polydipsia**). Sodium and potassium losses result in muscle weakness and fatigue. Because glucose cannot enter the cells, cellular starvation results. This leads to hunger and an increased appetite (**polyphagia**). Unless treatment is initiated, ketoacidosis, which appears in advanced stages of hyperglycemia, will develop.

Ketoacidosis, also referred to as diabetic acidosis or diabetic coma, may develop over several days or weeks. It can be caused by too little insulin, failure to follow a prescribed diet, physical or emotional stress, or undiagnosed diabetes. Low blood sugar (**hypoglycemia**) occurs when the level of insulin in the blood is out of proportion to that of available glucose. Hyperinsulinism may also be due to a tumor involving the islet cells, but similar symptoms occur if a person with diabetes receives too large a dosage of insulin. In either case, the condition is referred to as insulin shock. Treatment includes administering glucose intravenously, which usually brings the patient out of shock within a few minutes.

Table 14–7   CLINICAL MANIFESTATIONS OF
INSULIN-DEPENDENT DIABETES

Insulin-dependent diabetes is characterized by the sudden appearance of:

Constant urination (polyuria) and glycosuria
Abnormal thirst (polydipsia)
Unusual hunger (polyphagia)
The rapid loss of weight
Irritability
Obvious weakness and fatigue
Nausea and vomiting

Any one of these signals can indicate diabetes. Children usually exhibit dramatic, sudden symptoms and must receive prompt treatment.

Source: American Diabetes Association, New York.

Table 14–8 CLINICAL MANIFESTATIONS OF
NON–INSULIN-DEPENDENT DIABETES

Non–insulin-dependent diabetes may include any of the signs of insulin-dependent diabetes or:
Drowsiness
Itching
A family history of diabetes
Blurred vision
Excessive weight
Tingling, numbness, pain in the extremities
Easily fatigued
Skin infections and slow healing of cuts and scratches, especially of the feet
Many adults may have diabetes with none of these symptoms. The disease is often discovered during a routine physical examination.

Source: American Diabetes Association, New York.

Long-standing diabetes is a leading cause of blindness, as it causes diabetic retinopathy. Diabetes in pregnant women (**gestational diabetes**) usually subsides after the child is born (**parturition**). Some pancreatic disorders are summarized in Table 14–6.

Oncology

Pancreatic Cancer

Most carcinomas of the pancreas arise as epithelial tumors (**adenocarcinomas**) and make their presence known by obstruction and local invasion. Because the pancreas is richly supplied with nerves, pain is a prominent feature of pancreatic cancer, whether it arises in the head, the body, or the tail of the organ.

The prognosis of this tumor is poor, with only a 2 percent survival rate for 5 years. Pancreatic cancer is the fourth leading cause of cancer deaths in the United States. The highest incidence is among people 60 to 70 years of age. The etiology is unknown, but cigarette smoking, exposure to occupational chemicals, a diet high in fats, and heavy coffee intake are associated with an increased incidence of pancreatic cancer.

Pituitary Tumors

Pituitary tumors are generally not malignant, but because their growth is invasive, they are considered neoplastic and are usually treated as such. Initial signs and symptoms include headache, blurred vision, and oftentimes personality changes, dementia, and seizures. Tomography, skull radiographs, pneumoencephalography, angiography, and computed tomography scans assist in diagnosis. Depending on the size of the tumor and its location, different treatment modalities are employed. Treatments include surgical removal, radiation, or a combination of both.

Thyroid Cancer

There are a variety of thyroid cancers, classified according to the specific tissue that is affected. In general, however, all share many predisposing factors, including radiation, prolonged TSH stimulation, familial disposition, and chronic goiter. The malignancy usually begins with a painless, often hard nodule, or a nodule in the adjacent lymph nodes accompanied with an enlarged thyroid. When the tumor is excessively large, it frequently destroys thyroid tissue, which results in symptoms of hypothyroidism. Sometimes the tumor stimulates the production of thyroid hormone, resulting in symptoms of hyperthyroidism. Treatments include surgical removal, radiation, or a combination of both.

DIAGNOSTIC, SYMPTOMATIC, AND THERAPEUTIC TERMS

Term	Meaning
acromegaly ăk-rō-MĔG-ă-lē	disease characterized by enlarged features, particularly the face and hands, the result of oversecretion of the pituitary growth hormone after puberty (Fig. 14–3)
diuresis dī-ū-RĒ-sĭs	increased excretion of urine, as occurs in diabetes mellitus; can also be early sign of chronic interstitial nephritis
glucagon GLOO-kă-gŏn	hormone secreted by the pancreatic alpha cells that increases blood glucose concentration
glucose GLOO-kōs	simple sugar
glucosuria, glycosuria gloo-kō-SŪ-rē-ă, glī-kō-SŪ-rē-ă	presence of glucose in the urine; abnormal amount of sugar in the urine
hirsutism HŬR-sūt-ĭzm	abnormal hairiness, especially in women
homeostasis hō-mē-ō-STĀ-sĭs	state of equilibrium in the internal environment of the body
hypercalcemia hī-pĕr-kăl-SĒ-mē-ă	excessive amount of calcium in the blood
hyperkalemia hī-pĕr-kă-LĒ-mē-ă	excessive amount of potassium in the blood, most often because of defective renal excretion
hypervolemia hī-pĕr-vŏl-Ē-mē-ă	an abnormal increase in the volume of circulating fluid (plasma) in the body. It often is caused when the kidneys retain large amounts of sodium and water. Manifestations include weight gain, edema, dyspnea, tachycardia, and pulmonary congestion
hyponatremia hī-pō-nă-TRĒ-mē-ă	abnormal condition of low sodium in the blood
insulinoma ĭn-sū-lĭn-Ō-mă	tumor of the islets of Langerhans of the pancreas
obesity ō-BĒ-sĭ-tē	excessive accumulation of fat in the body
panhypopituitarism păn-hī-pō-pĭ-TŪ-ĭ-tăr-ĭzm	total pituitary impairment that brings about a progressive and general loss of hormonal activity
pheochromocytoma fē-ō-krō-mō-sī-TŌ-mă	small chromaffin cell tumor, usually located in the adrenal medulla
storm	an exacerbation of symptoms or a crisis in the course of a disease
thyroid THĪ-royd	thyrotoxic crisis. There is an abrupt onset of fever, sweating, tachycardia, pulmonary edema or congestive heart failure (CHF), and excessive restlessness. If left untreated, it may be fatal
virile VĬR-ĭl	masculine; having characteristics of a man, especially copulative powers
virilism VĬR-ĭl-ĭzm	masculinization in a woman; development of male secondary sex characteristics in the woman

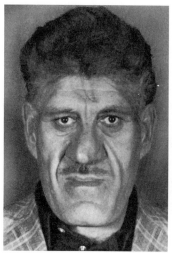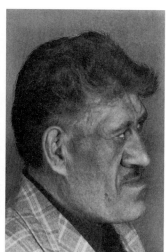

Figure 14–3 Acromegaly in a 56-year-old man. (From Martin, JB, Reichlin, S, and Brown, GM: Clinical Neuroendocrinology. F.A. Davis, Philadelphia, 1977, p 353, with permission.)

DIAGNOSTIC PROCEDURES

Imaging Procedure	Description
CT scan (pancreas, thyroid, adrenal glands)	used to detect disease in soft body tissues, such as the pancreas, thyroid, and adrenal glands; may also involve the use of radiographic contrast media
radioactive iodine uptake (RAIU)	radioactive iodine is administered either orally (PO) or intravenously (IV) to measure thyroid function and monitor the ability of the gland to take up iodine from the blood; used to detect thyroid nodules or tumors
thyroid echogram (ultrasound examination of thyroid)	valuable for distinguishing cystic from solid nodules. If the nodule is found to be purely cystic and fluid filled, it is aspirated and surgery is avoided. However, if the nodule has a mixed or solid appearance, carcinoma is a likely possibility and surgery is usually necessary. A nonfunctioning thyroid nodule can be evaluated with the use of reflected sound waves

Laboratory Procedure	Description
fasting blood sugar (FBS)	measures circulating glucose level after a 12-hour fast
glucose tolerance test (GTT)	performed by giving a certain amount of glucose (sugar) orally or intravenously, drawing blood samples at specified intervals, and determining the blood glucose level in each sample; most often used to assist in the diagnosis of diabetes or other disorders that affect carbohydrate metabolism
insulin tolerance test	determines insulin levels in serum (blood). Insulin is administered and blood glucose is measured at timed intervals. In hypoglycemia, the glucose levels may be lower and slower to return to normal
protein-bound iodine (PBI)	test that measures the concentration of thyroxine in a blood sample; result furnishes an index of thyroid activity
thyroid function test	a test for evidence of increased or decreased thyroid function, including a physical examination and laboratory tests. Some of the more common tests are based on determination of the two thyroid hormones, triiodothyronine (T_3) and tetraiodothyronine (T_4). Also frequently used are tests that assess radioactive iodine uptake by the thyroid
total calcium	measures calcium to detect bone and parathyroid disorders: hypercalcemia can indicate primary hyperparathyroidism; hypocalcemia can indicate hypoparathyroidism

SURGICAL AND THERAPEUTIC PROCEDURES

Procedure	Description
microneurosurgery of pituitary gland mī-krō-nū-rō-SĔR-jĕr-ē pĭ-TŪ-ĭ-tār-ē	microdissection of a tumor using a binocular surgical microscope for magnification
parathyroidectomy păr-ă-thī-royd-ĔK-tō-mē	excision of one or more of the parathyroid glands, usually done to control hyperparathyroidism
partial thyroidectomy thī-royd-ĔK-tō-mē	method of choice for removal of a fibrous nodular thyroid
pinealectomy pĭn-ē-ăl-ĔK-tō-mē	removal of the pineal body
thymectomy thī-MĔK-tō-mē	excision of the thymus gland
subtotal thyroidectomy thī-royd-ĔK-tō-mē	removal of most of the thyroid to relieve hyperthyroidism

PHARMACOLOGY

Medication	Action
anabolic agent	testosterone, or a steroid hormone resembling testosterone, which stimulates body tissue building. Anabolic steroids have been used, sometimes in large doses, by male and female athletes to improve performance, especially in events requiring strength. The use has been judged to be illegal by various organizations that supervise sports, including the International Olympic Committee and the U.S. Olympic Committee
antihyperlipidemics	lower cholesterol levels in the bloodstream; help prevent atherosclerosis (fatty build-up in the blood vessels)

PHARMACOLOGY (Continued)

Medication	Action
corticosteroids	replacement hormones for adrenal insufficiency (Addison's disease); widely used to suppress inflammation, control allergic reactions, reduce rejection in transplantation, and treat some cancers
insulin	major drug for treating diabetes; administered by injection to lower blood glucose (sugar) level
oral hypoglycemics	used with certain types of diabetes mellitus patients, mainly those who are overweight and have developed the condition as adults. These drugs are unrelated to insulin and are used in cases where the pancreas is already producing some insulin. Their effect is to stimulate the pancreas to secrete more insulin and make the body cells more receptive to the action of insulin
vasopressin	controls diabetes insipidus and subsequent polyuria due to ADH deficiency; replaces pituitary ADH and promotes reabsorption of water in the kidneys

ABBREVIATIONS

Abbreviation	Meaning
ACTH	adrenocorticotropic hormone
ADH	antidiuretic hormone (vasopressin)
DI	diabetes insipidus; diagnostic imaging
DM	diabetes mellitus
ECF	extracellular fluid
FBS	fasting blood sugar
FSH	follicle-stimulating hormone
GH	growth hormone
GTT	glucose tolerance test
ICF	intracellular fluid
ICSH	interstitial cell-stimulating hormone
IDDM	insulin-dependent diabetes mellitus
LDL	low-density lipoproteins
LH	luteinizing hormone
MSH	melanocyte-stimulating hormone
NIDDM	non-insulin-dependent diabetes mellitus
NPH	neutral protamine Hagedorn (insulin)
PBI	protein-bound iodine
PGH	pituitary growth hormone
PTH	parathyroid hormone
RAI	radioactive iodine
RAIU	radioactive iodine uptake
T_3	triiodothyronine
T_4	thyroxine
TSH	thyroid-stimulating hormone

MEDICAL RECORD

Hyperparathyroidism and Diabetes Mellitus

A 66-year-old former blackjack dealer is under evaluation for hyperparathyroidism (see Table 14–4). Surgery evidently has been recommended, but there is confusion as to how urgent this is. She has a 14-year history of type 1 diabetes mellitus, a history of shoulder pain, osteoarthritis of the spine, and peripheral vascular disease with claudication. She states her 548-pack-year smoking history ended 3.5 years ago. Her first knowledge of parathyroid disease was about 3 years ago when laboratory findings revealed an elevated calcium level. This subsequently led to the diagnosis of hyperparathyroidism. She was further evaluated by an endocrinologist in the Lake Tahoe area, who determined that she also had hypercalciuria, although there is nothing to suggest a history of kidney stones.

Impression   Hyperparathyroidism and hypercalciuria, probably a parathyroid adenoma.

Worksheet 5 provides a dictionary and reading application and an analysis of this medical record.

WORSHEET 1

■ ■ ■ ■ ■ ■ ■ ■ ■ ■ ■ ■ ■

Use glyc/o (sugar) to build a medical word meaning:

1. condition of excessive sugar in the blood _____

2. condition of deficiency of sugar in the blood _____

3. formation of glycogen _____

Use pancreat/o (pancreas) to build a medical word meaning:

4. inflammation of the pancreas _____

5. destruction of the pancreas _____

6. any pancreatic disease _____

Use thyr/o or thyroid/o (thyroid) to build a medical word meaning:

7. inflammation of the thyroid gland _____

8. enlargement of the thyroid _____

WORKSHEET 2

■ ■ ■ ■ ■ ■ ■ ■ ■ ■ ■ ■ ■

Build a surgical term meaning:

1. excision of the thyroid _____

2. incision of thyroid cartilage _____

3. excision of a parathyroid gland _____

4. removal of the adrenal _____

5. excision of the adrenal glands on both sides _____

WORKSHEET 3

■ ■ ■ ■ ■ ■ ■ ■ ■ ■ ■ ■

Match the following words with the definitions in the numbered list.

Addison's disease	hirsutism	myxedema
cretinism	hyperkalemia	pheochromocytoma
diuresis	hypokalemia	tetany
exophthalmic goiter	insulin	virile

1. _____ having characteristics of a man; masculine

2. _____ hypothyroidism that develops after puberty

3. _____ increased excretion of urine

4. _____ excessive growth of hair or the presence of hair in unusual places, especially in women

5. _____ hypothyroidism that develops in an infant

6. _____ hormone produced by beta cells of the pancreas

7. _____ disease resulting from deficiency in the secretion of adrenocortical hormones

8. _____ a condition marked by protrusion of the eyeballs, increased heart action, enlargement of the thyroid gland, weight loss, and nervousness

9. _____ excessive amount of potassium in the blood

10. _____ small chromaffin cell tumor, usually located in the adrenal medulla

WORKSHEET 4

* * * * * * * * * * * * *

Select the word that best describes the statements that follow:

antihyperlipidemics	insulin	T_4
corticosteroids	RAI	thyroid echogram
FBS	RAIU	toxicosis
GTT	T_3	vasopressin

1. _____ measures circulating glucose level after a 12-hour fast

2. _____ test based on the ability of the thyroid gland to trap and retain iodine, which provides an indirect measure of thyroid activity

3. _____ replacement hormones for adrenal insufficiency

4. _____ drug that controls diabetes insipidus and subsequent polyuria due to ADH deficiency

5. _____ ultrasound examination of the thyroid

6. _____ thyroxine

7. _____ major drug that lowers glucose level and is administered by injection

8. _____ diagnostic test to determine hypoglycemia, hyperglycemia, and adjustments of insulin dosages

9. _____ lowers cholesterol levels in the bloodstream

10. _____ radioactive iodine

11. _____ triiodothyronine

WORKSHEET 5

∎ ∎ ∎ ∎ ∎ ∎ ∎ ∎ ∎ ∎ ∎ ∎ ∎

MEDICAL RECORD: HYPERPARATHYROIDISM AND DIABETES MELLITUS

Underline the following terms in the medical record (see p. 286). Use a medical dictionary and other resources to define the terms and to determine their pronunciation; then practice reading the medical record aloud.

adenoma _____

type 1 diabetes mellitus _____

endocrinologist _____

hypercalciuria _____

hyperparathyroidism _____

parathyroid _____

MEDICAL RECORD EVALUATION: HYPERPARATHYROIDISM AND DIABETES MELLITUS

1. *Referring to Figure 14–2, designate the location of the parathyroid glands.*

2. *How many parathyroid glands are there?*

3. *What is an adenoma?*

4. *What body system(s) was involved in her condition?*

5. *Define endocrinologist.*

6. *What is hypercalciuria?*

7. *If she smoked 548 packs of cigarettes a year, how many packs did she smoke in an average day?*

WORKSHEET 6

- - - - - - - - - - - - - -

Label the following diagram. Check your answers by referring to Figure 14–2.

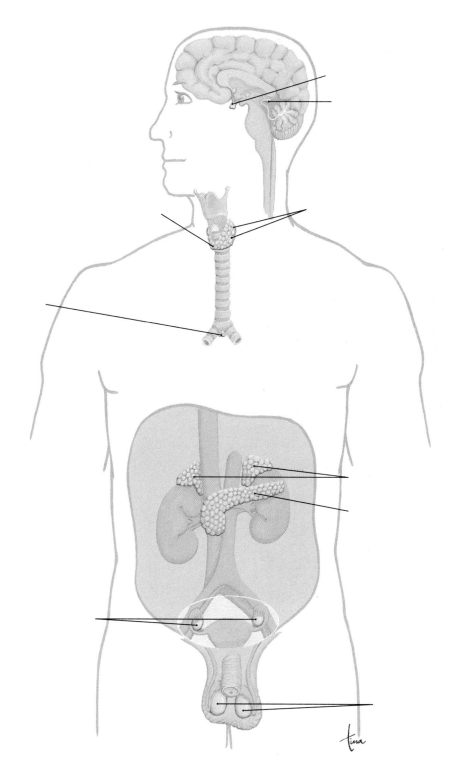

Adrenal (Suprarenal) glands	Parathyroid glands	Testes
Ovaries	Pineal gland	Thyroid gland
Pancreas	Pituitary (Hypophysis) gland	Thymus gland

NERVOUS SYSTEM

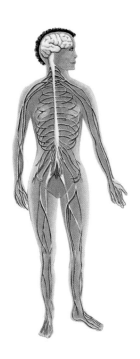

Chapter Outline

Student Objectives

Anatomy and Physiology
Nervous Tissue
  Neurons
  Neuroglia
Subdivisions of the Nervous System
Brain
Spinal Cord
Meninges

Combining Forms

Suffixes

Prefixes

Pathology
Bell's Palsy
Cerebrovascular Disease
Seizure Disorders

Parkinson's Disease
Multiple Sclerosis
Alzheimer's Disease
Oncology

Diagnostic, Symptomatic, and Therapeutic Terms

Diagnostic Procedures
Imaging Procedures

Surgical and Therapeutic Procedures

Pharmacology

Abbreviations

Medical Record
Subarachnoid Hemorrhage

Worksheets

Student Objectives

Upon completion of this chapter, you will be able to do the following:

1. Describe the structure and functions of neurons.

2. List and briefly describe the functions of four types of neuroglial cells.

3. List and briefly describe the subdivisions of the nervous system.

4. Describe the function of four major parts of the brain.

5. Discuss the structure and function of the spinal cord.

6. List the three meninges and describe their function.

7. Identify combining forms, suffixes, and prefixes related to the nervous system.

8. Identify and discuss pathology related to the nervous system.

9. Identify diagnostic, symptomatic, and therapeutic terms related to the nervous system.

10. Identify diagnostic procedures associated with the nervous system.

11. Identify surgical and therapeutic procedures related to the nervous system.

Student Objectives (Continued)

12. Discuss pharmacology related to the treatment of nervous disorders.
13. Define abbreviations related to the nervous system.
14. Demonstrate your knowledge of the chapter by completing the worksheets.

ANATOMY AND PHYSIOLOGY

The nervous system is one of the most complicated systems of the body. Along with the endocrine system, it controls many bodily activities. The nervous system senses changes in both the internal and external environments, interprets these changes, and then coordinates appropriate responses in order to maintain homeostasis.

Nervous Tissue

In spite of its complexity, the nervous system is composed of two principal types of cells: **neurons** and **neuroglia**. Neurons are cells that transmit impulses. **Sensory neurons**, also called **afferent nerves**, transmit stimuli to the brain and spinal cord; **motor neurons**, also called **efferent nerves**, transmit impulses from the brain or spinal cord to muscles and glands. Neuroglia are cells that primarily support neurons and play an important role when there is injury or infection in the nervous system

Neurons

Refer to Figure 15–1 as you read the following material.
Neurons consist of three major structures:

- (1) **Dendrites**, the branching cytoplasmic projections that receive impulses and transmit them to the cell body
- (2) **Cell body**, the structure containing the (3) **nucleus**
- (4) **Axon**, the long single projection that transmits the impulse from the cell body

Many axons in both the peripheral nervous system and the autonomic nervous system possess a white, lipoid covering called a (5) **myelin sheath**. This wrapping acts as an electrical insulator that reduces the possibility of an impulse stimulating adjacent nerves. It also accelerates impulse transmission through the axon. The myelin on axons in the brain and spinal cord gives these structures a white appearance and constitutes the white matter of the central nervous system. Unmyelinated fibers, dendrites, and nerve cell bodies make up the gray matter of the brain and spinal cord.

On peripheral nerves, the myelin sheath is formed by a neuroglial cell called a Schwann cell that wraps tightly around the axon. The (6) **Schwann cell** is pushed to the outer surface to form a thin cellular membrane called (7) **neurolemma**, or **neurolemmal sheath**. The neurolemmal sheath (myelin sheath) permits a damaged axon to regenerate. Because neurolemma is not found in the central nervous system, severed central nervous system nerves cannot regenerate. Therefore, function of severed nerves is permanently lost unless alternate neural pathways are established. The space between adjacent Schwann cells is called (8) **node of Ranvier**.

Neurons are not continuous with one another. Instead, a small space, known as a **synapse**, is found between the axon of one neuron and the dendrite or cell body of another. In order for an impulse to travel along a nerve path, it must cross the synapse. The electric current within the neuron causes the release of a chemical substance called a **neurotransmitter**. The neurotransmitter is released at the **synaptic knob** located at the terminal end of the axon. The neurotransmitter

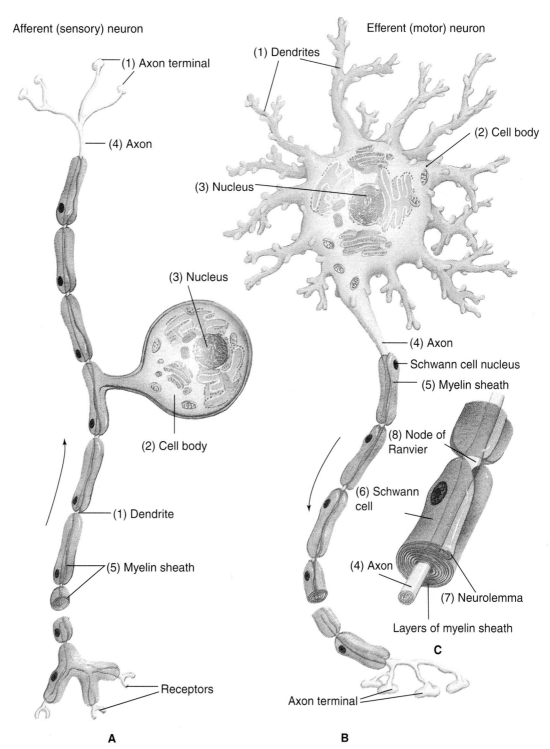

Figure 15–1   Neuron structure. (*A*) A typical sensory neuron. (*B*) A typical motor neuron. The arrows indicate the direction of impulse transmission. (*C*) Details of the myelin sheath and neurolemma formed by Schwann cells. (From Scanlon, VC, and Sanders, T: Understanding Human Structure and Function. F.A. Davis, Philadelphia, 1997, p 131, with permission.)

diffuses across the synapse to receptor sites on the dendrite of the next neuron. Here it generates the next electrical stimulus. The receiving neuron immediately inactivates the neurotransmitter, thereby preventing an unwanted continued stimulation and preparing the site for another stimulus by a neurotransmitter. Thus, impulses travel through neural pathways.

Neuroglia

The term **neuroglia** literally means "nerve glue." It was once believed that neuroglia served only a supporting role for neurons, but it is now known that neuroglia cells perform many functions.

Astrocytes, as their name suggests, are star-shaped neuroglia. They form tight sheaths around the capillaries of the brain. These sheaths keep large molecules from entering the delicate tissue of the brain and constitute the phenomenon called the **blood-brain barrier**. However, small molecules such as water, carbon dioxide, oxygen, and alcohol readily pass from blood vessels through the barrier and enter the interstitial spaces of the brain. Researchers must take the blood-brain barrier into consideration when developing drugs for treatment of brain disorders.

Oligodendrocytes, also called oligodendroglia, help in the development of myelin on neurons of the central nervous system.

Microglia, the smallest of the neuroglia, possess phagocytic properties and may become very active during times of infection.

Ependyma are ciliated cells that line fluid-filled cavities of the central nervous system, especially the ventricles of the brain. They assist in cerebrospinal fluid (CSF) circulation.

Subdivisions of the Nervous System

Figure 15–2 illustrates the subdivisions of the nervous system. Refer to this figure as you read the following paragraphs. The nervous system includes the **central nervous system (CNS)**, consisting of the brain and the spinal cord, and the **peripheral nervous system (PNS)**, consisting of all other neural elements of the body. The PNS includes 12 pairs of **cranial nerves**, which emerge from the base of the skull, and 31 pairs of **spinal nerves**, which emerge from the spinal cord. The cranial nerves and their distribution are shown in Figure 15–3. Figure 15–4 shows the spinal cord and identifies the 31 pairs of spinal nerves. All peripheral nerves consist of fibers that may be **sensory** or **motor**, or a mixture of both. Sensory nerves receive impulses from the sense organs,

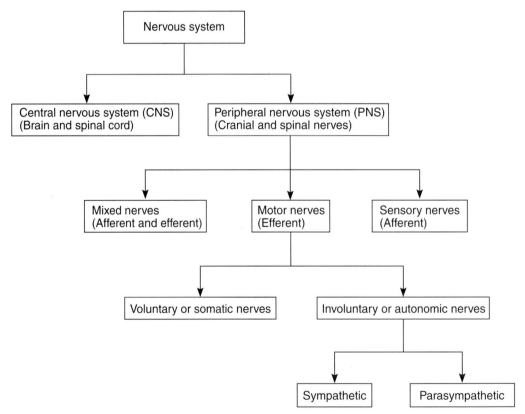

Figure 15–2 Subdivisions of the nervous system.

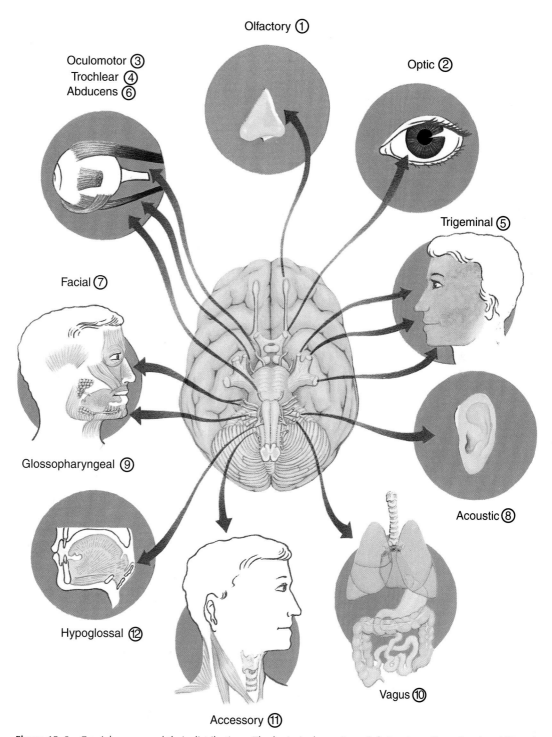

Figure 15–3 Cranial nerves and their distributions. The brain is shown in an inferior view. (From Scanlon, VC, and Sanders, T: Understanding Human Structure and Function. F.A. Davis, Philadelphia, 1997, p 148, with permission.)

including the eyes, ears, nose, tongue, and skin, and transmit them to the CNS. As noted previously, because the sensory nerves conduct impulses *toward* the CNS, they are also known as afferent nerves. Motor nerves, which conduct impulses *away from* the CNS, are known as efferent nerves. Motor impulses travel primarily to muscles, causing them to contract, or to glands, causing them to secrete.

Nerves composed of both sensory and motor fibers are called **mixed nerves**. An example of a mixed nerve is the facial nerve. When the facial nerve transmits an impulse to the face for smiling

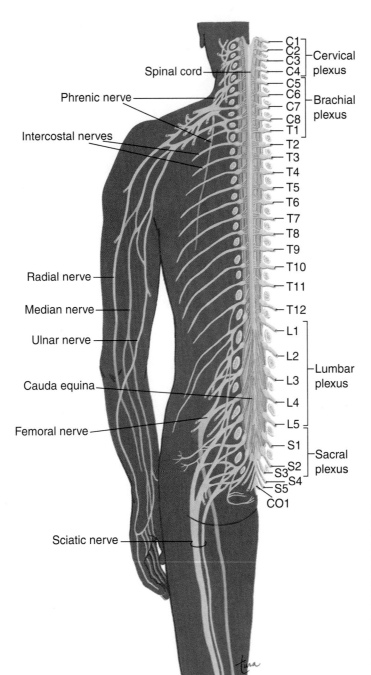

Figure 15–4 The spinal cord and spinal nerves. The distribution of spinal nerves is shown only on the left side. The nerve plexuses are labeled on the right side. A nerve plexus is a network of neurons from several segments of the spinal cord that combine to form nerves to specific parts of the body. For example, the radial and ulnar nerves of the arm emerge from the brachial plexus. (From Scanlon, VC, and Sanders, T: Understanding Human Structure and Function. F.A. Davis, Philadelphia, 1997, p 137, with permission.)

or frowning, it functions as a motor nerve. When it transmits a taste impulse from the tongue to the brain, it functions as a sensory nerve. Cranial nerves may be sensory, motor, or mixed, but all spinal nerves are mixed nerves.

Spinal nerves have two points of attachment to the spinal cord: an anterior root and a posterior root. The anterior root contains motor fibers and the posterior root contains sensory fibers. These two roots unite to form the spinal nerve.

Functionally, the PNS is subdivided into two specialized systems: the **somatic nervous system (SNS)** and the **autonomic nervous system (ANS)**. The SNS primarily enervates (supplies with nerves) skeletal muscles. It is associated with voluntary movement. Examples of voluntary activities include walking, talking, and playing tennis. However, the ANS sends impulses to glands, smooth muscles, and cardiac muscles. This system is considered involuntary, as it operates without conscious control. Examples of autonomic activities include digestion, heart contraction, and vasoconstriction.

The ANS is further subdivided into the **sympathetic** and **parasympathetic** systems. To a large extent, these subdivisions each oppose the action of the other, although in certain instances, they may exhibit independent action. In general, sympathetic nerve fibers produce vasoconstriction, increased heart rate, elevated blood pressure, and slowing of gastrointestinal activity. Sympathetic functions are evident in "fight-or-flight"situations. Blood flow increases in skeletal muscles to prepare an individual to either fight or run away from a threatening situation.

The parasympathetic system generally transmits impulses that bring about vasodilation, a slower heart rate, a decrease in blood pressure, and a return to normal gastrointestinal activity. When danger passes, more blood is directed to internal organs. The parasympathetic system is associated with "rest and relaxation."

Brain

In addition to being one of the largest organs of the body, the brain is also the most complex in structure and function. It integrates almost every physical and mental activity of the body. This organ is also the center for memory, emotion, thought, judgment, reasoning, and consciousness. It is composed of four major structures:

- Cerebrum
- Cerebellum
- Diencephalon
- Brainstem

In order to develop a better understanding of the anatomy of the brain, refer to Figure 15–5 as you read the following material.

The (1) **cerebrum** is the largest and uppermost portion of the brain. It consists of two hemispheres divided by a deep longitudinal fissure, or groove. The fissure does not completely

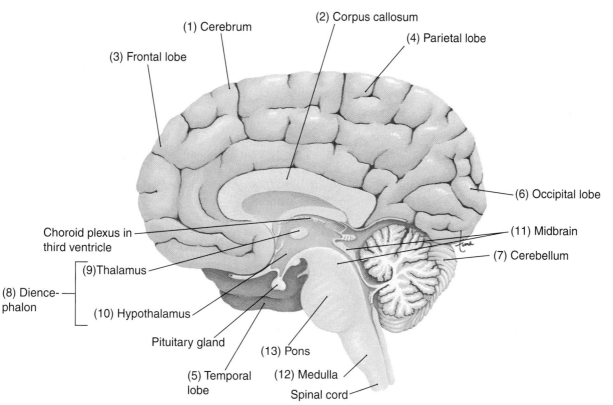

Figure 15–5   Midsagittal section of the brain as seen from the left side. The medial plane shows internal anatomy as well as the lobes of the cerebrum. (From Scanlon, VC, and Sanders, T: Understanding Human Structure and Function. F.A. Davis, Philadelphia, 1997, p 141, with permission.)

separate the hemispheres. A structure called the (2) **corpus callosum** joins these hemispheres, permitting communication between the right and left sides of the brain. Each hemisphere is divided into five lobes. Four of these lobes are named for the bones that lie directly above them: (3) **frontal**, (4) **parietal**, (5) **temporal**, and (6) **occipital**. The fifth lobe, the **insula** (not shown in figure), is hidden from view and can be seen only upon dissection.

The cerebral surface consists of numerous folds, or convolutions, called **gyri**. They are separated by furrows or fissures called **sulci**. A thin gray layer called the **cerebral cortex** covers the entire cerebrum. It is composed of millions of cell bodies that are responsible for its gray color.

The remainder of the cerebrum is composed primarily of white matter (myelinated axons). Major functions of the cerebrum include sensory perception and interpretation, muscular movement, and the emotional aspects of behavior and memory.

The second largest part of the brain, the (7) **cerebellum**, occupies the posterior portion of the brain. All functions of the cerebellum are concerned with movement. When the cerebrum initiates muscular movement, the cerebellum coordinates and refines it. The cerebellum also aids in maintaining equilibrium and balance.

The (8) **diencephalon (interbrain)** is composed of many smaller structures, two of which are the (9) **thalamus** and the (10) **hypothalamus**. The thalamus receives all sensory stimuli except olfactory. It processes and transmits them to the cerebral cortex. In addition, the thalamus receives impulses from the cerebrum and relays them to efferent nerves. The hypothalamus integrates autonomic nerve impulses and regulates certain endocrine functions.

The brainstem completes the last major section of the brain. It is composed of three structures: the (11) **midbrain** (mesencephalon), separating the cerebrum from the brainstem; the (12) **medulla**, which attaches to the spinal cord; and (13) the **pons**, or "bridge," connecting the midbrain to the medulla. In general, the brainstem serves as a pathway for impulse conduction between the brain and spinal cord. The brainstem serves as the origin for 10 of the 12 pairs of cranial nerves and controls respiration, blood pressure, and heart rate. This section is sometimes called the primary brain because it is the site where life begins and ends.

Spinal Cord

The spinal cord transmits sensory impulses from different parts of the body to the brain and also transmits motor impulses from the brain to muscles and organs of the body. The sensory nerve tracts are called **ascending tracts** because the direction of the impulse is upward. Conversely, motor nerve tracts are called **descending tracts** because they carry impulses in a downward direction to muscles and organs. A cross-section of the spinal cord reveals an inner gray area composed of cell bodies and dendrites, with a white outer area composed of myelinated tissue of the ascending and descending tracts.

The entire spinal cord is located within the spinal cavity of the vertebral column. Thirty-one pairs of spinal nerves exit between the intervertebral spaces almost throughout the entire length of the spinal column. Unlike the cranial nerves, which have specific names, the spinal nerves are known by the region of the vertebral column from which they exit.

Meninges

Both the brain and the spinal cord receive limited protection from three coverings called **meninges** (singular, **meninx**). The outermost coat, the **dura mater**, is tough and fibrous, composed primarily of connective tissue. Beneath the dura mater is a cavity called the **subdural space**, filled with serous fluid. The next layer of the meninges is the **arachnoid**. As its name suggests, the arachnoid has a spiderweb appearance. A **subarachnoid space**, which contains CSF, provides additional protection for the brain and spinal cord by acting as a shock absorber. Finally, the innermost layer, the **pia mater**, contains numerous blood vessels and lymphatics that nourish the underlying tissues.

Cerebrospinal fluid circulates around the spinal cord and brain and through spaces called **ventricles**, located within the inner portion of the brain. This colorless fluid contains proteins, glucose, urea, salts, and some white blood cells. It provides nutritive substances to the CNS.

Normally, CSF is absorbed as rapidly as it is formed, maintaining a constant fluid volume. Any interference with absorption results in a collection of fluid in the brain, a condition called **hydrocephalus**.

COMBINING FORMS

Combining Form	Meaning	Example	Pronunciation
cerebr/o	cerebrum	cerebr/o/malacia softening	sĕr-ĕ-brō-mă-LĀ-shē-ă
crani/o	cranium (skull)	crani/o/tomy incision	krā-nē-ŎT-ō-mē
encephal/o	brain	encephal/o/tomy incision	ĕn-sĕf-ă-LŎT-ō-mē
gli/o	glue, neuroglia	gli/oma tumor	glī-Ō-mă
kinesi/o	movement	kinesi/o/logy study of	kĭ-nē-sē-ŎL-ō-jē
mening/o	meninges	mening/o/cyte cell	mĕ-NĬNG-gō-sīt
myel/o	spinal cord, bone marrow	myel/o/gram record	MĪ-ĕ-lō-grăm
narc/o	stupor, numbing	narc/o/tic pertaining to	năr-KŎ-tĭk
neur/o	nerve, nervous system	neur/algia pain	nū-RĂL-jē-ă
thalam/o	thalamus, chamber	thalam/ectomy excision	thăl-ĕm-ĔK-tō-mē
ton/o	tone, tension, pressure	ton/o/meter instrument for measuring	tōn-ŎM-ĕ-tĕr
ventricul/o	ventricle (of heart or brain)	ventricul/o/stomy forming an opening	vĕn-trĭk-ū-LŎS-tō-mē

SUFFIXES

Suffix	Meaning	Example	Pronunciation
-algesia	pain	an/algesia without	ăn-ăl-JĒ-zē-ă
-algia		syn/algia together	sĭn-ĂL-jē-ă
-esthesia	feeling, sensation	hyper/esthesia excessive	hī-pĕr-ĕs-THĒ-zē-ă
-lepsy	seizure	narc/o/lepsy stupor, numbing	NĂR-kō-lĕp-sē
-phasia	speech	tachy/phasia rapid	tăk-ē-FĀ-zē-ă

PREFIXES

Prefix	Meaning	Example	Pronunciation
a-, an-	not, without	a/phasia speech	ă-FĀ-zē-ă
brady-	slow	brady/kinesia movement	brăd-ē-kī-NĒ-sē-ă

PATHOLOGY

Bell's Palsy

Bell's palsy is a facial paralysis caused by a functional disorder of the seventh cranial nerve and any or all of its branches. It may be unilateral, bilateral, transient, or permanent. Symptoms include weakness (**asthenia**) and numbness of the face, distortion of taste perception, facial disfigurement, and facial spasms. The cornea becomes dry owing to the lack of the blink reflex, often leading to corneal infections (**keratitis**). Speech difficulties (**dysphasia**) and pain behind the ear or in the face are also symptomatic of this disease.

Anti-inflammatory drugs and the application of heat help to promote circulation. Spontaneous recovery can be expected in about 3 to 5 weeks.

Cerebrovascular Disease

Cerebrovascular disease (CVD) refers to any functional abnormality of the cerebrum caused by disorders of the blood vessels that vascularize the brain. These disorders include hemorrhage, an impairment of cerebral circulation due to hardening of blood vessels (**arteriosclerosis**), cerebral thromboses, or emboli. Both hemorrhage and occlusion may lead to stroke (**cerebrovascular accident [CVA]; apoplexy**). During a CVA, blood supply is decreased (**ischemia**) or absent. If the CVA is mild, the individual may experience a brief "blackout," blurred vision, or dizziness and may not be aware of the "minor stroke" (**transient ischemic attack [TIA]**). In more serious cases, signs and symptoms include weakness in one half of the body (**hemiparesis**), paralysis in one half of the body (**hemiplegia**), inability to speak (**aphasia**), lack of muscular coordination (**ataxia**), stupor, or coma. Treatment involves speech, physical, and/or occupational therapy.

Seizure Disorders

Chronic or recurring seizure disorders are called **epilepsies**. These disorders involve electrical disturbances (**dysrhythmias**) in the brain, which result in abnormal, recurrent, and uncontrolled electrical discharges. Causes of epilepsy include brain injury, congenital anomalies, metabolic disorders, brain tumors, vascular disturbances, and genetic disorders.

Epilepsies are characterized by sudden bursts of abnormal electrical activity in neurons, resulting in temporary changes in brain function. These bursts may be mild and cause only slight changes in the level of consciousness, motor control, and sensory perception, or they may be severe and cause spastic, involuntary muscle contractions (**convulsions**) and, occasionally, loss of consciousness. Different classifications of epilepsy are based on the location and duration of changes in electrical activity in the brain. Two major types of epilepsies are petit mal and grand mal.

In **petit mal epilepsy**, there are brief episodes (10 to 30 seconds) in change of level of consciousness. Eye or muscle flutterings, mouth movement, and occasionally loss of muscle tone frequently characterize the seizures. If untreated, seizures can recur as often as 100 times a day.

In **grand mal seizures**, there is a loss of consciousness, with firm and violent (**tonic**) spasms, followed by episodes that alternate between muscular rigidity and relaxation (**clonic**) spasms, involuntary convulsive movements, labored breathing, tongue biting, and incontinence.

Diagnosis and evaluation often rely on measuring brain waves (**electroencephalography [EEG]**) to locate the affected area of the brain. Epilepsy can often be effectively controlled by antiepileptic medications.

Parkinson's Disease

Parkinson's disease, also called "shaking palsy," is a progressive neurological disorder affecting the portion of the brain responsible for controlling movement. As neurons degenerate, the patient develops a nodding of the head, slowness of movement (**bradykinesia, hypokinesia**), tremors, stiffness of large joints, and a shuffling gait. Muscle rigidity causes facial expressions to appear fixed and masklike. The eyes are unblinking. Sometimes the patient exhibits "pill rolling," in which he or she inadvertently rubs the thumb against the index finger.

In patients with Parkinson's disease, dopamine, a neurotransmitter that facilitates the transmission of impulses at synapses, is lacking in the brain. Management involves the administration of L-dopa, which can cross the blood-brain barrier. L-dopa is converted in the brain to dopamine. However, this treatment only reduces the symptoms.

Multiple Sclerosis

Multiple sclerosis (MS) is a progressive degenerative disease of the CNS. MS is characterized by inflammation, hardening, and, finally, loss of myelin (**demyelination**) throughout the spinal cord and brain. As myelin deteriorates, the transmission of electrical impulses from one neuron to another is impeded. In effect, the conduction pathway develops "short circuits."

Signs and symptoms include tremors, muscle weakness, and slowness of movement. Occasionally, visual disturbances exist. During remissions, symptoms temporarily disappear, but progressive hardening of myelin areas leads to other attacks.

Ultimately, most voluntary motor control is lost and the patient becomes bedridden. Death occurs anywhere from 7 to 30 years after the onset of the disease. Young adults, usually women, between the ages of 20 and 40 years are the most frequent victims of MS. The etiology of the disease is uncertain, but autoimmune disease or a slow virus infection is believed to be the most probable cause.

Alzheimer's Disease

Alzheimer's disease is a progressive neurological disorder that causes memory loss and serious mental deterioration. Small lesions called **plaques** that develop in the cerebral cortex disrupt the passage of electrochemical signals between cells. The clinical manifestations include memory loss and cognitive decline. There is also a decline in social and daily function skills. Most patients undergo personality, emotional, and behavioral changes. As the disease progresses, there may be a loss of concentration, fatigue, restlessness, and anxiety. This disorder was once considered a rare disease, but it is now identified as a leading cause of senile dementia.

Although there is no specific treatment, some relief is often associated with medications that prevent a breakdown of brain chemicals that are required for neurotransmission.

Oncology

Intracranial tumors can arise from any structure within the cranial cavity, including the pituitary, pineal region, cranial nerves, and the arachnoid and pia mater (**leptomeninges**). However, most intracranial tumors originate directly in brain tissue. In addition, all of these tissues may be the site of metastatic spread from primary malignancies that occur outside of the nervous system. Metastatic tumors of the cranial cavity tend to exhibit growth characteristics similar to those of the primary malignancy but tend to grow more slowly than the parent tumor. Metastatic tumors of the cranial cavity are usually easier to remove than primary intracranial tumors.

Primary intracranial tumors are often classified according to histological type and include those that originate in neurons and those that develop in glial tissue.

The signs and symptoms of intracranial neoplasms include headaches, especially upon arising in the morning, during coughing episodes, and upon bending or sudden movement. Occasionally the optic nerve swells (**papilledema**) in the back of the eyeball because of increased intracranial pressure. Often there are personality changes, which include depression, anxiety, and irritability.

Computed tomography (CT) scans and magnetic resonance imaging (MRI) help to establish a diagnosis but are not definitive. Surgical removal relieves pressure and confirms or rules out malignancy. Even after surgery, most intracranial neoplasms require radiation therapy (RT) as a second line of treatment. Chemotherapy, when added to RT, provides the best chance for survival and quality of life.

DIAGNOSTIC, SYMPTOMATIC, AND THERAPEUTIC TERMS

Term	Meaning
agnosia ăg-NŌ-zē-ă	loss of comprehension of auditory, visual, or other sensations even though the sensory sphere is intact
asthenia ăs-THĒ-nē-ă	weakness or debility
ataxia ă-TĂK-sē-ă	lack of muscular coordination in the execution of voluntary movement
aura AW-ră	premonitory awareness of an approaching physical or mental disorder; peculiar sensation that precedes epileptic seizures
autism AW-tĭzm	a self-centered mental state from which reality tends to be excluded
cerebral palsy sĕ-RĒ-brăl PAWL-zē	a self-limiting paralysis due to developmental defects in the brain or trauma during the birthing process
clonic spasm KLŎN-ĭk spăzm	alternate contraction and relaxation of muscles
closed head trauma TRAW-mă	traumatic injury to the head, in which the dura mater remains intact and brain tissue is not exposed. The injury site may occur at the impact site where the brain hits the inside of the skull (coup), or at the rebound site where the opposite side of the brain strikes the skull (contrecoup)
coma KŌ-mă	abnormally deep unconsciousness with absence of voluntary response to stimuli
concussion kŏn-KŬSH-ŭn	injury (usually to the brain) resulting from impact with an object
dementia dē-MĔN-shē-ă	a broad term that refers to cognitive deficit, including memory impairment
Guillain-Barré syndrome gē-YĂ băr-RĀ SĬN-drōm	acute polyneuritis with progressive muscular weakness of extremities; most commonly occurs in people aged 30 to 50 years; spontaneous and complete recovery in about 95 percent of cases
herpes zoster (shingles) HĔR-pēz ZŎS-tĕr (SHĬNG-lz)	a painful acute infectious disease of the posterior root ganglia of only a few segments of the spinal or cranial nerves. The disease is caused by the same organism (varicella-zoster) that causes chickenpox in children. The disease is self-limiting and usually resolves in 10 days to 5 weeks (Fig. 15–6)

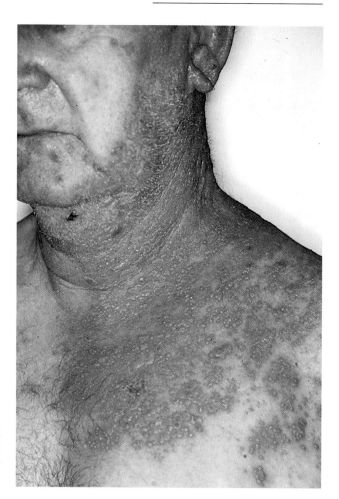

Figure 15–6 Herpes zoster (shingles). (From Reeves, JRT, and Maibach, HI: Clinical Dermatology Illustrated: A Regional Approach, ed 3. MacLennan & Petty, Rosebery, Australia, 1998 [distributed in America by F.A. Davis, Philadelphia], p 255, with permission.)

DIAGNOSTIC, SYMPTOMATIC, AND THERAPEUTIC TERMS (Continued)

Term	Meaning
Huntington's chorea HŬNT-ĭng-tŭnz kō-RĒ-ă	inherited disease of the CNS that usually has its onset in people between 30 and 50 years of age. This disease is characterized by quick, involuntary movements, speech disturbances, and mental deterioration
hydrocephalus hī-drō-SĚF-ă-lŭs	accumulation of fluid in the ventricles of the brain, causing thinning of brain tissue and separation of cranial bones
lethargy LĔTH-ăr-jē	abnormal activity or lack of response to normal stimuli; sluggishness
neural tube NŪ-răl TŪB	tube formed by the fusion of the neural folds from which the brain and spinal cord arise
defect	a defective closure of the neural tube during embryogenesis. Included are fetal anencephaly, spina bifida, lumbar meningomyelocele, and meningocele (Fig. 15–7)
paraplegia păr-ă-PLĒ-jē-ă	paralysis of the lower portion of the trunk and both legs
paresis PĂR-ē-sĭs/pă-RĒ-sĭs	partial or incomplete paralysis

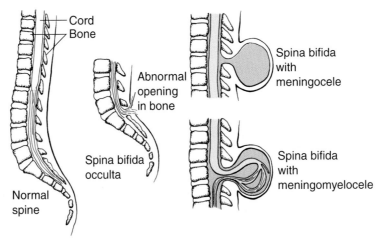

Figure 15–7 Neural tube defects. (From Rothstein et al: The Rehabilitation Specialist's Handbook, ed 2. F.A. Davis, Philadelphia, 1998, p 704, with permission.)

DIAGNOSTIC, SYMPTOMATIC, AND THERAPEUTIC TERMS (Continued)

Term	Meaning
paresthesia păr-ĕs-THĒ-zē-ă	sensation of numbness, prickling, or tingling; heightened sensitivity
poliomyelitis pōl-ē-ō-mī-ĕl-Ī-tĭs	inflammation of the gray matter of the spinal cord caused by a virus, often resulting in spinal and muscle deformity and paralysis
quadriplegia kwŏd-rĭ-PLĒ-jē-ă	paralysis of all four extremities and usually the trunk
Reye's syndrome RĪZ SĬN-drōm	acute encephalopathy and fatty infiltration of the liver and possibly pancreas, heart, kidney, spleen, and lymph nodes; usually seen in children younger than 15 years of age who had an acute viral infection. The mortality may be as high as 80 percent. The use of aspirin by children experiencing chickenpox or influenza may induce Reye's syndrome
sciatica sī-ĂT-ĭ-kă	severe pain in the leg along the course of the sciatic nerve felt at the base of the spine, down the thigh, and radiating down the leg, because of a compressed nerve
syncope SĬN-kō-pē	fainting
vasovagal văs-ō-VĀ-găl	sudden fainting due to a drop in blood pressure brought on by the response of the nervous system to abrupt emotional stress, pain, or trauma
transient ischemic attack (TIA) TRĂN-zē-ĕnt ĭs-KĒ-mĭk	temporary interference with blood supply to the brain lasting from a few minutes to a few hours

DIAGNOSTIC PROCEDURES

Imaging Procedures

Imaging Procedure	Description
cerebral angiography, cerebral arteriography	visualization of the cerebrovascular system after injection of radiopaque dye into the carotid or vertebral artery to visualize abnormalities of the cerebrovascular circulation, vascular tumors, aneurysms, and occlusions. Abscesses, nonvascular tumors, and hematomas are often identified because they distort the normal vascular image
echoencephalography	ultrasound technique used to study the intracranial structures of the brain and especially to diagnose conditions that cause a shift in the midline structures of the brain
electroencephalography (EEG)	recording of electric activity in the brain by placing electrodes on the skull; produces graphic tracing called an electroencephalogram
electromyography	graphic recording of muscle contractions as a result of electrical stimulation
myelography	radiography of the spinal cord after injection of a contrast medium
tomography (cranial)	procedure that provides a three-dimensional visual "slice" of an organ or structure by blurring out material above and below the plane to be examined; helps to differentiate intracranial pathologies such as tumors, cysts, edema, hemorrhage, and cerebral aneurysms
computed (CT scan)	a cross-sectional transverse plane of an organ or structure, produced as an image generated by computer analysis
positron emission (PET) scan	a cross-sectional transverse plane that identifies metabolic and physiological function in tissues. The image is formed by computer analysis of data transmitted by positron-emitting radionuclides. These radioactive substances emit positrons, which form images of the brain. They measure regional cerebral blood flow, blood volume, oxygen uptake, and glucose transport and metabolism and locate neurotransmitter receptors. The images that are produced are in colors that indicate the degree of metabolism or blood flow. The highest rates appear red, those lower appear yellow, then green and the lowest rates appear blue (Fig. 15–8)

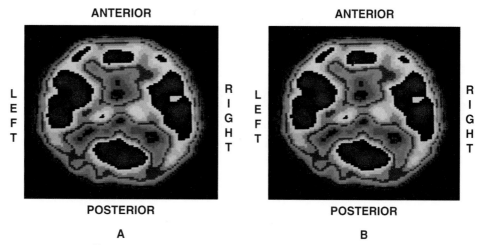

ANTERIOR   ANTERIOR

LEFT   RIGHT   LEFT   RIGHT

POSTERIOR   POSTERIOR

A   B

Figure 15–8 PET scan of brain. Transverse section in (A) normal young patient, (B) normal aging patient. (From Mazziotta, JC, and Gilman, S: Brain Imaging: Principles and Applications. Oxford University Press, Oxford, 1992, p 1964, with permission.)

SURGICAL AND THERAPEUTIC PROCEDURES

Procedure	Description
cryosurgery krī-ō-SĔR-jĕr-ē	technique of exposing tissues to extreme cold, sometimes used to destroy portions of the brain (e.g., the thalamus)
spinal puncture, spinal tap, CSF analysis	needle puncture of the spinal cavity to extract spinal fluid for diagnostic purposes, to introduce anesthetic agents into the spinal canal, or to remove fluid to allow other fluids (e.g., radiopaque substances) to be injected
stereotaxy STĔR-ē-ō-tăk-sē	precise method of locating and destroying deep-seated brain structures using three-dimensional coordinates generated by CT scan
thalamotomy thăl-ă-MŎT-ō-mē	partial destruction of the thalamus to treat psychosis or intractable pain
tractotomy trăk-TŎT-ō-mē	transection of a nerve tract in the brainstem or spinal cord, sometimes used to relieve intractable pain
trephination trĕf-ĭn-Ā-shŭn	cutting a circular opening into the skull to reveal brain tissue and decrease intracranial pressure
vagotomy vă-GŎT-ō-mē	interruption of the function of the vagus nerve to relieve peptic ulcer

PHARMACOLOGY

Medication	Action
analgesics	reduce or relieve pain (e.g., aspirin, codeine, morphine)
anticonvulsants	prevent or reduce the severity of epileptic or other convulsive seizures
antidepressants	alleviate mental depression
hypnotics	induce sleep or hypnosis
opiates	narcotic drugs that contain opium or its derivatives; used as an analgesic, as a hypnotic, and to control diarrhea and spasmodic conditions; also elevate mood and relieve tension and anxiety
psychotropic drugs	alter psychic function, behavior, or experience; often used in management of psychotic disorders
sedatives	exert a soothing or tranquilizing effect by depressing CNS activity; tend to cause lassitude and reduced mental activity
tranquilizers	calm anxiety or agitation, without decreasing level of consciousness

ABBREVIATIONS

Abbreviation	Term
ALS	amyotrophic lateral sclerosis
ANS	autonomic nervous system
AVMs	arteriovenous malformations
CNS	central nervous system
CP	cerebral palsy
CSF	cerebrospinal fluid
CT scan, CAT scan	computed tomography scan, computed axial tomography scan
CVA	cerebrovascular accident
CVD	cerebrovascular disease

ABBREVIATIONS (Continued)

Abbreviation	Term
EEG	electroencephalogram
EMG	electromyogram
HNP	herniated nucleus pulposus (herniated disk)
ICP	intracranial pressure
LP	lumbar puncture
MRI	magnetic resonance imaging
MS	multiple sclerosis
PET	positron emission tomography
PNS	peripheral nervous system
R/O	rule out
RT	radiation therapy
SAH	subarachnoid hemorrhage
SNS	somatic nervous system
TIA	transient ischemic attack

MEDICAL RECORD

Subarachnoid Hemorrhage

History of Present Illness   The patient is a 61-year-old woman with a history of developing sudden onset of "extremely severe headaches" while swimming. She had associated neck pain, occipital pain, nausea, and vomiting.

A CT scan was obtained that showed blood in the cisterna subarachnoidalis consistent with subarachnoid hemorrhage. The patient also had mild acute hydrocephalus. Neurologically, the patient was found to be within normal limits. A cerebral angiogram was performed and no aneurysm was noted. The patient was hospitalized on 7/5/xx. On 7/7/xx, she had sudden worsening of her headache associated with nausea and vomiting. Also, she was noted to have meningismus on examination. A lumbar puncture was performed in order R/O possible rebleed. At the time of the lumbar puncture, CSF in four tubes was read as consistent with recurrent subarachnoid hemorrhage. An MRI was performed without evidence of an aneurysm.

Disposition   On 7/16/xx, the patient underwent repeat angiogram, which again showed no aneurysm. The patient was deemed stable for discharge on 7/16/xx.

Activity   She was instructed to avoid any type of activity that could result in raised pressure in the head (i.e., Valsalva's maneuvers associated with constipation, coughing, sneezing, or vomiting). The patient was advised that she should undergo no activity more vigorous than walking.

Discharge Diagnosis   Subarachnoid hemorrhage.

Worksheet 5 provides a dictionary and reading application and an analysis of this medical record.

WORKSHEET 1

■ ■ ■ ■ ■ ■ ■ ■ ■ ■ ■ ■ ■

*Use **encephal/o** (brain) to build a medical word meaning:*

1. disease of the brain _____

2. herniation of the brain _____

*Use **cerebr/o** (cerebrum) to build a medical word meaning:*

3. pertaining to the cerebrum and spinal cord _____

4. abnormal condition of hardening of the cerebrum _____

5. disease of the cerebrum _____

*Use **crani/o** (cranium, skull) to build a medical word meaning:*

6. herniation (through the) cranium _____

7. softening of the cranium _____

8. condition of hardening of the skull _____

9. instrument for measuring the skull _____

*Use **neur/o** (nerve) to build a medical word meaning:*

10. embryonic nerve (cell) _____

11. nerve pain _____

12. specialist in the study of the nervous system _____

*Use **myel/o** (spinal cord) to build a medical word meaning:*

13. radiograph of the spinal cord _____

14. herniation of the spinal cord _____

15. paralysis of the spinal cord _____

*Use **mening/o** (meninges) to build a medical word meaning:*

16. herniation of the meninges _____

17. herniation of the meninges and spinal cord _____

*Use the suffix **-plegia** (paralysis) to build a medical word meaning:*

18. paralysis of one half (of the body) _____

19. paralysis of four (limbs) _____

Use the suffix -lepsy (seizure) to build a medical word meaning:

20. seizure of sleep _____

Use the suffix -algesia (pain) to build a medical word meaning:

21. without pain _____

Use the suffix -phasia (speech) to build a medical word meaning:

22. difficult speech _____

23. lacking or without speech _____

Use the suffix -trophy (nourishment) to build a medical word meaning:

24. excessive nourishment _____

25. lacking nourishment _____

WORKSHEET 2

■ ■ ■ ■ ■ ■ ■ ■ ■ ■ ■ ■ ■ ■

Build a surgical term meaning:

1. destruction of a nerve _____

2. incision of the skull _____

3. surgical repair of the skull _____

4. suture of a nerve _____

5. incision of the brain _____

6. incision of the thalamus _____

WORKSHEET 3

■ ■ ■ ■ ■ ■ ■ ■ ■ ■ ■ ■ ■

Match the following medical words with the definitions in the numbered list.

asthenia   herpes zoster   poliomyelitis
aura   Huntington's chorea   Reye's syndrome
coma   lethargy   syncope
concussion   paraplegia   TIA

1. _____ head injury resulting from an impact with an object

2. _____ acute infectious disease of posterior root ganglia by same organism responsible for chickenpox in children

3. _____ inherited disease of the CNS, characterized by quick involuntary movements, speech disturbances, and mental deterioration

4. _____ premonitory awareness of an approaching mental disorder; the peculiar sensation that precedes an epileptic seizure

5. _____ paralysis of the lower portion of the trunk and both legs

6. _____ inflammation of the gray matter of spinal cord often resulting in muscle deformity and paralysis

7. _____ temporary interference with blood supply to the brain

8. _____ acute encephalopathy seen in children, often associated with the use of aspirin to relieve symptoms of chickenpox, influenza

9. _____ sluggishness, abnormal inactivity, or lack of response to normal stimuli

10. _____ weakness or debility

WORKSHEET 4

■ ■ ■ ■ ■ ■ ■ ■ ■ ■ ■ ■ ■

Match the following medical words with the definitions in the numbered list.

analgesic   echoencephalography   spinal puncture

cerebral angiography   electromyography   tranquilizer

CT scan (cranial)   myelography   trephination

cryosurgery   positron emission tomography vagotomy

1. _____ visualization of the cerebrovascular system after injection of a radiopaque dye into the vertebral or carotid artery

2. _____ technique of destroying tissue by exposure to extreme cold; frequently used in brain surgery

3. _____ surgical procedure to create a circular opening into the skull

4. _____ needle puncture to extract spinal fluid for diagnostic purposes or to introduce an anesthetic

5. _____ graphic recording of muscular contraction owing to electrical stimulation

6. _____ medication that reduces or relieves pain

7. _____ calms anxiousness or agitation without decreasing level of consciousness

8. _____ produces cross-sectional images of brain by using radioactive substances to measure blood flow and blood volume and locate neurotransmitter receptors

9. _____ provides a three-dimensional visual "slice" of the cranial contents that helps differentiate intracranial pathologies

10. _____ ultrasound technique used to study the intracranial structures of the brain, especially a shift in the midline structures of the brain

WORKSHEET 5

■ ■ ■ ■ ■ ■ ■ ■ ■ ■ ■ ■ ■ ■

MEDICAL RECORD: SUBARACHNOID HEMORRHAGE

Underline the following terms in the medical record (see p. 309). Use a medical dictionary and other resources to define the terms and to determine their pronunciation; then practice reading the medical record aloud.

aneurysm _____

angiogram _____

cerebral angiogram _____

cisterna subarachnoidalis _____

CSF _____

CT scan _____

hydrocephalus _____

lumbar puncture _____

meningismus _____

MRI _____

occipital _____

R/O _____

subarachnoid hemorrhage _____

Valsalva's maneuver _____

MEDICAL RECORD EVALUATION: SUBARACHNOID HEMORRHAGE

1. *In what part of the head did the patient feel pain?*

2. *List the radiological tests performed on the patient and the finding each provided.*

3. *How does meningismus differ from meningitis?*

4. *Did the lumbar puncture rule out or confirm a second subarachnoid hemorrhage?*

5. *Which two tests ruled out an aneurysm?*

6. *What is the Valsalva's maneuver?*

WORKSHEET 6

■ ■ ■ ■ ■ ■ ■ ■ ■ ■ ■ ■ ■

Label the following diagram. Check your answers by referring to Figure 15–5.

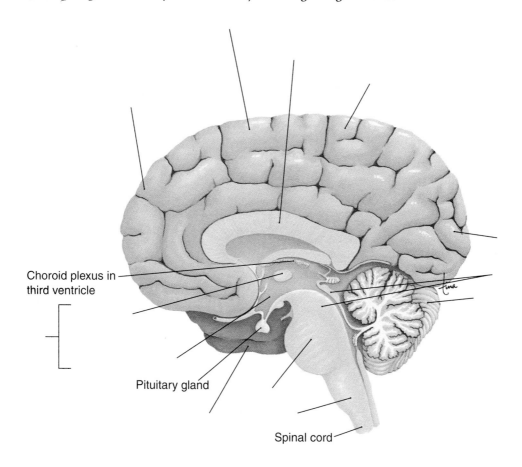

Choroid plexus in third ventricle

Pituitary gland

Spinal cord

Cerebellum	Hypothalamus	Parietal lobe
Cerebrum	Medulla	Pons
Corpus callosum	Midbrain	Temporal lobe
Diencephalon	Occipital lobe	Thalamus
Frontal lobe		

Chapter 16

SPECIAL SENSES

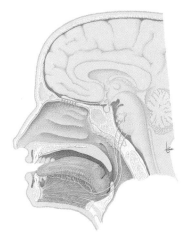

Chapter Outline

Student Objectives

Anatomy and Physiology
The Eye
The Ear
Hearing
Equilibrium

Combining Forms

Suffixes

Prefixes

Pathology
Errors of Refraction
Cataracts
Glaucoma
Strabismus
Macular Degeneration

Otitis Media
Otosclerosis
Oncology

Diagnostic, Symptomatic, and Therapeutic Terms

Diagnostic Procedures
Endoscopic Procedures
Imaging Procedures
Clinical Procedures

Surgical and Therapeutic Procedures

Pharmacology

Abbreviations

Medical Record
Operative Report

Worksheets

Student Objectives

Upon completion of this chapter, you will be able to do the following:

1. Identify major structures and functions of the eye.
2. List and describe accessory structures associated with the eye.
3. Identify major structures and functions of the ear.
4. Explain the physiology of hearing.
5. Describe the structures and functions of the ear related to the sense of equilibrium.
6. Identify combining forms, suffixes, and prefixes related to the eye and ear.
7. Identify and discuss pathology related to the eye and ear.
8. Identify diagnostic, symptomatic, and surgical terms related to the eye and ear.
9. Identify diagnostic procedures related to the eye and ear.
10. Identify surgical and therapeutic procedures related to the eye and ear.
11. Discuss pharmacology related to the treatment of eye and ear disorders.
12. Define abbreviations related to the eye and ear.
13. Demonstrate your knowledge of the chapter by completing the worksheets.

ANATOMY AND PHYSIOLOGY

The special senses include taste, smell, sight, hearing, and equilibrium. The senses of taste and smell have been covered in previous chapters. This chapter presents information on the eye, the sense organ for sight, and the ear, the sense organ for hearing and equilibrium.

The Eye

The eye (Fig. 16–1) is a globe-shaped organ composed of three distinct layers. Its outermost layer, the (1) **sclera**, is a tough fibrous tissue that serves as a protective shield for more sensitive structures beneath. The sclera is also known as the white of the eye. A membrane, the (2) **conjunctiva**, lines the eyelids and is reflected onto the eyeball. A highly vascular middle layer, the (3) **choroid**, provides the blood supply for the entire eye. It contains pigmented cells that prevent extraneous light from entering the inside of the eye. The innermost layer of the eye, the (4) **retina**, is composed of nerve endings that are responsible for the reception and transmission of light impulses.

A specialized portion of the sclera, the (5) **cornea**, passes in front of the (6) **lens**. Rather than being opaque, the cornea is transparent, allowing light to enter the interior of the eye. The cornea is one of the few body structures that does not contain capillaries.

The lens is a crystalline structure held between the (7) **ciliary body (muscles)** by the (8) **suspensory ligaments**. As these muscles relax or contract, they alter the shape of the lens, making it thicker or thinner. This enables light rays to focus on the retina, a process called **accommodation**.

One of two major fluids (humors) of the eye is **aqueous humor**. It is found in the (9) **anterior cavity** and provides nourishment for the lens and the cornea. Aqueous humor is continually produced by the ciliary body and is drained from the eye by way of a small opening called the

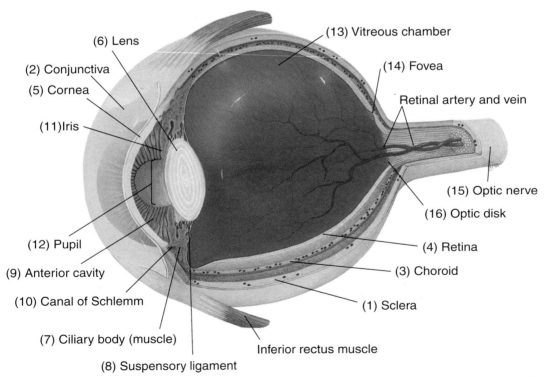

Figure 16–1   Internal anatomy of the eyeball. (From Scanlon, VC, and Sanders, T: Understanding Human Structure and Function. F.A. Davis, Philadelphia, 1997, p 164, with permission.)

(10) **canal of Schlemm**. If aqueous humor fails to drain from the eye at the rate at which it is produced, a condition called glaucoma results.

A colored contractile membrane, the (11) **iris**, functions as a sphincter. Its perforated center is the (12) **pupil**. By changing its size, the pupil regulates the amount of light entering the eye. As environmental light increases, the pupil constricts; as light decreases, the pupil dilates.

The second major humor of the eye is **vitreous humor**, a jellylike substance that fills the entire (13) **vitreous chamber**. The vitreous humor, lens, and aqueous humor are the refractive structures of the eye. They bend light rays, focusing them sharply on the retina. If any one of these structures does not function properly, vision is impaired.

The retina is an extremely delicate eye membrane. It is continuous with the optic nerve and has two types of visual receptors, **rods** and **cones**. Rods function in dim light, producing black-and-white vision. Cones function in bright light, producing color vision. The (14) **fovea** is in the center of the retina. All of its receptors are cones that lie very close to each other. It provides the greatest acuity for color vision. When the eye focuses on an object, light rays from that object are directed to the fovea.

Rods and cones contain chemicals called **photopigments**. As light strikes the photopigments, a chemical change occurs that stimulates rods and cones. The impulses they produce are transmitted through the (15) **optic nerve** to the brain, where they are interpreted as vision.

Both the optic nerve and blood vessels of the eye enter the eyeball at the (16) **optic disc**. Its center is referred to as the **blind spot** because the area has neither rods nor cones.

Six muscles control the movement of the eye: the superior, inferior, lateral, and medial rectus muscles and the superior and inferior oblique muscles. These muscles are coordinated to move both eyes in a synchronized manner.

Refer to Figure 16–2 as you read the following paragraphs.

Two movable folds of skin constitute the eyelids, each with eyelashes that protect the front of the eye. A thin mucous membrane called the (1) **conjunctiva** lines the inner surface of the eyelids and the cornea. Lying superior and to the outer edge of each eye are the (2) **lacrimal glands**, which produce tears that bathe and lubricate the eyes. The tears collect at the inner edges of the eyes, the **canthi** (singular, **canthus**), and pass through pinpoint openings, the (3) **lacrimal canals**, to the mucous membranes that line the inside of the (4) **nasal cavity**.

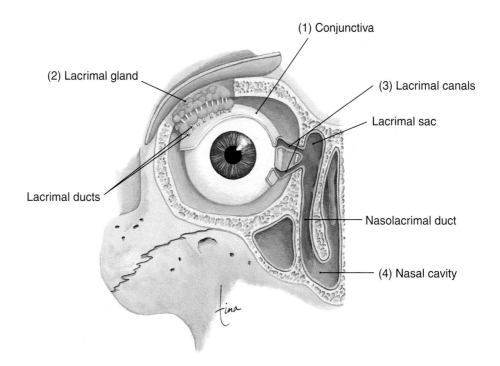

Figure 16–2 Lacrimal apparatus shown in an anterior view of the right eye. (From Scanlon, VC, and Sanders, T: Understanding Human Structure and Function. F.A. Davis, Philadelphia, 1997, p 162, with permission.)

The Ear

The ear is the sense organ receptor for hearing and equilibrium. Hearing is a function of the cochlea, whereas the semicircular canals and vestibule control equilibrium.

Hearing

The ear consists of three major sections: the outer or **external ear**, the middle ear or **tympanic cavity**, and the inner ear or **labyrinth**. Each of these sections transmits sound waves, but in different ways. The external ear conducts sound waves through air; the middle ear, through bone; and the inner ear, through fluid. This series of transmissions plays an integral part in hearing.

Refer to Figure 16–3 and identify the following structures associated with hearing.

An (1) **auricle** (or **pinna**) collects waves traveling through air and channels them to the (2) **external auditory meatus** (ear canal). This canal is a slender tube lined with glands that produce a waxy secretion called **cerumen**. Its stickiness prevents tiny foreign particles from entering the deeper areas of the canal. A flat membranous structure, the (3) **tympanic membrane** (**tympanum**, or eardrum), is drawn over the end of the ear canal. Sound waves that enter the ear canal strike against the tympanum, causing it to vibrate. Three tiny articulating bones called ossicles, located in the middle ear, pick up the tympanic vibrations. These bones, the (4) **malleus** (hammer), the (5) **incus** (anvil), and the (6) **stapes** (stirrups), are responsible for transmitting sound waves through the middle ear. These ossicles form a chain that stretches from the inner surface of the tympanum to a snail-shaped structure, the (7) **cochlea**, located in the inner ear. The cochlea is filled with fluid. Lining its inner surface are tiny nerve endings called the **hairs of Corti**.

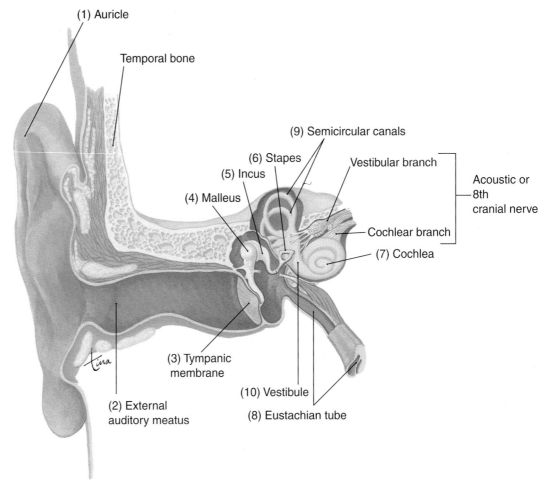

Figure 16–3   Outer, middle, and inner ear structures as shown in a frontal section through the right temporal bone. (From Scanlon, VC, and Sanders, T: Understanding Human Structure and Function. F.A. Davis, Philadelphia, 1997, p 169, with permission.)

A membrane-covered opening on the external surface of the cochlea, the **oval window**, is the place of attachment for the stapes. Transmission of sound along the ossicles in the middle ear causes the stapes to exert a gentle pumping action against the oval window. The pumping action forces the cochlear fluid to move. Disturbance of the fluid stimulates the hairs of Corti, generating impulses that are transmitted to the brain by way of the auditory nerve, where they are interpreted as sound.

The (8) **eustachian tube** connects the middle ear to the pharynx. Its purpose is to equalize pressure on the outer and inner surfaces of the eardrum. When sudden pressure changes occur, pressure can be equalized on either side of the tympanic membrane by deliberately swallowing.

Equilibrium

Besides the cochlea, the inner ear contains the (9) **semicircular canals** and the (10) **vestibule**. The vestibule joins the cochlea and the semicircular canals. The inner ear is sometimes referred to as the labyrinth because of its complicated mazelike design. Complex structures located in this maze are responsible for maintaining a sense of equilibrium. Both **static** and **dynamic equilibrium** are provided by these structures. Static equilibrium refers to the orientation of the body relative to gravity. It allows an individual to maintain posture and orientation while at rest. Dynamic equilibrium refers to maintaining body position in response to movement.

COMBINING FORMS

Combining Form	Meaning	Example	Pronunciation
Eye			
ambly/o	dull, dim	ambly/opia vision	ăm-blē-Ō-pē-ă
aque/o	water	aque/ous pertaining to	Ā-kwē-ŭs

blephar/o	eyelid	blephar/o/ptosis
		    prolapse, downward
		    displacement
			blĕf-ă-rō-TŌ-sĭs

choroid/o	choroid	choroid/o/pathy disease	kō-roy-DŎP-ă-thē
corne/o	cornea, horny tissue	corne/itis inflammation	kor-nē-Ī-tĭs
kerat/o		kerat/o/meter instrument for measuring	kĕr-ă-TŎM-ĕ-tĕr
cycl/o	ciliary body	cycl/o/plegia paralysis	sī-klō-PLĒ-jē-ă
dacry/o	tear, lacrimal sac	dacry/o/genic producing	dăk-rē-ō-JĔN-ĭk
dacryocyst/o	tear sac, lacrimal sac	dacryocyst/o/cele hernia, swelling	dăk-rē-ō-SĬS-tō-sēl
irid/o	iris	irid/o/plegia paralysis	ĭr-ĭd-ō-PLĒ-jē-ă
ocul/o	eye	ocul/o/nas/ al nose pertaining to	ŏk-ū-lō-NĀ-săl
ophthalm/o		ophthalm/o/logist specialist in the study (of)	ŏf-thăl-MŎL-ō-jĭst
opt/o	vision, eye	opt/ic pertaining to	ŎP-tĭk

COMBINING FORMS (Continued)

Combining Form	Meaning	Example	Pronunciation
phac/o	lens	phac/o/cele herniation	FĂK-ō-sēl
presby/o	old age	presby/opia vision	prĕz-bē-Ō-pē-ă
core/o		core/o/plasty surgical repair	KŌ-rē-ō-plăs-tē
pupill/o	pupil	pupill/o/scopy examination	pū-pĭl-ŎS-kō-pē
retin/o	retina	retin/o/pathy disease	rĕt-ĭn-ŎP-ă-thē
scler/o	sclera, hardening	scler/ectomy excision	sklĕ-RĔK-tō-mē
Ear			
audi/o	hearing	audi/o/logy study of	aw-dē-ŎL-ō-jē
labyrinth/o	labyrinth, inner ear	labyrinth/itis inflammation	lăb-ĭ-rĭn-THĪ-tĭs
ot/o	ear	ot/o/rrhea discharge	ō-tō-RĒ-ă
salping/o	eustachian tube, oviduct	salping/itis inflammation	săl-pĭn-JĪ-tĭs
staped/o	stapes	staped/ectomy excision	stā-pĕ-DĔK-tō-mē
myring/o		myring/o/tomy incision	mĭr-ĭn-GŎT-ō-mē
tympan/o	tympanic membrane, eardrum	tympan/o/centesis puncture	tĭm-pă-nō-sĕn-TĒ-sĭs

SUFFIXES

Suffix	Meaning	Example	Pronunciation
-opia	vision	dipl/opia double	dĭp-LŌ-pē-ă
-tropia	turning	hyper/tropia excessive	hī-pĕr-TRŌ-pē-ă

PREFIXES

Prefix	Meaning	Example	Pronunciation
eso-	inward	eso/tropia turning	ĕs-ō-TRŌ-pē-ă
exo-	outside, outward	exo/trop/ ic turning pertaining to	ĕks-ō-TRŌ-pĭk

PATHOLOGY

Errors of Refraction

An error of refraction, also called **ametropia**, exists when light rays fail to focus sharply on the retina. This may be due to a defect in the lens, cornea, or the shape of the eyeball. If the eyeball is too long, the image falls in front of the retina, causing nearsightedness, or **myopia** (Fig. 16–4). Correction is made using a concave lens. In farsightedness (**hyperopia, hypermetropia**), which is the opposite of myopia, the eyeball is too short and the image falls behind the retina. A form of farsightedness is **presbyopia**, a defect associated with the aging process. The onset usually

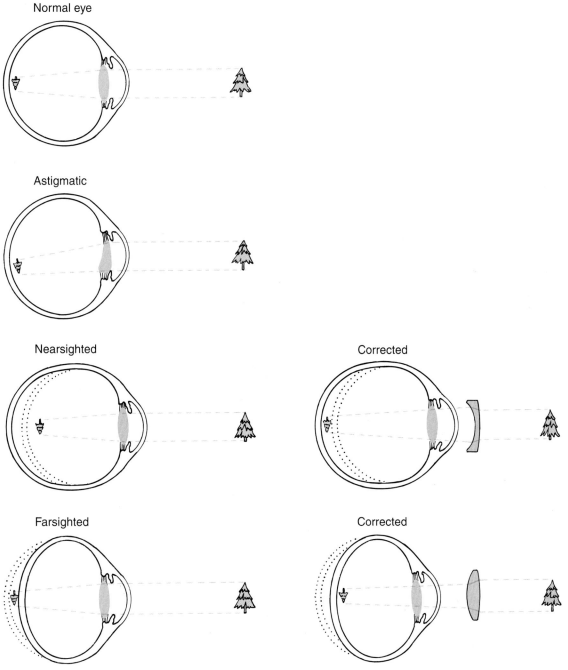

Figure 16–4   Refraction in the eye. The normal eye focuses light rays on the retina. Errors of refraction include astigmatism, nearsightedness, and farsightedness. (From Scanlon, VC, and Sanders, T: Understanding Human Structure and Function. F.A. Davis, Philadelphia, 1997, p 167, with permission.)

occurs between 40 and 45 years of age. The individual can see distant objects clearly but cannot see near objects in proper focus. Correction involves the use of a convex lens.

In another form of ametropia called **astigmatism**, the cornea or lens has a defective curvature. This causes light rays to diffuse over a large area of the retina, rather than being focused sharply on a given point. Corrective lenses that compensate for the imperfect curvature of the cornea or lens are used for astigmatism.

Cataracts

Cataracts are opacities that form on the lens or on the capsule containing the lens. These opacities are frequently produced by protein that slowly builds up until vision is lost. The only effective treatment is removal of the lens or capsule.

Several techniques may be employed for cataract removal. In one method, a super-cooled metal probe (**cryoprobe**) is placed on the cataract. The cataract bonds to the cold probe, and the cataract and lens are gently lifted from the eye. This method of treatment is known as **intracapsular extraction**. It is usually the method of choice when the cataract develops as a result of old age (**senescent** or **senile cataract**).

Cataracts found in children are usually a result of genetic defects or maternal rubella during the first trimester of pregnancy. In children and young adults, the surgery of choice is **extracapsular extraction**. Both the cortex and lens are removed, but the posterior lens capsule is retained.

In **phacoemulsification**, the capsule is fragmented using ultrasonic vibrations. Prognosis is good in most patients, with vision improvement in 95 percent of all patients.

Glaucoma

Glaucoma is characterized by increased pressure within the eyeball (**intraocular pressure**) caused by the failure of aqueous humor to drain from the eye through a tiny duct called the canal of Schlemm. The increased pressure on the optic nerve destroys it, and vision is permanently lost.

Medications that cause the pupils to constrict (**miotics**) permit aqueous humor to escape from the eye, thereby relieving pressure. If miotics are ineffective, surgery may be necessary. Surgery for glaucoma includes **paracentesis** of the cornea, excision of a small portion of the iris (**partial iridectomy**), and separation of the iris from its attachment (**iridodialysis, coredialysis**).

Glaucoma is diagnosed by using an instrument that measures the internal pressure of the eye (**tonometer**). This procedure should be performed in all patients older than 35 years of age during routine eye examinations.

Strabismus

Strabismus is a condition in which the eyes turn from the normal position so that they deviate in different directions (Fig. 16–5). If the eyes turn outward (**exotropia**), causing a divergent

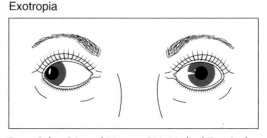

Esotropia   Exotropia

Figure 16–5   Strabismus: esotropia (left); exotropia (right). (From Gylys, BA, and Masters, RM: Medical Terminology Simplified: A Programmed Learning Approach by Body Systems, ed 2. F.A. Davis, Philadelphia, 1998, p 439, with permission.)

squint, the individual is said to be wall-eyed. If the eyes turn toward each other (**esotropia**), causing a convergent squint, the individual is said to be cross-eyed. Strabismus may be due to poor vision, unequal ocular muscle tone, or an oculomotor nerve lesion.

In children, strabismus is associated with "lazy eye syndrome" (**amblyopia**). Vision is suppressed in one eye so that the child uses only the other eye for vision. The suppression of vision in the "lazy" eye is usually due to extreme nearsightedness (**unilateral myopia**) or double vision that develops because of strabismus.

Methods of treatment include corrective lenses, eye exercises to correct vision (**orthoptic training**), and surgery (**strabotomy**) in which the ocular tendons are cut.

Macular Degeneration

Macular degeneration is the deterioration of the macula of the retina. The macula is much more sensitive to visual detail than any other portion of the retina. It is responsible for central, or straight ahead vision required for reading, driving, detail work, and recognizing faces. Although deterioration of the macula is associated with the toxic effects of some drugs, the most common type is age-related macular degeneration (ARMD or AMD). ARMD is a leading cause of visual loss in the United States.

Two forms of ARMD are identified: wet and dry. The less common, but more severe, form is wet or **neovascular** ARMD. It affects about 10 percent of those afflicted with the disease. Small blood vessels form under the macula. Blood and other fluids leak from these vessels and destroy the visual cells, leading to permanent visual loss. If identified in its early stages, laser surgery can be employed to destroy the new forming vessels. This treatment is called laser **photocoagulation**. It proves successful in about one half of the patients with wet ARMD.

The more common form of the disease is dry ARMD. Small yellow patches called **drusen** develop on the macula and interfere with central vision. Although some vision is lost, this disease rarely leads to total blindness. Patients with this disorder are encouraged to see their ophthalmologist frequently and perform a simple at-home test that identifies visual changes that may indicate the development of the more serious neovascular ARMD.

Otitis Media

Otitis media is an inflammation of the middle ear. It is found most commonly in infants and young children, especially in the presence of an upper respiratory infection (URI). Symptoms may include earache, draining of pus from the ear (**otopyorrhea**), or rupturing of the eardrum (**tympanorrhexis, myringorrhexis**). Treatment consists of bedrest, medications to relieve pain (**analgesics**), and antibiotics. Occasionally, an incision of the eardrum (**myringotomy, tympanotomy**) may be necessary to relieve pressure and to promote draining of pus from the middle ear.

Recurrent episodes of otitis media may cause scarring of the tympanic membrane, leading to hearing loss. Treatment in children involves the placing of pressure-equalizing tubes through the tympanic membrane. This helps to drain fluid from the middle ear. If left untreated, otitis media may lead to infection of the mastoid process (**mastoiditis**) or inflammation of brain tissue near the middle ear (**otoencephalitis**).

Otosclerosis

Otosclerosis is characterized by an abnormal hardening (**ankylosis**) of spongy bone around the oval window. This decreases the ability of the stapes to move the oval window, causing hearing loss. Occasionally, the individual perceives a ringing sound (**tinnitus**) within the ear. Surgical correction involves the removal of the stapes (**stapedectomy**) and reconstruction of the oval window.

Oncology

Two major neoplastic diseases account for more than 90 percent of all primary intraocular diseases: **retinoblastoma**, found primarily in children, and **melanoma**, found primarily in adults.

Most retinoblastomas tend to be familial. The cell involved is the retinal neuron. Vision is impaired, and in about 30 percent of the patients, the disease is found in both eyes **(bilateral)**. Treatment usually involves the removal of the affected eye(s) **(enucleation)**, followed by radiation.

Intraorbital melanoma frequently arises in the pigmented cells of the choroid. Sometimes, however, it may originate in the iris or ciliary body. The disease is usually asymptomatic until there is a hemorrhage into the anterior chamber. Any discrete, fleshy mass on the iris should be examined by an ophthalmologist. If malignancy occurs in the choroid, it usually appears as a brown or gray mushroom-shaped lesion. If the lesion is on the iris, an iridectomy is performed. For melanoma of the choroid, enucleation is necessary. Many eye tumors are noninvasive and are not necessarily life-threatening.

DIAGNOSTIC, SYMPTOMATIC, AND THERAPEUTIC TERMS

Term	Meaning
Eye	
achromatopsia ă-krō-mă-TŎP-sē-ă	severe congenital deficiency in color perception; complete color blindness
adnexa	accessory parts of a structure
ocular	the structures surrounding the eye, including the extraocular muscles, orbit, eyelids, conjunctiva, and lacrimal system
chalazion kă-LĀ-zē-ōn	meibomian cyst; steatoma; a small hard tumor developing on the eyelid, somewhat similar to a sebaceous cyst
conjunctivitis kŏn-jŭnk-tĭ-VĪ-tĭs	inflammation of the conjunctiva with vascular congestion, producing a red or pink eye; may be secondary to viral, chlamydial, bacterial, or fungal infections or allergy
convergence kŏn-VĔR-jĕns	medial movement of the two eyeballs so that they are both directed at the object being viewed
ectropion ĕk-TRŌ-pē-ŏn	eversion of the edge of the eyelid
entropion ĕn-TRŌ-pē-ŏn	inversion or turning inward of the edge of the lower eyelid
epiphora ĕ-PĬF-ō-ră	abnormal overflow of tears, sometimes because of obstruction of the tear ducts
exophthalmos ĕks-ŏf-THĂL-mŏs	protrusion of one or both eyeballs frequently caused by hyperactive thyroid, trauma, or tumors
hordeolum, sty hor-DĒ-ō-lŭm	a localized, circumscribed, inflammatory swelling of one of the several sebaceous glands of the eyelid, generally caused by a bacterial infection
metamorphopsia mĕt-ă-mor-FŎP-sē-ă	visual distortion of objects, often associated with errors of refraction, retinal disease, choroiditis, detachment of the retina, or tumors of the retina or choroid
nyctalopia nĭk-tă-LŌ-pē-ă	night blindness; an inability to see well in dim light. Frequently associated with vitamin A deficiency
nystagmus nĭs-TĂG-mŭs	involuntary eye movements that appear jerky
papilledema, choked disc păp-ĭl-ĕ-DĒ-mă	edema and hyperemia of the optic disc usually associated with increased ocular pressure resulting from intracranial pressure
photophobia	unusual intolerance and sensitivity to light. Occurs in diseases such as meningitis, inflammation of the eyes, measles, and rubella

DIAGNOSTIC, SYMPTOMATIC, AND THERAPEUTIC TERMS
(Continued)

Term	Meaning
retinopathy	any disorder of the retina
diabetic	retinal blood vessel disorder that occurs in patients with diabetes, manifested by small hemorrhages, edema, and formation of new vessels, leading to scarring and eventual loss of vision
trachoma trā-KŌ-mă	chronic contagious form of conjunctivitis found frequently in the southwestern states; often leads to blindness
visual field	area within which objects may be seen when the eye is fixed
Ear	
anacusis ăn-ă-KŪ-sĭs	deafness
conduction impairment kŏn-DŬK-shŭn	blocking of sound waves as they are conducted through the external and middle ear (conduction pathway)
labyrinthitis lăb-ĭ-rĭn-THĪ-tĭs	inflammation of the inner ear that usually results from an acute febrile process; may cause progressive vertigo
Ménière's disease mān-ē-ĀRZ	disorder of the labyrinth that leads to progressive loss of hearing, characterized by vertigo, sensorineural hearing loss, and tinnitus
otitis externa ō-TĪ-tĭs ĕks-TĔR-nă	infection of the external auditory canal
presbyacusia, presbycusis prĕz-bē-ă-KŪ-sē-ă, prĕs-bĭ-KŪ-sĭs	impairment of hearing resulting from old age
pressure-equalizing tubes (PE tubes)	tubes that are inserted through the tympanic membrane, often used in the treatment of chronic otitis media
tinnitus tĭn-Ī-tŭs	a subjective ringing or tinkling in the ears
vertigo VĔR-tĭ-gō	hallucination of movement; a feeling of spinning or dizziness

DIAGNOSTIC PROCEDURES

Procedure	Description
Eye	
gonioscopy gō-nē-ŎS-kō-pē	the examination of the angle of the anterior chamber of the eye in order to determine ocular motility and rotation
ophthalmoscopy ŏf-thăl-MŎS-kō-pē	visual examination of the interior of the eye using an ophthalmoscope; useful in detecting eye disorders as well as disorders of other organs that cause changes in the eye
retinoscopy rĕt-ĭn-ŎS-kō-pē	visual examination to evaluate refractive errors of the eye
Ear	
otoscopy ō-TŎS-kŏ-pē	visual examination of the external auditory canal and the tympanic membrane using an otoscope
pneumatic	a procedure that assesses the ability of the tympanic membrane to move in response to a change in air pressure. The fluctuation in air pressure causes movement of a normal tympanic membrane

Procedure	Description
Eye	
dacryocystography dăk-rē-ō-sĭs-TŎG-ră-fē	radiographic imaging procedures of the nasolacrimal (tear) glands and ducts
fluorescein angiography floo-ō-RĔS-ē-ĭn ăn-jē-ŎG-ră-fē	assesses blood vessels and their leakage in and beneath the retina by the injection of colored dye (i.e., diabetic retinopathy)
Ear	
eustachianography ū-STĀ-shĕn-ŏg-ră-fē	radiographic imaging procedure of the eustachian tube and the middle ear
tympanography tĭm-păn-ŎG-ră-fē	radiographic imaging procedure of the tympanic membrane and the middle ear

Procedure	Description
Eye	
electronystagmography ē-lĕk-trō-nĭs-tăg-MŎG-ră-fē	method of recording nystagmus activity by detecting the electrical activity of the extraocular muscles
tonometry tōn-ŎM-ĕ-trē	measurement of tension and pressure, especially of the eye for detection of glaucoma
visual acuity test ă-KŪ-ĭ-tē	part of an eye examination that evaluates the patient's ability to distinguish the form and detail of an object
Ear	
audiometry aw-dē-ŎM-ĕ-trē	measurement of the acuity of hearing for the various frequencies of sound waves

SURGICAL AND THERAPEUTIC PROCEDURES

Procedure	Description
Eye	
blepharectomy blĕf-ă-RĔK-tō-mē	excision of a lesion of the eyelid
blepharoplasty BLĔF-ă-rō-plăs-tē	cosmetic surgery that removes fatty tissue called "bags" above and below the eye, which frequently form as a result of the aging process
cyclodialysis sī-klō-dī-ĂL-ĭ-sĭs	formation of an opening between the anterior chamber and the suprachoroidal space for the draining of aqueous humor in glaucoma
enucleation ē-nū-klē-Ā-shŭn	removal of an organ or other mass intact from its supporting tissues; removal of the eyeball from the orbit
evisceration ē-vĭs-ĕr-Ā-shŭn	removal of the contents of the eye while leaving the sclera and cornea
keratocentesis kĕr-ă-tō-sĕn-TĒ-sĭs	surgical puncture of the cornea
keratotomy kĕr-ă-TŎT-ō-mē	incision of the cornea
radial	surgical treatment for nearsightedness. Hairline radial incisions of the outer portion of the cornea allows it to flatten, thus correcting nearsightedness
phacoemulsification făk-ō-ē-MŬL-sĭ-fĭ-kā-shŭn	method of treating cataracts by using ultrasonic waves to disintegrate the cataract, which is then aspirated and removed
sclerostomy sklĕ-RŎS-tō-mē	surgical formation of an opening in the sclera

SURGICAL AND THERAPEUTIC PROCEDURES (Continued)

Procedure	Description
Ear	
mastoid antrotomy MĂS-toyd ăn-TRŎT-ō-mē	surgical opening of a cavity within the mastoid process
myringoplasty, tympanoplasty mĭr-ĬN-gō-plăs-tē, tĭm-păn-ō-PLĂS-tē	reconstruction of the eardrum
otoplasty Ō-tō-plăs-tē	corrective surgery for a deformed or excessively large or small pinna

PHARMACOLOGY

Medication	Action
beta-adrenergics	agents that lower intraocular pressure by reducing the production of aqueous humor; used in treatment of glaucoma
cycloplegics	agents that paralyze the ciliary muscles, thereby dilating pupils; used to facilitate certain eye examinations
miotics	substances that constrict the pupils; used in treatment of glaucoma
mydriatics	agents that dilate the pupils. In certain eye diseases, the pupil must be dilated during treatment to prevent adhesions of the pupils

ABBREVIATIONS

Abbreviation	Term
Eye	
Acc	accommodation
ARMD, AMD	age-related macular degeneration
As, Ast, astig	astigmatism
D	diopter (lens strength)
EM, em	emmetropia
EENT	eyes, ears, nose, and throat
EOM	extraocular movement
IOP	intraocular pressure
mix astig	mixed astigmatism
OD	right eye (oculus dexter)
OS	left eye (oculus sinister)
OU	both eyes (oculi unitas); each eye (oculus uterque)
REM	rapid eye movement
ST	esotropia
VA	visual acuity
VF	visual field
XT	exotropia

ABBREVIATIONS (Continued)

Abbreviation	Term
Ear	
ABLB	alternate binaural loudness balance
ABR	auditory brainstem response
AC	air conduction
AD	right ear (auris dextra)
AS	left ear (auris sinistra)
AU	both ears (auris uterque)
PTS	permanent threshold shift
TTS	temporary threshold shift

MEDICAL RECORD

Operative Report

Preoperative Diagnosis   Foreign body, ears.

Postoperative Diagnosis   Foreign body, ears.

Procedure   Removal of foreign bodies from ears with placement of paper patches.

Anesthesia   General.

Operative Indications   The patient is a 9-year-old girl who presents with bilateral retained tympanostomy tubes. The tubes had been placed for more than 2.5 years.
     The risks and alternatives were explained to the mother, and she agreed to the surgery.

Operative Findings   Retained tympanostomy tubes, bilateral.

Operative Description   In the supine position under satisfactory general anesthesia via mask, the patient was draped in a routine fashion.
     The operating microscope was used to inspect the right ear. A previously placed tympanostomy tube was found to be in position and was surrounded with hard cerumen. The cerumen and the tube were removed, resulting in a very large perforation. The edges of the perforation were freshened sharply with a pick, and a paper patch was applied.

     Worksheet 5 provides a dictionary and reading application and an analysis of this medical record.

WORSHEET 1

Use **ophthalm/o** *(eye) to build a medical word meaning:*

1. paralysis of the eye _____

2. instrument to examine the eye _____

3. study of the eye _____

Use **pupill/o** *(pupil) to build a medical word meaning:*

4. examination of the pupil _____

5. instrument to measure the pupil _____

Use **kerat/o** *(cornea) to build a medical word meaning:*

6. instrument to incise the cornea _____

7. instrument for measuring the cornea _____

Use **scler/o** *(sclera) to build a medical word meaning:*

8. inflammation of the sclera _____

9. softening of the sclera _____

Use **irid/o** *(iris) to build a medical word meaning:*

10. paralysis of the iris _____

11. herniation of the iris _____

12. softening of the iris _____

Use **retin/o** *(retina) to build a medical word meaning:*

13. disease of the retina _____

14. inflammation of the retina _____

Use **blephar/o** *(eyelid) to build a medical word meaning:*

15. paralysis of the eyelid _____

16. inflammation of the eyelid and the conjunctiva _____

17. tumor of the gland of the eyelid _____

Use the suffix **-opia** *(vision) to build a medical word meaning:*

18. excessive (farsighted) vision _____

19. dim or dull vision _____

Use ot/o (ear) to build a medical word meaning:

20. pain in the ear _____

21. discharge from the ear _____

22. flow of pus from the ear _____

Use audi/o (hearing) to build a medical word meaning:

23. instrument for measuring hearing _____

24. study of hearing _____

Use myring/o (eardrum) to build a medical word meaning:

25. instrument for cutting the eardrum _____

WORKSHEET 2

■ ■ ■ ■ ■ ■ ■ ■ ■ ■ ■ ■

Build a surgical term meaning:

1. removal of the stapes _____

2. incision of the labyrinth _____

3. removal of the mastoid process _____

4. surgical repair of the eardrum _____

5. puncture of the eardrum _____

6. incision of the cornea _____

7. surgical repair of an ear (deformity) _____

8. suture of the eyelid _____

WORKSHEET 3

■ ■ ■ ■ ■ ■ ■ ■ ■ ■ ■ ■ ■

Match the following medical words with the definitions in the numbered list.

achromatopsia   hordeolum   nystagmus

anacusis   labyrinthitis   otitis externa

aphakia   metamorphopsia   spina bifida

exophthalmos   nyctalopia   visual field

1. _____ inflammatory swelling of one of the sebaceous glands of the eyelid

2. _____ inflammation of the inner ear; may cause progressive vertigo

3. _____ infection of the external auditory canal

4. _____ area within which objects may be seen when the eye is fixed

5. _____ deficiency in color perception; color blind

6. _____ deafness

7. _____ distortion of shapes

8. _____ night blindness

9. _____ protrusion of one or both eyes

10. _____ involuntary eye movement that appears jerky

WORKSHEET 4

■ ■ ■ ■ ■ ■ ■ ■ ■ ■ ■ ■ ■ ■

Match the following medical words with the definitions in the numbered list.

AD	electronystagmography	OD
ARMD	enucleation	OS
AS	evisceration	otoplasty
audiometry	mastoid antrotomy	otoscopy
cyclodialysis	miotics	phacoemulsification
cycloplegics	mydriatics	retinoscopy

1. _____ medications that dilate pupils

2. _____ formation of an opening in the anterior chamber for draining of aqueous humor

3. _____ deterioration of the macula, often associated with the aging process

4. _____ evaluating refractive errors of the eye by projecting a beam of light into the eye

5. _____ right ear

6. _____ right eye

7. _____ measurement of the acuity of hearing for various sound wave frequencies

8. _____ recording nystagmus activity by detecting the electrical activity of the extraocular muscles

9. _____ treating cataracts by disintegrating them using ultrasonic waves

10. _____ drugs that constrict the pupils

11. _____ visual examination of the external auditory canal and tympanic membrane

12. _____ removal of the eyeball

13. _____ removal of the contents of the eye while leaving the sclera and cornea intact

14. _____ paralyzes the ciliary muscles, thereby dilating the pupils; used to facilitate certain eye examinations

15. _____ corrective surgery for a deformed pinna

WORKSHEET 5

■ ■ ■ ■ ■ ■ ■ ■ ■ ■ ■ ■ ■

MEDICAL RECORD: OPERATIVE REPORT

Underline the following terms in the medical record (see p. 330). Use a medical dictionary and other resources to define the terms and to determine their pronunciation; then practice reading the medical record aloud.

cerumen _____

perforation _____

supine _____

tympanostomy _____

MEDICAL RECORD EVALUATION: OPERATIVE REPORT

1. *Did the patient's surgery involve one or both ears?*

2. *What was the nature of the foreign body in the patient's ears?*

3. *What ear structure was involved?*

4. *What type of anesthetic was administered?*

5. *In what position was the face during surgery?*

6. *What instrument was used to locate the tubes?*

7. *What was the material in which the tubes were embedded?*

8. *What injury was caused by the tubes?*

WORSHEET 6

Label the following diagram. Check your answers by referring to Figure 16–1.

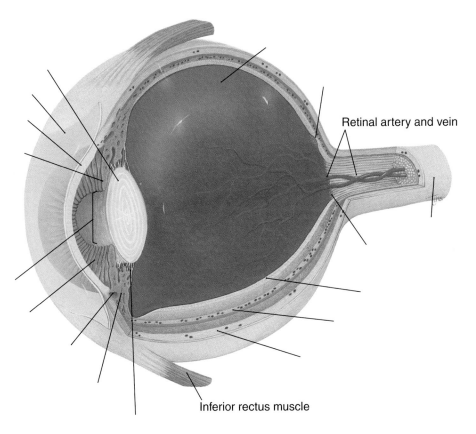

Retinal artery and vein

Inferior rectus muscle

Anterior cavity	Conjunctiva	Lens	Retina
Canal of Schlemm	Cornea	Optic disk	Sclera
Choroid	Fovea	Optic nerve	Suspensory ligament
Ciliary body (muscle)	Iris	Pupil	Vitreous chamber

WORSHEET 7

Label the following diagram. Check your answers by referring to Figure 16–3.

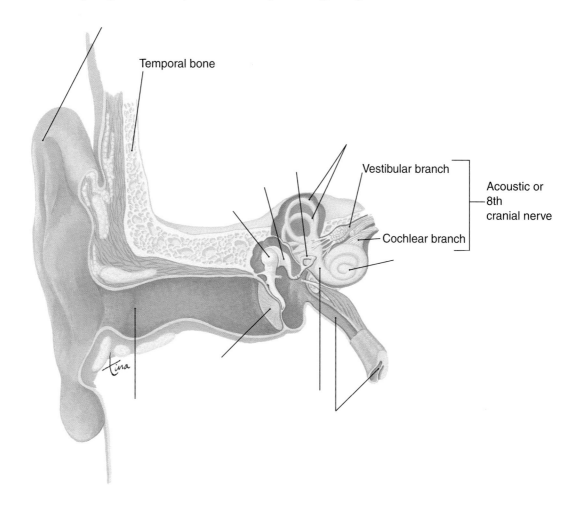

Temporal bone

Vestibular branch

Acoustic or
8th
cranial nerve

Cochlear branch

Auricle
Cochlea
Eustachian tube
External auditory meatus
Incus

Malleus
Semicircular canals
Stapes
Tympanic membrane
Vestibule

Appendix A

ANSWER KEY

Chapter 1 ▪ BASIC ELEMENTS OF A MEDICAL WORD

WORKSHEET 1

1. root, combining form, suffix, prefix.
2. teach.
3. False. A combining vowel is usually an "o."
4. True.
5. True.
6. False. A combining vowel is used before a suffix that begins with a consonant.
7. False. To define a medical word, first define the suffix or end of the word. Second, define the prefix or first part of the word. Last, define the middle of the word.

WORKSHEET 2

1. rhin/o
2. splen/o
3. hyster/o
4. enter/o
5. neur/o
6. ot/o
7. dermat/o
8. hydr/o
9. hepat/o
10. toxic/o

WORKSHEET 3

1. nephritis
2. arthrodesis
3. phlebotomy
4. dentist
5. gastrectomy
6. lumpectomy
7. hepatoma
8. cardi/o/logist
9. gastr/ia
10. therm/o/meter

WORKSHEET 4

3. cardi/o
4. oste/o
5. gastr/o
6. nephr/o
9. erythr/o
10. dent/o

NOTE: The rest of the elements listed in worksheets are word roots.

WORKSHEET 5

1. mast/o
2. hepat/o
3. arthr/o
4. cyst/o
5. phleb/o
6. thorac/o
7. abdomin/o
8. trache/o
9. leuk/o
10. gastr/o

Chapter 2 ▪ SUFFIXES: SURGICAL, DIAGNOSTIC, SYMPTOMATIC, AND RELATED

WORKSHEET 1

1. episiotomy
2. colectomy
3. arthrocentesis
4. splenectomy
5. colostomy
6. dermatome
7. tympanotomy
8. tracheostomy
9. mastectomy
10. lithotomy
11. hemorrhoidectomy
12. colostomy
13. colectomy
14. dermatome
15. arthrocentesis
16. lithotomy
17. mastectomy
18. tympanotomy
19. tracheostomy
20. splenectomy

WORKSHEET 2

1. arthrodesis
2. rhinoplasty
3. tenoplasty
4. myorrhaphy
5. mastopexy
6. cystorrhaphy
7. osteoclasis
8. lithotripsy
9. enterolysis
10. neurotripsy
11. rhinoplasty
12. arthrodesis
13. myorrhaphy
14. mastopexy
15. cystorrhaphy
16. tenoplasty
17. osteoclasis
18. lithotripsy
19. enterolysis
20. neurotripsy

WORKSHEET 3

1. bronchiectasis
2. gastrodynia
3. nephrosis
4. cholelith
5. carcinogen
6. psychology
7. osteomalacia
8. hepatomegaly
9. cholelithiasis
10. thermometer
11. hepatocele
12. lipoid
13. neuropathy
14. dermatosis
15. hemiplegia
16. proctoscopy
17. dysphagia
18. aphasia
19. cephalalgia
20. blepharospasm
21. angiorrhexis
22. hemopoiesis
23. hysteroptosis
24. hemiparesis
25. hyperplasia, hypertrophy

WORKSHEET 4

1. lithotripsy
2. arthrocentesis
3. splenectomy
4. colostomy
5. dermatome
6. tracheostomy
7. lithotomy
8. mastectomy
9. hemorrhoidectomy
10. tracheotomy
11. mastopexy
12. colectomy
13. gastrorrhaphy
14. hysteropexy
15. rhinoplasty
16. arthrodesis
17. osteoclasis
18. neurolysis
19. myorrhaphy
20. tympanotomy

WORKSHEET 5

1. bronchiectasis
2. neuralgia, neurodynia
3. gastritis
4. cephalodynia
5. hepatoma
6. carcinogenesis
7. dermatosis
8. lipoid
9. nephromegaly
10. pylorostenosis
11. otorrhea

12. hemopoiesis
13. hysterorrhexis
14. blepharospasm
15. cystocele
16. hemorrhage
17. lithiasis
18. hemiplegia

19. myopathy
20. dysphagia
21. osteomalacia
22. aphasia
23. leukemia
24. erythropenia
25. pelvimetry

Chapter 3 ▪ SUFFIXES: ADJECTIVE, NOUN, DIMINUTIVE, SINGULAR, PLURAL

WORKSHEET 1

1. thoracic
2. gastric, gastral
3. bacterial
4. aquatic
5. axillary
6. cardiac, cardial
7. spinal, spinous
8. membranous

WORKSHEET 2

1. internist
2. leukemia
3. sigmoidoscopy
4. alcoholism
5. allergist
6. senilism
7. mania
8. orthopedist

WORKSHEET 3

Plural	Rule
1. diagnoses	Drop is and add es.
2. fornices	Drop ix and add ices.
3. bursae	Retain a and add e.
4. vertebrae	Retain a and add e.
5. keratoses	Drop is and add es.
6. bronchi	Drop us and add i.
7. spermatozoa	Drop on and add a.
8. septa	Drop um and add a.
9. cocci	Drop us and add i.
10. apices	Drop ex and add ices.
11. ganglia	Drop on and add a.
12. prognoses	Drop is and add es.
13. thrombi	Drop us and add i.
14. appendices	Drop ix and add ices.
15. bacteria	Drop um and add a.
16. radii	Drop us and add i.
17. testes	Drop is and add es.
18. nevi	Drop us and add i.

Chapter 4 ▪ PREFIXES

WORKSHEET 1

Word	Definition of Prefix
1. inter/dental	between
2. hypo/dermic	under, below
3. epi/gastrium	above, upon
4. retro/active	backward, behind
5. sub/nasal	under, below
6. medi/al	middle
7. infra/patellar	under, below
8. post/natal	after, behind
9. quadri/plegia	four
10. hyper/lipidemia	excessive, above normal
11. primi/para	first
12. micro/cephaly	small
13. tri/ceps	three
14. poly/dipsia	many, much
15. im/potent	not
16. an/aerobic	without, not
17. macro/cephaly	large

Word	Definition of Prefix
18. intra/muscular	in, within
19. supra/renal	above, excessive
20. dia/rrhea	through, across
21. circum/renal	around
22. ad/hesion	toward
23. peri/renal	around
24. brady/cardia	slow
25. tachy/pnea	rapid, fast
26. dys/pnea	bad, painful, difficult
27. eu/pnea	good, normal
28. hetero/graft	different
29. mal/function	bad
30. peri/osteum	around

WORKSHEET 2

1. retroperitoneal
2. hypodermic

3. preoperative
4. subnasal
5. postoperative
6. intercostal
7. medial
8. periosteum
9. diarrhea
10. ectoderm
11. suprarenal
12. hemiplegia
13. quadriplegia
14. macrocephaly
15. microscope
16. polyphobia
17. primigravida

WORKSHEET 3

1. dyspepsia
2. heterosexual
3. pseudomembranous
4. antibacterial
5. bradycardia
6. malnutrition
7. amastia
8. anesthesia
9. eupnea
10. synarthrosis
11. tachycardia
12. contraception
13. homosexual

Chapter 5 ■ BODY STRUCTURE

WORKSHEET 1

1. hist/o
2. -gram
3. ultra-
4. ventr/o
5. home/o
6. -cyte
7. infra-
8. -graphy
9. peri-
10. later/o

WORKSHEET 2

1. lateral
2. medial
3. distal
4. proximal
5. supine
6. prone
7. adduction
8. abduction
9. superior
10. inferior
11. anterior
12. posterior
13. inversion
14. eversion

WORKSHEET 3

1. etiology
2. radiologist
3. pathologist
4. morbid
5. pathogenesis
6. sign

7. symptom
8. prognosis
9. diagnosis
10. homeostasis
11. radiopaque material
12. tomography
13. MRI
14. ultrasonography
15. x-ray

WORKSHEET 4

1. sepsis
2. adhesion
3. ablation
4. suppurative
5. radiopharmaceutical
6. nuclear medicine
7. dehiscence
8. curettage
9. laser surgery
10. I&D
11. resection
12. radical surgery
13. ligation
14. anastomosis
15. cauterize

WORKSHEET 5

1. To determine cervical curvature.
2. No, there was no evidence of recent body disease or injury.
3. The first cervical vertebra (atlas) and the second cervical vertebra (axis).
4. No, it was intact.
5. A muscle spasm.

Chapter 6 ▪ INTEGUMENTARY SYSTEM

WORKSHEET 1

1. mastodynia, mastalgia
2. mastitis
3. mastopathy
4. amastia
5. mammogram
6. mammary
7. adipoma, lipoma
8. adipocele, lipocele
9. adipoid, lipoid
10. lipocyte, adipocyte
11. dermatitis
12. dermatologist
13. onychitis
14. onychoma
15. onychopathy
16. onychomycosis
17. onychomalacia
18. onychocryptosis
19. trichopathy
20. trichomycosis

WORKSHEET 2

1. mastectomy, mammectomy
2. mammoplasty, mastoplasty
3. adipectomy, lipectomy
4. onychectomy
5. onychotomy
6. dermatoplasty, dermoplasty

WORKSHEET 3

1. pediculosis
2. vitiligo
3. tinea
4. scabies
5. impetigo
6. urticaria
7. chloasma
8. ecchymosis
9. petechiae
10. alopecia

WORKSHEET 4

1. antipruritics
2. antiseptics, antibacterials
3. astringents
4. dermabrasion
5. parasiticides
6. keratolytics
7. desquamation
8. patch test
9. protectives
10. pruritus

WORKSHEET 5

1. Stratum germinativum
2. Papillary dermis
3. Nodular and infiltrating basal cell carcinoma near the elbow
4. Bowen's disease

Chapter 7 ▪ GASTROINTESTINAL SYSTEM

WORKSHEET 1

1. esophagodynia, esophagalgia
2. esophagospasm
3. esophagostenosis
4. gastritis
5. gastrodynia, gastralgia
6. gastropathy
7. gastromegaly, megalogastria
8. duodenal
9. ileitis
10. jejunoileal, jejunoiliac
11. enteritis
12. enteropathy
13. colitis
14. coloscopy
15. coloenteritis, enterocolitis
16. coloptosis
17. colopathy
18. proctostenosis, rectostenosis
19. rectocele, proctocele
20. proctoplegia, proctoparalysis
21. cholecystitis
22. cholelithiasis
23. hepatoma
24. hepatomegaly
25. pancreatitis

WORKSHEET 2

1. gingivectomy
2. glossectomy
3. esophagoplasty
4. gastrectomy
5. gastrojejunostomy
6. esophagectomy
7. gastroenterocolostomy
8. enteroplasty
9. enteropexy

10. choledochorrhaphy
11. colostomy
12. hepatopexy
13. proctoplasty, rectoplasty
14. cholecystectomy
15. choledochoplasty

WORKSHEET 3

1. hematemesis
2. dysphagia
3. fecalith
4. halitosis
5. anorexia
6. dyspepsia
7. melena
8. cachexia
9. obstipation
10. bulimia

WORKSHEET 4

1. pc, pp
2. occult blood
3. emetics

4. bid
5. choledochoplasty
6. lower GI
7. gastroscopy
8. stomatoplasty
9. cathartics
10. anastomosis
11. cholecystography
12. Crohn's disease
13. antiflatulents
14. antacids
15. FBS
16. alkaline phosphatase
17. qid
18. stat
19. proctosigmoidoscopy
20. upper GI

WORKSHEET 5

1. Posteriorly and inferiorly.
2. Yes.
3. Appendectomy and cholecystectomy.
4. Continuous deep right-sided pain, which took a crescendo pattern and then a decrescendo pattern. The initial pain was intermittent and sharp.

Chapter 8 ■ RESPIRATORY SYSTEM

WORKSHEET 1

1. rhinopathy
2. rhinitis
3. rhinorrhea
4. laryngitis
5. laryngoscopy
6. laryngospasm
7. laryngostenosis
8. laryngotracheal, tracheolaryngeal
9. laryngopathy
10. bronchoscope
11. bronchitis
12. bronchiectasis
13. bronchiospasm, bronchospasm
14. bronchopathy
15. pneumonitis, pneumonia
16. pneumonography
17. thoracic
18. thoracomyodynia, thoracomyalgia
19. dyspnea
20. orthopnea
21. apnea
22. eupnea
23. bradypnea
24. pneumothorax
25. hemothorax

WORKSHEET 2

1. laryngostomy
2. pneumonocentesis, pneumocentesis
3. lobectomy
4. rhinoplasty
5. thoracocentesis, thoracentesis
6. laryngorrhaphy
7. pneumonopexy, pneumopexy
8. bronchoplasty
9. tracheostomy
10. pleurectomy

WORKSHEET 3

1. sputum
2. rales, crackles
3. compliance
4. mucus
5. pertussis
6. Cheyne-Stokes respiration
7. anosmia
8. anoxemia
9. stridor
10. coryza

WORKSHEET 4

1. spirometry
2. bronchography
3. CT scan (thoracic)
4. antral irrigation
5. AP
6. COPD
7. antitussives
8. antihistamines
9. mucolytics
10. arterial blood gases
11. thoracentesis
12. sweat test
13. Mantoux test
14. CXR
15. FEV

WORKSHEET 5

1. Shortness of breath
2. Difficult breathing, high blood pressure, chronic obstructive pulmonary disease, and peripheral vascular disease
3. Bilateral wheezes and rhonchi heard anteriorly and posteriorly
4. Interstitial vascular congestion, superimposed inflammatory change, possibly some pleural reactive change
5. Acute exacerbation of chronic obstructive pulmonary disease; congestive heart failure; hypertension; peripheral vascular disease
6. Congestive heart failure
7. CHF

Chapter 9 ■ CARDIOVASCULAR SYSTEM

WORKSHEET 1

1. atheroma
2. atherosclerosis
3. phlebitis
4. phlebosclerosis
5. phlebothrombosis
6. venosclerosis
7. venospasm
8. venous
9. venostenosis
10. cardiomegaly, megalocardia
11. endocarditis
12. epicarditis
13. cardiopulmonary
14. cardiovascular
15. myocarditis
16. cardiomyopathy, myocardiopathy
17. arteriosclerosis
18. arteriospasm
19. arteriorrhexis
20. arterial

3. hypertension
4. Adams-Stokes syndrome
5. patent
6. tetralogy of Fallot
7. ischemia
8. fibrillations
9. hyperlipidemia
10. aneurysm

WORKSHEET 2

1. cardiotomy
2. cardiocentesis
3. phlebopexy, venopexy
4. arteriorrhaphy
5. pericardiectomy
6. phlebotomy, venotomy
7. arterioplasty
8. angioplasty
9. embolectomy
10. venorrhaphy, phleborrhaphy

WORKSHEET 4

1. echocardiography
2. electrocardiography (ECG, EKG)
3. pericardiocentesis
4. MS
5. antianginals
6. inotropics, cardiotonics
7. cardiac enzyme studies
8. phlebotomy, venotomy
9. beta blockers
10. stress test
11. phonocardiography
12. MI
13. ligation and stripping
14. arterial anastomosis
15. arterial biopsy

WORKSHEET 5

1. Approximately 2 hours.
2. Yes.
3. SGOT, CPK, and LDH.
4. Streptokinase and heparin.
5. The front side of the heart.
6. No. In the earlier admission, the damage was to the lower part of the heart.

WORKSHEET 3

1. coarctation
2. cardiac arrest

Chapter 10 ■ BLOOD AND LYMPHATIC SYSTEMS

WORKSHEET 1

1. erythrocytosis
2. leukocytosis
3. granulocytosis
4. thrombocytosis
5. lymphocytosis
6. reticulocytosis
7. erythrocytopenia, erythropenia
8. leukocytopenia, leukopenia
9. thrombocytopenia, thrombopenia
10. granulocytopenia, granulopenia
11. lymphocytopenia
12. hematopoiesis, hemopoiesis
13. erythropoiesis, erythrocytopoiesis
14. leukopoiesis, leukocytopoiesis
15. lymphopoiesis, lymphocytopoiesis
16. immunologist
17. immunology
18. splenocele
19. splenitis
20. splenolysis

WORKSHEET 2

1. splenectomy
2. splenotomy
3. thymectomy
4. thymolysis
5. splenolaparotomy, laparosplenotomy
6. splenopexy

WORKSHEET 3

1. serology
2. antigen

3. hemolysis
4. hemostasis
5. septicemia
6. antibody
7. lymphosarcoma
8. dyscrasia
9. ascites
10. lymphadenopathy

WORKSHEET 4

1. hemostatics
2. hemoglobin
3. ESR
4. hematocrit
5. Ig
6. poly, seg
7. transfusion
8. Monospot
9. aspiration
10. CBC
11. fibrinolytics
12. anticoagulants
13. prothrombin time
14. EBV
15. splenography

WORKSHEET 5

1. Cobe Spectra.
2. Blood pressure, which fell to 90 mm Hg systolic.
3. Approximately 12 cups.
4. −253 mL.
5. All were within the reference range, except platelets, which were low.
6. 1 hour and 50 minutes.

Chapter 11 ■ MUSCULOSKELETAL SYSTEM

WORKSHEET 1

1. osteocytes
2. ostealgia, osteodynia
3. osteoarthropathy
4. osteogenesis
5. cervical
6. cervicobrachial
7. cervicofacial
8. myelocele
9. myelosarcoma
10. myelomalacia
11. myeloblastoma
12. suprasternal
13. sternoid
14. chondroblast
15. arthritis

16. osteoarthritis
17. pelvimeter
18. myoma
19. myosclerosis
20. myorrhexis

WORKSHEET 2

1. phalangectomy
2. thoracotomy
3. vertebrectomy
4. arthrodesis
5. osteoplasty
6. myoplasty
7. laminectomy

WORKSHEET 3

1. subluxation
2. rickets
3. spondylolisthesis
4. claudication
5. muscular dystrophy
6. talipes
7. sequestrum
8. myasthenia gravis
9. prosthesis
10. ganglion cyst
11. hypotonia

WORKSHEET 4

1. myelography
2. open reduction

3. chrysotherapy
4. corticosteroids
5. laminectomy
6. arthrography
7. arthrodesis
8. amputation
9. HNP

WORKSHEET 5

1. AP.
2. The fracture caused damage to surrounding tissue.
3. To determine whether the elbow was fractured.
4. The distal shafts of the radius and ulna.
5. A single view of the left elbow was obtained in the lateral projection.

Chapter 12 ■ GENITOURINARY SYSTEM

WORKSHEET 1

1. nephrolith
2. nephrologist
3. nephropyosis
4. nephrohydrosis
5. pyelectasis, pyelectasia
6. pyelopathy
7. ureterectasis, ureterectasia
8. ureterolith
9. ureteromegaly
10. cystitis
11. cystoscope
12. vesicocele
13. vesicoprostatic
14. urethrostenosis
15. urethrotome
16. urograph
17. uropathy
18. hematuria
19. dysuria
20. oliguria
21. orchiopathy
22. orchialgia, orchiodynia, orchidalgia
23. vesiculopathy
24. prostatorrhea
25. balanorrhea

WORKSHEET 2

1. vasectomy
2. urethrorrhaphy
3. ureteropyeloplasty
4. nephroureterectomy, ureteronephrectomy
5. cystolithectomy
6. cystoplasty
7. urethrostenosis
8. prostatectomy
9. prostatolithotomy
10. orchidectomy, orchiectomy

WORKSHEET 3

1. incontinence
2. oliguria
3. epispadias
4. impotence
5. varicocele
6. hypospadias
7. urolithiasis
8. frequency
9. aspermia
10. urgency

WORKSHEET 4

1. intravenous pyelogram (IVP)
2. urinalysis (UA)
3. blood urea nitrogen (BUN)
4. uricosuric agents
5. gonadotropins
6. pH
7. circumcision
8. diuretics
9. spermicidal preparations
10. semen analysis
11. UTI
12. nephrotomography
13. estrogenic hormones
14. urethroscopy
15. cystography

WORKSHEET 5

1. To examine the bladder
2. #26 French Van Buren
3. To dilate the urethra
4. Longitudinally
5. No, because there was minimal bleeding

Chapter 13 ■ FEMALE REPRODUCTIVE SYSTEM

WORKSHEET 1

1. gynecopathy
2. gynecology
3. gynecologist
4. cervicovaginitis
5. cervicovesical
6. colposcope
7. colposcopy
8. vaginitis
9. vaginal
10. vaginomycosis
11. vaginolabial
12. hysteromyoma
13. hysteropathy
14. hysterosalpingography
15. metrorrhagia
16. parametritis
17. uterocele
18. uterocervical
19. uterorectal
20. uterovesical
21. oophoritis
22. oophoralgia, oophorodynia
23. oophorosalpingitis
24. salpingocele
25. salpingography

WORKSHEET 2

1. oophoropexy, ovariopexy
2. oophorrhaphy
3. colpoplasty, vaginoplasty
4. hystero-oophorectomy
5. colpoperineoplasty, vaginoperineoplasty
6. episiorrhaphy, perineorrhaphy
7. hysterosalpingo-oophorectomy
8. amniocentesis

WORKSHEET 3

1. pyosalpinx
2. primipara
3. gestation
4. cerclage
5. retroversion
6. corpus luteum
7. dystocia
8. atresia
9. Down syndrome
10. pruritus vulvae

WORKSHEET 4

1. Pap smear
2. hysterosalpingography
3. amniocentesis
4. cryosurgery
5. colpocleisis
6. D&C
7. total abdominal hysterectomy (TAH)
8. tubal ligation
9. CPD
10. laparoscopy
11. spermicidals
12. ultrasonography
13. chorionic villus sampling
14. estrogens
15. oxytocin

WORKSHEET 5

1. A brownish discharge
2. Severe itching and pain
3. Yes
4. The ulcerlike lesion on the right
5. Probably from the cold sore when having oral-genital sex

Chapter 14 ■ ENDOCRINE SYSTEM

WORKSHEET 1

1. hyperglycemia
2. hypoglycemia
3. glycogenesis
4. pancreatitis
5. pancreatolysis
6. pancreatopathy
7. thyroiditis
8. thyromegaly

WORKSHEET 2

1. thyroidectomy
2. thyrochondrotomy
3. parathyroidectomy
4. adrenalectomy
5. bilateral adrenalectomy

WORKSHEET 3

1. virile
2. myxedema
3. diuresis
4. hirsutism
5. cretinism
6. insulin
7. Addison's disease
8. exophthalmic goiter

9. hyperkalemia
10. pheochromocytoma

10. RAI
11. T$_3$

WORKSHEET 4

1. FBS
2. RAIU
3. corticosteroids
4. vasopressin
5. thyroid echogram
6. T$_4$
7. insulin
8. GTT
9. antihyperlipidemics

WORKSHEET 5

1. The four parathyroid glands are located bilaterally on the thyroid gland.
2. Four.
3. A benign tumor of a gland.
4. Endocrine, circulatory.
5. Physician who specializes in treating diseases of the endocrine system.
6. Excessive amount of calcium in the urine.
7. Approximately 1.5 packs per day.

Chapter 15 ■ NERVOUS SYSTEM

WORKSHEET 1

1. encephalopathy
2. encephalocele
3. cerebrospinal
4. cerebrosclerosis
5. cerebropathy
6. craniocele
7. craniomalacia
8. craniosclerosis
9. craniometer
10. neuroblast
11. neuralgia, neurodynia
12. neurologist
13. myelography, myelogram
14. myelocele
15. myeloplegia, myeloparalysis
16. meningocele
17. meningomyelocele
18. hemiplegia
19. quadriplegia
20. narcolepsy
21. analgesia
22. dysphasia
23. aphasia
24. hypertrophy
25. atrophy

WORKSHEET 2

1. neurolysis
2. craniotomy
3. cranioplasty
4. neurorrhaphy
5. encephalotomy
6. thalamotomy

WORKSHEET 3

1. concussion
2. herpes zoster
3. Huntington's chorea
4. aura
5. paraplegia
6. poliomyelitis
7. TIA
8. Reye's syndrome
9. lethargy
10. asthenia

WORKSHEET 4

1. cerebral angiography
2. cryosurgery
3. trephination
4. spinal puncture
5. electromyography
6. analgesic
7. tranquilizer
8. positron emission tomography
9. CT scan (cranial)
10. echoencephalography

WORKSHEET 5

1. Occipital, the back part of the head.
2. CT scan: blood in the cisterna subarachnoidalis and mild acute hydrocephalus; cerebroangiogram: no aneurysm.
3. There is no inflammation in meningismus.
4. It confirmed another subarachnoid hemorrhage.
5. MRI and angiogram.
6. An attempt to exhale forcibly with the glottis, nose, and mouth closed.

Chapter 16 ■ SPECIAL SENSES

WORKSHEET 1

1. ophthalmoplegia
2. ophthalmoscope
3. ophthalmology
4. pupilloscopy
5. pupillometer
6. keratome, keratotome
7. keratometer
8. scleritis
9. scleromalacia
10. iridoplegia, iridoparalysis
11. iridocele
12. iridomalacia
13. retinopathy
14. retinitis
15. blepharoplegia
16. blepharoconjunctivitis
17. blepharoadenoma
18. hyperopia
19. amblyopia
20. otalgia, otodynia
21. otorrhea
22. otopyorrhea
23. audiometer
24. audiology
25. myringotome

WORKSHEET 2

1. stapedectomy
2. labyrinthotomy
3. mastoidectomy
4. myringoplasty, tympanoplasty
5. tympanocentesis, myringocentesis
6. corneotomy, keratotomy
7. otoplasty
8. blepharorrhaphy

WORKSHEET 3

1. hordeolum
2. labyrinthitis
3. otitis externa
4. visual field
5. achromatopsia
6. anacusis
7. metamorphopsia
8. nyctalopia
9. exophthalmos
10. nystagmus

WORKSHEET 4

1. mydriatic
2. cyclodialysis
3. ARMD
4. retinoscopy
5. AD
6. OD
7. audiometry
8. electronystagmography
9. phacoemulsification
10. miotics
11. otoscopy
12. enucleation
13. evisceration
14. cycloplegics
15. otoplasty

WORKSHEET 5

1. Both ears.
2. Tympanostomy tubes inserted 2.5 years ago.
3. Eardrum.
4. General anesthetic.
5. The face was upward.
6. Operating microscope.
7. Cerumen, earwax.
8. Perforation of the eardrums.

ABBREVIATIONS

The use of medical and scientific abbreviations is timesaving and often a standard practice in the health care industry. Note the use of capital and lowercase letters. This is a comprehensive list, and consequently, some abbreviations may not appear in any of the chapters.

Abbreviation

A, Acc	accommodation
AB, ab	abortion
Ab	antibody
ABC	aspiration biopsy cytology
ABGs	arterial blood gases
ABLB	alternate binaural loudness balance
ABR	auditory brainstem response
ac	before meals (ante cibum)
AC	air conduction; anticoagulant
ACG	angiocardiography
ACS	American Cancer Society
ACTH	adrenocorticotropic hormone
AD	right ear (auris dextra)
ad lib	as desired
adeno-CA	adenocarcinoma
ADH	antidiuretic hormone (vasopressin)
AE	above the elbow
AF	atrial fibrillation
AFB	acid-fast bacillus (TB organism)
AFP	alpha-fetoprotein
A/G	albumin-globulin ratio
Ag	antigen
AGN	acute glomerulonephritis
AHF	antihemophilic factor VIII
AHG	antihemophilic globulin factor VIII
AI	artificial insemination
AIDS	acquired immunodeficiency syndrome
AK	above the knee
AKA	above-knee amputation
alk phos	alkaline phosphatase
ALL	acute lymphocytic leukemia
ALS	amyotrophic lateral sclerosis
AMA	American Medical Association
AMD, ARMD	age-related macular degeneration

AMI	acute myocardial infarction
AML	acute myelogenous leukemia
ANS	autonomic nervous system
A&P	auscultation and percussion
AP	anteroposterior
APTT	activated partial thromboplastin time
ARDS	adult respiratory distress syndrome
ARF	acute renal failure
AS	aortic stenosis; left ear (auris sinistra)
As, Ast, astigm	astigmatism
ASD	atrial septal defect
ASHD	arteriosclerotic heart disease
AST	aspartate transaminase
ATN	acute tubular necrosis
AU	both ears (auris uterque)
AV	atrioventricular; arteriovenous
AVMs	arteriovenous malformations
AVR	aortic valve replacement
Ba	barium
BaE	barium enema
baso	basophil
BBB	bundle branch block
BE	below the elbow
bid	twice a day
BIN, bin	twice a night
BK	below the knee
BKA	below-knee amputation
BM	bowel movement
BMR	basal metabolic rate
BNO	bladder neck obstruction
BP	blood pressure
BPH	benign prostatic hyperplasia, benign prostatic hypertrophy
BT	bleeding time
BUN	blood urea nitrogen
Bx	biopsy
c̄	with (cum)
C1, C2, etc.	first cervical vertebra, second cervical vertebra, etc.
C&S	culture and sensitivity
CA	cancer
Ca	calcium
CAD	coronary artery disease
cath	catheterization, catheter
CBC	complete blood count
cc	cubic centimeter
CC	cardiac catheterization; chief complaint
CCU	coronary care unit
CDC	Centers for Disease Control and Prevention
CDH	congenital dislocation of the hip
CEA	carcinoembryonic antigen
CHD	coronary heart disease
CHF	congestive heart failure
CK	creatine kinase
Cl	chlorine
CLL	chronic lymphocytic leukemia
cm	centimeter
CML	chronic myelogenous leukemia
CNS	central nervous system
c/o	complains of
CO_2	carbon dioxide

COLD	chronic obstructive lung disease
COPD	chronic obstructive pulmonary disease
CP	cerebral palsy
CPD	cephalopelvic disproportion
CPK	creatine phosphokinase
CPR	cardiopulmonary resuscitation
CR	computerized radiography
CS, C-section	cesarean section
CSF	cerebrospinal fluid
CTS	carpal tunnel syndrome
CT scan, CAT scan	computed tomography scan, computed axial tomography scan
CV	cardiovascular
CVA	cerebrovascular accident
CVD	cerebrovascular disease
CVS	chorionic villus sampling
CWP	childbirth without pain
CXR	chest x-ray film, chest radiograph
cysto	cystoscopy
/d	per day
D	diopter (lens strength)
D&C	dilatation and curettage
D&E	dilation and evacuation
dc	discontinue
DC	discharge
DDS	Doctor of Dental Surgery
decub	decubitus
derm	dermatology
DI	diabetes insipidus; diagnostic imaging
diff	differential count (white blood cells)
DJD	degenerative joint disease
DM	diabetes mellitus
DO	doctor of osteopathy
DOA	dead on arrival
DOB	date of birth
DPT	diphtheria, pertussis, tetanus
DRE	digital rectal examination
DRGs	diagnosis-related groups
DSA	digital subtraction angiography
DUB	dysfunctional uterine bleeding
DVT	deep vein thrombosis
Dx	diagnosis
EBV	Epstein-Barr virus
ECF	extracellular fluid; extended care facility
ECG, EKG	electrocardiogram
ECHO	echocardiogram
EDC	estimated date of confinement
EEG	electroencephalogram, electroencephalograph
EENT	eye, ear, nose, and throat
EGD	esophagogastroduodenoscopy
EM, em	emmetropia
EMG	electromyogram
ENT	ear, nose, and throat
EOM	extraocular movement
eos, eosin	eosinophil
ERCP	endoscopic retrograde cholangiopancreatography
ERT	estrogen replacement therapy
ESL, ESWL	extracorporeal shock-wave lithotripsy
ESR; SR, sed rate	erythrocyte sedimentation rate; sedimentation rate
EST	electroshock therapy
ET	esotropia

F	Fahrenheit
FACP	Fellow, American College of Physicians
FACS	Fellow, American College of Surgeons
FBS	fasting blood sugar
FDA	Food and Drug Administration
FEF	forced expiratory flow
FEKG	fetal electrocardiogram
FEV	forced expiratory volume
FH	family history
FHR	fetal heart rate
FHT	fetal heart tone
FS	frozen section
FSH	follicle-stimulating hormone
FTND	full-term normal delivery
FUO	fever of undetermined origin
FVC	forced vital capacity
Fx	fracture
g	gram
GB	gallbladder
GC	gonorrhea
GCSF	granulocyte colony-stimulating factor
GERD	gastroesophageal reflux disease
GH	growth hormone
GI	gastrointestinal
GOT	glutamic oxaloacetic transaminase (AST)
GPT	glutamic pyruvic transaminase (ALT)
gr	grain
GTT	glucose tolerance test
gtt	drops (guttae)
GU	genitourinary
GYN	gynecology
h	hour
H	hypodermic; hydrogen
HAV	hepatitis A virus
HBV	hepatitis B virus
HCG	human chorionic gonadotropin
HCl	hydrochloric acid
HCO	bicarbonate
HCT, Hct	hematocrit
HD	hip disarticulation; hemodialysis; hearing distance
HDL	high-density lipoprotein
HDN	hemolytic disease of the newborn
HEENT	head, eyes, ears, nose, and throat
Hg	mercury
HGB, Hgb, Hb	hemoglobin
HIV	human immunodeficiency virus
HMD	hyaline membrane disease
HNP	herniated nucleus pulposus (herniated disk)
HP	hemipelvectomy
hs	at bedtime
HSG	hysterosalpingography
HSV	herpes simplex virus
Hx	history
hypo	hypodermically
IAS	interatrial septum
IBS	irritable bowel syndrome
ICF	intracellular fluid
ICP	intracranial pressure

ICSH	interstitial cell-stimulating hormone
ICU	intensive care unit
ID	intradermal
I&D	incision and drainage
IDDM	insulin-dependent diabetes mellitus
Ig	immunoglobulin
IH	infectious hepatitis
IM	intramuscular
inj	injection
IOP	intraocular pressure
IPPB	intermittent positive-pressure breathing
IQ	intelligence quotient
IRDS	infant respiratory distress syndrome
IS	intercostal space
ITP	idiopathic thrombocytopenia purpura
IUD	intrauterine device
IUGR	intrauterine growth rate; intrauterine growth retardation
IV	intravenous
IVC	inferior vena cava; intravenous cholangiography
IVF	in vitro fertilization
IVP	intravenous pyelogram
IVS	interventricular septum
K^+	potassium (an electrolyte)
KD	knee disarticulation
kg	kilogram
KUB	kidney, ureter, and bladder
L, l	liter
L1, L2, etc.	first lumbar vertebra, second lumbar vertebra, etc.
LA	left atrium
L&A	light and accommodation
LAT, lat	lateral
LB	large bowel
LD	lactate dehydrogenase
LDL	low-density lipoprotein
LE	lupus erythematosus; lower extremity
LH	luteinizing hormone
LLQ	left lower quadrant
LMP	last menstrual period
LP	lumbar puncture
LPN	licensed practical nurse
LRQ	lower right quadrant
L, lt	left
LUQ	left upper quadrant
LV	left ventricle
lymphs	lymphocytes
MCH	mean corpuscular hemoglobin
MCHC	mean corpuscular hemoglobin concentration
MCV	mean corpuscular volume
MD	medical doctor
mets	metastases
MG	myasthenia gravis
mg	milligram (0.001 gram)
MH	marital history
MI	myocardial infarction; mitral insufficiency
mix astig	mixed astigmatism
mL, ml	milliliter (0.001 liter)
mm	millimeter (0.001 meter; 0.039 inch)
mono	monocyte

MRI	magnetic resonance imaging
MS	mitral stenosis; multiple sclerosis; musculoskeletal
MSH	melanocyte-stimulating hormone
MVP	mitral valve prolapse
myop	myopia
Na^+	sodium (an electrolyte)
NB	newborn
NIDDM	non–insulin-dependent diabetes mellitus
NPH	neutral protamine Hagedorn (insulin)
NPO, npo	nothing by mouth (nulla per os)
NSAID	nonsteroidal anti-inflammatory drug
O_2	oxygen
OA	osteoarthritis
OB	obstetrics
OB-GYN	obstetrics and gynecology
OCPs	oral contraceptive pills
od	once a day
OD	right eye (oculus dexter); overdose
OHS	open heart surgery
OR	operating room
ORTH, ortho	orthopedics, orthopaedics
os	mouth; opening; bone
OS	left eye (oculus sinister)
OTC	over the counter
oto	otology
OU	both eyes (oculi unitas); each eye (oculus uterque)
OV	office visit
oz	ounce
P	pulse; phosphorus
PA	posteroanterior; pernicious anemia
PAC	premature arterial contraction
Pap smear	Papanicolaou's smear
paren	parenterally
PAT	paroxysmal atrial tachycardia
Path	pathology
PBI	protein-bound iodine
pc, pp	after meals
PCP	*Pneumocystis carinii* pneumonia
PCV	packed cell volume (hematocrit)
PD	peritoneal dialysis
PDR	*Physician's Desk Reference*
PE	physical examination
PET	positron emission tomography
PFT	pulmonary function test
PGH	pituitary growth hormone
pH	hydrogen ion concentration, degree of acidity
PH	past history
PID	pelvic inflammatory disease
PKU	phenylketonuria
PMH	past medical history
PMN, seg, poly	polymorphonuclear neutrophil
PMP	previous menstrual period
PMS	premenstrual syndrome
PND	paroxysmal nocturnal dyspnea
PNS	peripheral nervous system
PO, po	orally, by mouth
pp	postprandial (after meals)

prn	as required
PSA	prostate-specific antigen
PT, pro time	prothrombin time
pt	patient
PT	physical therapy
PTCA	percutaneous transluminal coronary angiography
PTH	parathyroid hormone
PTS	permanent threshold shift
PTT	partial thromboplastin time
PUD	peptic ulcer disease
PVC	premature ventricular contraction
PVD	peripheral vascular disease
q	every
qam, qm	every morning
qd	every day (quaque die)
qh	every hour
q2h	every 2 hours
qid	four times a day
qns	quantity not sufficient
qpm, qn	every night
R, rt	right
RA	right atrium; rheumatoid arthritis
rad	radiation absorbed dose
RAI	radioactive iodine
RAIU	radioactive iodine uptake
RBC	red blood cell; red blood cell (count)
RD	respiratory disease
RDS	respiratory distress syndrome
REM	rapid eye movement
RLQ	right lower quadrant
RN	registered nurse
RNA	ribonucleic acid
R/O	rule out
ROM	range of motion
RP	retrograde pyelogram
RT	radiation therapy
RUQ	right upper quadrant
RV	right ventricle
Rx	prescription, treatment, therapy
s̄	without
S1, S2, etc	first sacral vertebra, second sacral vertebra, etc
SA	sinoatrial (node)
SAH	subarachnoid hemorrhage
SC, sc, subcu, subq	subcutaneous
SD	shoulder disarticulation
seg, poly	polymorphonuclear neutrophil
SGOT, SGPT	liver function enzyme tests
SH	serum hepatitis
SIDS	sudden infant death syndrome
SK	streptokinase
SLE	systemic lupus erythematosus
SNS	somatic nervous system
SOB	shortness of breath
sono	sonogram, sonography
SOP	standard operating procedure
sos	if necessary
sp gr, SG	specific gravity
SR	sedimentation rate

ss	half
st	stage (of a disease)
ST	esotropia
staph	staphylococcus
stat	immediately
STDs	sexually transmitted diseases
strep	streptococcus
subcu, subq	subcutaneous
SVC	superior vena cava
SVD	spontaneous vaginal delivery
Sx	signs, symptoms
T	temperature
T1, T2, etc.	first thoracic vertebra, second thoracic vertebra, etc.
T_3	triiodothyronine
T_4	thyroxine
T&A	tonsillectomy and adenoidectomy
TAH	total abdominal hysterectomy
TB	tuberculosis
THA	total hip arthroplasty
THR	total hip replacement
TIA	transient ischemic attack
tid	three times a day
TKA	total knee arthroplasty
TMJ	temporomandibular joint
TKR	total knee replacement
TNM	tumor, nodes, metastasis
top	topically
TPA, tPA	tissue plasminogen activator
TPN	total parenteral nutrition
TPR	temperature, pulse, and respiration
tr, tinct	tincture
TSH	thyroid-stimulating hormone
TSS	toxic shock syndrome
TTH	thyrotropic hormone
TTS	temporary threshold shift
TUR, TURP	transurethral resection of prostate
Tx	tumor cannot be assessed
U	units
UA	urinalysis
UC	uterine contractions
UGI	upper gastrointestinal
U&L, U/L	upper and lower
ULQ	upper left quadrant
ung	ointment
URI	upper respiratory infection
URQ	upper right quadrant
UTI	urinary tract infection
UV	ultraviolet
VA	visual acuity
VC	vital capacity
VCU, VCUG	voiding cystourethrogram
VD	venereal disease
VF	visual field
VHD	ventricular heart disease
VLDL	very-low-density lipoprotein
VSD	ventricular septal defect
VT	ventricular tachycardia

WBC	white blood cell; white blood cell (count)
wt	weight
w/v	weight by volume
✕	multiplied by
XP	xeroderma pigmentosa
XT	exotropia
XX	female sex chromosomes
XY	male sex chromosomes
YOB	year of birth

Appendix C

PREFIXES • ABBREVIATIONS • PRONUNCIATION

ROOTS • COMBINING FORMS • SUFFIXES

INDEX OF MEDICAL WORD ELEMENTS

Part I ■ MEDICAL WORD ELEMENT TO ENGLISH TERM

Medical Word Element	Pronunciation	Meaning	Page Numbers
a-	ă	without, not	34, 175, 302
ab-	ăb	from, away from	34, 52
abdomin/o	ăb-dŏm-ĭ-nō	abdomen	50
-ac	ăk	pertaining to	26
acr/o	ăk-rō	extremity	50, 277
acromi/o	ă-krō-mē-ō	acromion (projection of scapula)	200
ad-	ăd	toward	34, 52
aden/o	ăd-ē-nō	gland	66, 173
adenoid/o	ăd-ē-noyd-ō	adenoid	118
adip/o	ăd-ĭ-pō	fat	66
adren/o	ăd-rē-nō	adrenal glands	277
adrenal/o	ă-drĕn-ăl-ō	adrenal glands	277
-al	ăl	pertaining to	26
albin/o	ăl-bĭn-ō	white	50
albumin/o	al-bū-mĭn-ō	albumin (protein)	226
-algesia	ăl-gē-zē-ă	pain	301
-algia	ăl-jē-ă	pain	12, 14, 301
all-	ăl	other, differing from the usual	52
alveol/o	ăl-vē-ōl-ō	alveolus (pl. alveoli)	119
ambly/o	ăm-blē-ō	dull, dim	321
amni/o	ăm-nē-ō	amnion (amniotic sac)	249
an-	ăn	without, not	34, 302
an/o	ā-nō	anus	92
andr/o	ăn-drō	male	225, 277
angi/o	ăn-jē-ō	vessel	145
aniso-	ăn-ī-sō	unequal, dissimilar	175
ankyl/o	ăng-kĭ-lō	stiffness, bent, crooked	200
ante-	ăn-tē	before, in front	32
anter/o	ăn-tĕr-ō	anterior, front	49
anthrac/o	ăn-thră-kō	black, coal	50, 119

361

Medical Word Element	Pronunciation	Meaning	Page Numbers
anti-	ăn-tĭ	against	35
aort/o	ā-or-tō	aorta	145
append/o	ăp-ĕn-dō	appendix	92
appendic/o	ăp-ĕn-dĭk-ō	appendix	92
aque/o	ā-kwē-ō	water	321
-ar	ĕr	pertaining to	26
-arche	ăr-kē	beginning	250
arteri/o	ăr-tē-rē-ō	artery	145
arteriol/o	ăr-tĕr-ĭ-ōl-ō	arteriole	145
arthr/o	ăr-thrō	joint	3, 12, 200
-ary	ĕr-ē	pertaining to	26
atel/o	ăt-ĕ-lō	incomplete, imperfect	119
ather/o	ăth-ĕr-ō	fatty plaque	145
atri/o	ā-trē-ō	atrium	145
audi/o	aw-dē-ō	hearing	322
bacteri/o	băk-tē-rē-ō	bacteria	226
balan/o	bă-lăn-ō	glans penis	226
bi-	bī	two	33
-blast	blăst	embryonic cell	175, 201
blast/o	blăs-tō	embryonic cell	173
blephar/o	blĕf-ă-rō	eyelid	321
brachi/o	brăk-ē-ō	arm	199
brady-	brăd-ē	slow	35, 120, 301
bronch/o	brŏng-kō	bronchus (pl. bronchi)	119
bronchi/o	brŏng-kē-ō	bronchus (pl. bronchi)	119
bucc/o	bŭk-ō	cheek	91
calc/o	kăl-kō	calcium	277
calcane/o	kăl-kā-nē-ō	calcaneum (heel bone)	199
-capnia	kăp-nē-ă	carbon dioxide (CO_2)	120
cardi/o	kăr-dē-ō	heart	2, 145
carp/o	kăr-pō	carpus, wrist bones	199
caud/o	kaw-dō	tail	49
-cele	sēl	hernia, swelling	14
-centesis	sĕn-tē-sĭs	puncture	3, 12, 13
cephal/o	sĕf-ăl-ō	head	199
cerebr/o	sĕr-ē-brō	cerebrum	301
cervic/o	sĕr-vĭ-kō	neck, cervix uteri (neck of uterus)	199, 249
cheil/o	kī-lō	lip	91
chlor/o	klor-ō	green	50
chol/e	kō-lē	bile, gall	92
cholangi/o	kō-lăn-jē-ō	bile vessel	92
cholecyst/o	kō-lē-sĭs-tō	gallbladder	92
choledoch/o	kō-lĕ-dō-kō	bile duct	92
chondr/o	kŏn-drō	cartilage	201
choroid/o	kō-royd-ō	choroid	321
chrom/o	krōm-ō	color	173
circum-	sĕr-kŭm	around	34
cirrh/o	sĭr-rō	yellow	50
-clasis	klă-sĭs	break, fracture, refracture	14, 201
col/o	kō-lō	colon	92
colon/o	kō-lŏn-ō	colon	4, 12, 92
colp/o	kŏl-pō	vagina	249
condyl/o	kŏn-dĭ-lō	condyle	200
coni/o	kō-nē-ō	dust	119
contra-	kŏn-tră	against	35
core/o	kō-rē-ō	pupil	322

Medical Word Element	Pronunciation	Meaning	Page Numbers
corne/o	kŏr-nē-ō	cornea	321
cost/o	kŏs-tō	ribs	199
crani/o	krā-nē-ō	cranium, skull	199, 301
-crine	krĭn/krīn	secrete	277
crypt/o	krĭp-tō	hidden	67, 226
cutane/o	kū-tā-nē-ō	skin	67
cyan/o	sī-ăn-ō	blue	50
cycl/o	sī-klō	ciliary body	321
-cyesis	sī-ē-sĭs	pregnancy	250
cyst/o	sĭs-tō	bladder	225
-cyte	sīt	cell	68
cyt/o	sī-tō	cell	49
dacry/o	dăk-rē-ō	tear, lacrimal sac	321
dacryocyst/o	dăk-rē-ō-sĭs-tō	lacrimal sac, tear sac	321
dactyl/o	dăk-tĭ-lō	digit (finger or toe)	200
dent/o	dĕnt-ō	teeth	91
-derma	dĕr-mă	skin	68
derm/o	dĕr-mō	skin	67
dermat/o	dĕr-mă-tō	skin	67
-desis	dē-sĭs	binding, fixation (of a bone or joint)	14, 201
dia-	dī-ă	through, across	34, 93
dipl-	dĭpl	double, twofold	33
diplo-	dĭp-lō	double, twofold	33
-dipsia	dĭp-sē-ă	thirst	277
dist/o	dĭs-tō	far, farthest	49
dors/o	dor-sō	back (of body)	49
duoden/o	dū-ŏd-ē-nō	duodenum	92
-dynia	dĭn-ē-ă	pain	14
dys-	dĭs	bad, painful, difficult	35, 93, 250
-eal	ē-ăl	pertaining to	26
ec-	ĕk	out, out from	34
-ectasis	ĕk-tă-sĭs	dilation, expansion	14
ecto-	ĕk-tō	outside	34
-ectomy	ĕk-tŏ-mē	excision, removal	12, 13
-emesis	ĕm-ĕ-sĭs	vomiting	14, 93
-emia	ē-mē-ă	blood condition	14, 175
encephal/o	ĕn-sĕf-ă-lō	brain	13, 301
endo-	ĕn-dō	in, within	34, 146, 250
enter/o	ĕn-tĕr-ō	intestine (usually small intestine)	92
eosin/o	ē-ō-sĭn-ō	dawn (rose colored)	174
epi-	ĕp-ĭ	above, upon	32, 68
epididym/o	ĕp-ĭ-dĭd-ĭ-mō	epididymis	226
episi/o	ē-pĭz-ē-ō	vulva	249
erythem/o	ĕr-ĭ-thē-mō	red	51
erythr/o	ē-rĭth-rō	red	51, 174
eso-	ĕ-sō	inward	322
esophag/o	ē-sŏf-ă-gō	esophagus	91
-esthesia	ĕs-thē-zē-ă	feeling, sensation	301
eu-	ū	good, normal	35, 120
ex-	ĕks	out, out from	34
exo-	ĕks-ō	outside, outward	34, 322
extra-	ĕks-tră	outside	34, 146
fasci/o	făsh-ē-ō	band	51
femor/o	fĕm-ō-rō	femur (thigh bone)	199
fibul/o	fĭb-ū-lō	fibula (smaller, outer bone of lower leg)	200

Medical Word Element	Pronunciation	Meaning	Page Numbers
galact/o	gă-lăk-tō	milk	249
gastr/o	găs-trō	stomach	2, 3, 13, 91
-gen	jĕn	forming, producing, origin	14
-genesis	jĕn-ĕ-sĭs	forming, producing, origin	14, 52, 226
gingiv/o	jĭn-jĭ-vō	gum(s)	91
gli/o	glī-ō	glue, neuroglia	301
-globin	glō-bĭn	protein	175
glomerul/o	glō-mĕr-ū-lō	glomerulus	225
gloss/o	glŏs-ō	tongue	91
gluc/o	gloo-kō	sugar, sweetness	277
glyc/o	glī-kō	sugar, sweetness	277
-gnosis	nō-sĭs	knowing	52
gonad/o	gō-năd-ō	gonads, sex glands	277
-gram	grăm	a writing, record	14, 52, 68, 145
granul/o	grăn-ū-lō	granule	174
-graph	grăf	instrument for recording	14, 52, 68, 145
-graphy	gră-fē	process of recording	14, 52, 68
-gravida	grăv-ĭ-dă	pregnancy	250
gynec/o	jĭn-ē-kō/gĭ-nē-kō	woman, female	249
hem/o	hēm-ō	blood	174
hemangi/o	hē-măn-jē-ō	blood vessel	145
hemat/o	hĕm-ă-tō	blood	174
hemi-	hĕm-ē	one half	33
hepat/o	hĕp-ă-tō	liver	2, 92
hetero-	hĕt-ĕr-ō	different	35, 175
hidr/o	hī-drō	sweat	67
hist/o	hĭs-tō	tissue	49
home/o	hō-mē-ō	same, alike	51, 277
homo-	hō-mō	same	35, 175
humer/o	hū-mĕr-ō	humerus	199
hyper-	hī-pĕr	excessive, above normal	3, 33, 68, 93
hypo-	hī-pō	under, below	32, 68
hyster/o	hĭs-tĕr-ō	uterus, womb	249
-ia	ē-ă	condition	3, 26
-iasis	ī-ă-sĭs	abnormal condition (produced by something specified)	15, 93, 226
-iatrics	ī-ăt-rĭks	medicine, medical profession, physicians	26
-iatry	ī-ă-trē	treatment, medicine	26
-ic	ĭk	pertaining to	26
-ical	ĭk-ăl	pertaining to	26
ichthy/o	ĭk-thē-ō	dry, scaly	67
-icle	ĭk-ăl	small, minute	27
idi/o	ĭd-ē-ō	unknown, peculiar	51
ile/o	ĭl-ē-ō	ileum	92
ili/o	ĭl-ē-ō	ilium (lateral, flaring portion of hip bone)	200
im-	ĭm	not	34
immun/o	ĭm-ū-nō	safe	174
in-	ĭn	in, not	34
infer/o	ĭn-fĕr-ō	lower, below	49
infra-	ĭn-fră	under, below	3, 32, 52
inguin/o	ĭng-gwĭ-nō	groin	50
inter-	ĭn-tĕr	between	33
intra-	ĭn-tră	in, within	34
irid/o	ĭr-ĭ-dō	iris	321
iso-	ī-sō	same, equal	175

Medical Word Element	**Pronunciation**	**Meaning**	**Page Numbers**
ischi/o	ĭs-kē-ō	ischium (lower portion of hip bone)	200
-ism	ĭzm	condition	26
-ist	ĭst	specialist	26
-itis	ī-tĭs	inflammation	12, 13, 15
jaund/o	jawn-dō	yellow	50
jejun/o	jĕ-joo-nō	jejunum	92
kary/o	kăr-ē-ō	nucleus	174
kerat/o	kĕr-ă-tō	horny tissue, hard, cornea	67, 321
kinesi/o	kĭ-nē-sē-ō	movement	301
labi/o	lā-bē-ō	lip	91, 249
labyrinth/o	lăb-ĭ-rĭn-thō	labyrinth, inner ear	322
lact/o	lăk-tō	milk	67, 249
lamin/o	lăm-ĭ-nō	lamina	200
lapar/o	lăp-ăr-ō	abdomen	249
laryng/o	lă-rĭng-ō	larynx (voice box)	118
later/o	lăt-ĕr-ō	side, to one side	49
leiomy/o	lī-ō-mī-ō	smooth muscle (visceral)	201
-lepsy	lĕp-sē	seizure	301
leuc/o	loo-kō	white	50
leuk/o	loo-kō	white	50, 174
lingu/o	lĭng-gwō	tongue	91
lip/o	lī-pō	fat	67
-lith	lĭth	stone, calculus	15, 93
lob/o	lō-bō	lobe	119
-logist	lō-jĭst	specialist in the study of	15, 68
-logy	lō-jē	study of	15, 68
lumb/o	lŭm-bō	loins	50, 200
lymph/o	lĭm-fō	lymph	174
-lysis	lī-sĭs	separation, destruction, loosening	14
macro-	măk-rō	large	3, 33, 175
mal-	măl	bad	35
-malacia	mă-lā-shē-ă	softening	15, 201
mamm/o	mă-mō	breast	67, 249
mast/o	măs-tō	breast	67, 249
medi-	mē-dē	middle	33
medi/o	mē-dē-ō	middle	49
-megaly	mĕg-ă-lē	enlargement	3, 15, 93
melan/o	mĕl-ă-nō	black	51
mening/o	mĕ-nĭng-gō	meninges	301
men/o	mĕn-ō	menses, menstruation	249
mes/o	mĕs-ō	middle	33
metacarp/o	mĕt-ă-kăr-pō	metacarpus (bones of the hand)	199
-meter	mē-tĕr	instrument for measuring	15
metr/o	mĕ-trō	uterus, womb	249
-metry	mĕt-rē	act of measuring	15
micro-	mī-krō	small	3, 33, 175
mono-	mŏn-ō	one	33, 175
morph/o	mor-fō	shape	174
multi-	mŭl-tē	many, much	33, 250
my/o	mī-ō	muscle	201
myc/o	mī-kō	fungus	67
myel/o	mī-ĕ-lō	bone marrow, spinal cord	174, 200, 301
myring/o	mĭr-ĭn-gō	tympanic membrane, eardrum	322

Medical Word Element	*Pronunciation*	*Meaning*	*Page Numbers*
narc/o	năr-kō	stupor, numbing	301
nas/o	nā-zō	nose	118
nat/a	nā-tă	birth	249
nephr/o	nĕf-rō	kidney	2, 225
neur/o	nū-rō	nerve, nervous system	301
noct/o	nŏk-tō	night	226
nucle/o	nū-klē-ō	nucleus	49, 174
ocul/o	ŏk-ū-lō	eye	321
odont/o	ō-dŏn-tō	teeth	91
-oid	oid	resembling	15
-ole	ŏl	small, minute	27
olig/o	ō-lĭ-gō	scanty	226
-oma	ō-mă	tumor	15
omphal/o	ŏm-fă-lō	navel (umbilicus)	50
onych/o	ŏn-ĭ-kō	nail	67
oophor/o	ō-ŏf-ō-rō	ovary	249
ophthalm/o	ŏf-thăl-mō	eye	321
-opia	ō-pē-ă	vision	322
opt/o	ŏp-tō	eye, vision	321
orch/i	or-kē	testes	226
orchi/o	or-kē-ō	testes	226
orchid/o	or-kĭ-dō	testes	226
-orexia	or-ĕks-ē-ă	appetite	93
or/o	or-ō	mouth	91
orth/o	or-thō	straight	119, 200
-ory	or-ē	pertaining to	26
-osis	ō-sĭs	abnormal condition, increase (used primarily with blood cells)	3, 15, 175
-osmia	ŏz-mē-ă	smell	120
oste/o	ŏs-tē-ō	bone	2, 3, 13, 200
ot/o	ō-tō	ear	322
-ous	ŭs	pertaining to	26
ovari/o	ō-văr-ē-ō	ovary	249
ox/o	ŏks-ō	oxygen (O_2)	119
pan-	păn	all	35
pancreat/o	păn-krē-ă-tō	pancreas	93, 277
para-	păr-ă	near, beside, beyond	34
-para	păr-ă	to bear (offspring)	15, 250
parathyroid/o	păr-ă-thī-royd-ō	parathyroid glands	277
-paresis	pă-rē-sĭs	partial paralysis	15
patell/o	pă-tĕl-ō	patella (kneecap)	200
path/o	păth-ō	disease	51
-pathy	pă-thē	disease	15, 52
pector/o	pĕk-tō-rō	chest	119
ped/i	pĕd-ē	foot	200
pelv/i	pĕl-vē	pelvis	50, 200
pelv/o	pĕl-vō	pelvis	50
-penia	pē-nē-ă	decrease, deficiency	15, 175
-pepsia	pĕp-sē-ă	digestion	93
peri-	pĕr-ē	around	34, 52, 93, 146
perine/o	pĕr-ĭ-nē-ō	perineum	249
-pexy	pĕk-sē	fixation (of an organ)	14
phac/o	fă-kō	lens	322
phag/o	făg-ō	swallowing, eating	174
-phagia	fă-jē-ă	eating, swallowing	15, 93, 277
phalang/o	făl-ăn-jō	phalanges (bones of fingers and toes)	199
pharyng/o	fă-rĭng-gō	pharynx, throat	91, 118

Medical Word Element	Pronunciation	Meaning	Page Numbers
-phasia	fā-zē-ă	speech	15, 301
-phil	fĭl	attraction to	175
-philia	fĭl-ē-ă	attraction for	15
phleb/o	flĕb-ō	vein	12, 145
-phobia	fō-bē-ă	fear	15
-phonia	fō-nē-ă	voice	120
-phoresis	fō-rē-sĭs	borne, carried	175
phren/o	frĕn-ō	diaphragm, mind	119
-physis	fĭ-sĭs	growth	201, 278
pil/o	pĭ-lō	hair	67
-plasia	plā-zē-ă	formation, growth	15
-plasty	plăs-tē	surgical repair	14, 93, 201
-plegia	plē-jē-ă	paralysis	15
pleur/o	ploo-rō	pleura	119
-pnea	nē-ă	breathing	120
pneum/o	nū-mō	air, lung	119
pneumon/o	nū-mŏn-ō	air, lung	119
pod/o	pō-dō	foot	200
-poiesis	poy-ē-sĭs	formation, production	16, 175
poikil/o	poy-kĭ-lō	varied, irregular	174
poli/o	pōl-ē-ō	gray	51
poly-	pŏl-ē	many, much	33, 175
-porosis	pō-rō-sĭs	porous	201
post-	pōst	after, behind	33
poster/o	pŏs-tĕr-ō	back (of body), behind, posterior	49
-prandial	prăn-dē-ăl	meal	93
pre-	prē	before, in front	32
presby/o	prĕz-bē-ō	old age	322
primi-	prĭ-mĭ	first	33, 250
pro-	prō	before, in front	32
proct/o	prŏk-tō	anus, rectum	92
prostat/o	prŏs-tă-tō	prostate	226
proxim/o	prŏk-sĭm-ō	near, nearest	49
pseudo-	soo-dō	false	35
-ptosis	tō-sĭs	prolapse, downward displacement	16
-ptysis	tĭ-sĭs	spitting	120
pub/o	pū-bō	pubis (part of hip bone)	200
pulmon/o	pŭl-mŏn-ō	lung	119
pupill/o	pū-pĭ-lō	pupil	322
py/o	pī-ō	pus	226
pylor/o	pī-lō-rō	pylorus	91
quadri-	kwŏd-rĭ	four	33
rachi/o	răk-ē-ō	spine	199
radi/o	rā-dē-ŏ	radiation, x-ray	51
rect/o	rĕk-tō	rectum	92
ren/o	rē-nō	kidney	225
reticul/o	rē-tĭk-ū-lō	net, mesh	174
retin/o	rĕt-ĭ-nō	retina	322
retro-	rĕt-rō	backward, behind	33
rhabd/o	răb-dō	rod-shaped (striated)	201
rhabdomy/o	răb-dō-mī-ō	rod-shaped muscle (striated)	201
rhin/o	rī-nō	nose	118
-rrhage	răj	bursting forth	16
-rrhagia	ră-jē-ă	bursting forth	16
-rrhaphy	ră-fē	suture	14
-rrhea	rē-ă	discharge, flow	16

Medical Word Element	*Pronunciation*	*Meaning*	*Page Numbers*
-rrhexis	rĕk-sĭs	rupture	16
rube/o	roo-bē-ō	red	51
salping/o	săl-pĭng-gō/săl-pĭn-jō	fallopian tubes, oviducts, uterine tubes, eustachian tubes	249, 322
-salpinx	săl-pĭnks	fallopian tubes, oviducts, uterine tubes	250
-schisis	skĭ-sĭs	a splitting	201
scler/o	sklĕ-rō	hardening, sclera	67, 322
-scope	skōp	instrument to view or examine	16
-scopy	skō-pē	visual examination	12, 16, 201
semi-	sĕm-ē	one half	33
sial/o	sī-ă-lō	saliva, salivary gland	93
sider/o	sĭd-ĕr-ō	iron	174
sigmoid/o	sĭg-moy-dō	sigmoid colon	92
somat/o	sō-măt-ō	body	51, 277
-spasm	spăzm	involuntary contraction, twitching	16
spermat/o	spĕr-mă-tō	sperm	226
sphygm/o	sfĭg-mō	pulse	145
spir/o	spī-rō	breathe	119
splen/o	splē-nō	spleen	174
spondyl/o	spŏn-dĭ-lō	vertebrae (backbone)	199
squam/o	skwā-mō	scaly	67
staped/o	stā-pē-dō	stapes	322
-stasis	stā-sĭs	standing still	16, 175
steat/o	stē-ă-tō	fat	67
-stenosis	stĕ-nō-sĭs	narrowing, stricture	16
stern/o	stĕr-nō	sternum (breastbone)	199
steth/o	stĕth-ō	chest	119
stomat/o	stō-mă-tō	mouth	91
-stomy	stō-mē	forming an opening (mouth)	13
sub-	sŭb	under, below	32, 68, 93
super-	soo-pĕr	above, excessive	34
super/o	soo-pĕr-ō	upper, above	49
supra-	soo-pră	above, excessive	34
sym-	sĭm	union, together, joined	35
syn-	sĭn	union, together, joined	35
tachy-	tăk-ē	rapid	35, 120
ten/o	tĕn-ō	tendon	201
tend/o	tĕnd-ō	tendon	201
tendin/o	tĕn-dĭn-ō	tendon	201
thalam/o	thăl-ă-mō	thalamus, chamber	301
thel/o	thē-lō	nipple	67
-therapy	thĕr-ă-pē	treatment	68
therm/o	thĕr-mō	heat	3
thorac/o	thō-răk-ō	chest	3, 12, 119, 199
-thorax	thō-răks	chest	120
thromb/o	thrŏm-bō	blood clot	145, 174
thym/o	thī-mō	thymus	174, 277
thyr/o	thī-rō	thyroid	277
thyroid/o	thī-royd-ō	thyroid	277
tibi/o	tĭb-ē-ō	tibia (larger, inner bone of lower leg)	200
-tic	tĭk	pertaining to	26
-tocia	tō-sē-ă	childbirth, labor	250
-tome	tōm	instrument to cut	13
-tomy	tō-mē	incision	3, 12, 13
ton/o	tŏn-ō	tone, tension, pressure	301
tonsill/o	tŏn-sĭ-lō	tonsils	118
-toxic	tŏks-ĭk	poison	16, 278

Medical Word Element	Pronunciation	Meaning	Page Numbers
trache/o	trā-kē-ō	trachea	119
trans-	trănz	through, across	34, 52, 146
tri-	trī	three	33
trich/o	trĭk-ō	hair	67
-tripsy	trĭp-sē	crushing	14
-trophy	trō-fē	development, nourishment	16, 278
-tropia	trō-pē-ă	turning	322
-tropin	trō-pĭn	stimulate	278
tympan/o	tĭm-pă-nō	tympanic membrane, eardrum	322
-ula	ū-lă	small, minute	27
-ule	yool	small, minute	27
ultra-	ŭl-tră	beyond, excess	52
ungu/o	ŭng-gwō	nail	67
uni-	yoo-nē	one	33
ur/o	ū-rō	urine, urinary	225
ureter/o	ū-rē-tĕr-ō	ureter	225
urethr/o	ū-rē-thrō	urethra	225
-uria	ū-rē-ă	urine	226, 278
uter/o	ū-tĕr-ō	uterus, womb	249
vagin/o	vă-jĭn-ō	vagina	249
vas/o	vās-ō	vessel, vas deferens, duct	145, 226
ven/o	vē-nō	vein	145
ventricul/o	vĕn-trĭk-ū-lō	ventricle (of heart or brain)	301
ventr/o	vĕn-trō	belly, belly-side	49
-version	vĕr-zhŭn	act of turning	250
vertebr/o	vĕr-tē-brō	vertebrae (backbone)	199
vesic/o	vĕs-ĭ-kō	bladder	225
vesicul/o	vĕ-sĭk-ū-lō	seminal vesicle	226
viscer/o	vĭs-ĕr-ō	internal organs	51
vulv/o	vŭl-vō	vulva	249
xanth/o	zăn-thō	yellow	50
xen/o	zĕn-ō	foreign, strange	51
xer/o	zē-rō	dry	51, 67
-y	ē	condition	26

Part II ■ ENGLISH TERM TO MEDICAL WORD ELEMENT

English Term	Medical Word Element	Pronunciation	Page Numbers
abdomen	abdomin/o	ăb-dŏm-ĭ-nō	50
	lapar/o	lăp-ăr-ō	249
abnormal condition	-iasis	ī-ă-sĭs	15, 93, 226
	-osis	ō-sĭs	15, 175
above	epi-	ĕp-ĭ	32, 68
	super-	soo-pĕr	34
	supra-	soo-pră	34
above normal	hyper-	hī-pĕr	3, 33, 68, 93
acromion	acromi/o	ă-krō-mē-ō	200
across	dia-	dī-ă	34, 93
	trans-	trănz	34, 52, 146
act of measuring	-metry	mĕt-rē	15

English Term	Medical Word Element	Pronunciation	Page Numbers
act of turning	-version	vĕr-zhŭn	250
adenoid	adenoid/o	ăd-ē-noyd-ō	118
adrenal glands	adren/o	ăd-rē-nō	277
	adrenal/o	ă-drĕn-ăl-ō	277
after	post-	pōst	33
against	anti-	ăn-tĭ	35
	contra-	kŏn-tră	35
air	pneum/o	nū-mō	119
albumin (protein)	albumin/o	ăl-bū-mĭn-ō	226
alike	home/o	hō-mē-ō	277
all	pan-	păn	35
alveolus (pl. alveoli)	alveol/o	ăl-vē-ōl-ō	119
amnion (amniotic sac)	amni/o	ăm-nē-ō	249
anterior	anter/o	ăn-tĕr-ō	49
anus	an/o	ā-nō	92
	proct/o	prŏk-tō	92
appendix	append/o	ăp-ĕn-dō	92
	appendic/o	ăp-ĕn-dĭk-ō	92
appetite	-orexia	or-ĕks-ē-ă	93
aorta	aort/o	ā-or-tō	145
arm	brachi/o	brăk-ē-ō	199
around	circum-	sĕr-kŭm	34
	peri-	pĕr-ē	34, 52, 93, 146
arteriole	arteriol/o	ăr-tĕr-ĭ-ōl-ō	145
artery	arteri/o	ăr-tĕ-rē-ō	145
atrium	atri/o	ā-trē-ō	145
attraction to (for)	-phil	fĭl	175
	-philia	fĭl-ē-ă	15
away from	ab-	ăb	34, 52
back	poster/o	pŏs-tĕr-ō	49
back (of body)	dors/o	dor-sō	49
backbone	spondyl/o	spŏn-dĭl-ō	199
	vertebr/o	vĕr-tĕ-brō	199
backward	retro-	rĕt-rō	33
bacteria	bacteri/o	băk-tē-rē-ō	226
bad	dys-	dĭs	35, 93, 250
	mal-	măl	35
band	fasci/o	făsh-ē-ō	51
bear (offspring), to	-para	păr-ă	15, 250
before	ante-	ăn-tē	32
	pre-	prē	32
	pro-	prō	32
beginning	-arche	ăr-kē	250
behind	post-	pōst	33
	postero-	pŏs-tĕr-ō	49
	retro-	rĕt-rō	33
belly	ventr/o	vĕn-trō	49
belly-side	ventr/o	vĕn-trō	49
below	hypo-	hī-pō	32, 68
	infer/o	ĭn-fĕr-ō	49
	infra-	ĭn-fră	32, 52
	sub-	sŭb	32, 68, 93
bent	ankyl/o	ăng-kĭ-lō	200
beside	para	păr-ă	34
between	inter-	ĭn-tĕr	33
beyond	para-	păr-ă	34
	ultra-	ŭl-tră	52
bile	chol/e	kō-lē	92
bile duct	choledoch/o	kō-lĕ-dō-kō	92

English Term	Medical Word Element	Pronunciation	Page Numbers
bile vessel	cholangi/o	kō-lăn-jē-ō	92
binding	-desis	dē-sĭs	14, 201
birth	nat/a	nā-tă	249
black	-anthrac/o	an-thră-kō	50, 119
	melan/o	mĕl-ă-nō	50
bladder	cyst/o	sĭs-tō	225
	vesic/o	vĕs-ĭ-kō	225
blood	hem/o	hēm-ō	174
	hemat/o	hĕm-ă-tō	174
blood clot	thromb/o	thrŏm-bō	145, 174
blood condition	-emia	ē-mē-ă	14, 175
blood vessel	hemangi/o	hē-măn-jē-ō	145
blue	cyan/o	sī-ăn-ō	50
body	somat/o	sō-măt-ō	51, 277
bone	oste/o	ŏs-tē-ō	2, 3, 13, 200
bone marrow	myel/o	mī-ĕ-lō	174, 200, 301
borne	-phoresis	fō-rē-sĭs	175
brain	encephal/o	ĕn-sĕf-ă-lō	13, 301
break	-clasis	klă-sĭs	14, 201
breast	mamm/o	mă-mō	67, 249
	mast/o	măs-tō	67, 249
breastbone	stern/o	stĕr-nō	199
breathe	spir/o	spī-rō	119
breathing	-pnea	nē-ă	120
bronchus (pl. bronchi)	bronch/o	brŏng-kō	119
	bronchi/o	brŏng-kē-ō	119
bursting forth	-rrhage	răj	16
	-rrhagia	rā-jē-ă	16
calcaneum (heel bone)	calcane/o	kăl-kā-nē-ō	199
calcium	calc/o	kăl-kō	277
calculus	-lith	lĭth	15, 93
carbon dioxide (CO_2)	-capnia	kăp-nē-ă	120
carpus	carp/o	kăr-pō	199
carried	-phoresis	fō-rē-sĭs	175
cartilage	chondr/o	kŏn-drō	201
cell	-cyte	sīt	68
	cyt/o	sī-tō	49
cerebrum	cerebr/o	sĕr-ē-brō	301
cervix uteri (neck of uterus)	cervic/o	sĕr-vĭ-kō	249
chamber	thalam/o	thăl-ă-mō	301
cheek	bucc/o	bŭk-ō	91
chest	pector/o	pĕk-tō-rō	119
	steth/o	stĕth-ō	119
	thorac/o	thō-răk-ō	3, 12, 119, 199
	-thorax	thō-răks	120
childbirth	-tocia	tō-sē-ă	250
choroid	choroid/o	kō-royd-ō	321
ciliary body	cycl/o	sī-klō	321
clot (blood)	thromb/o	thrŏm-bō	145, 174
coal	anthrac/o	ăn-thră-kō	119
colon	col/o	kō-lō	92
	colon/o	kō-lŏn-ō	4, 12, 92
color	chrom/o	krōm-ō	173
condition	-ia	ē-ă	3, 26
	-iasis	ī-ă-sĭs	15, 93, 226
	-ism	ĭzm	26
	-y	ē	26
condyle	condyl/o	kŏn-dĭ-lō	200

English Term	Medical Word Element	Pronunciation	Page Numbers
contraction, involuntary	-spasm	spăzm	16
control	-stasis	stā-sĭs	16, 175
cornea	corne/o	kor-nē-ō	321
	kerat/o	kĕr-ă-tō	67, 321
cranium	crani/o	krā-nē-ō	199, 301
crooked	ankyl/o	ăng-kĭ-lō	200
crushing	-tripsy	trĭp-sē	14
cut into	-tomy	tō-mē	3, 12, 13
dawn (rose colored)	eosin/o	ē-ō-sĭn-ō	173
decrease	-penia	pē-nē-ă	15, 175
deficiency	-penia	pē-nē-ă	15, 175
destruction	-lysis	lĭ-sĭs	14
development	-trophy	trō-fē	16, 277
diaphragm	phren/o	frĕn-ō	119
different	hetero-	hĕt-ĕr-ō	35, 175
differing from the usual	all-	ăl	52
difficult	dys-	dĭs	35, 250
digestion	-pepsia	pĕp-sē-ă	93
digit (finger or toe)	dactyl/o	dăk-tĭ-lō	200
dilation	-ectasis	ĕk-tă-sĭs	14
dim	ambly/o	ăm-blē-ō	321
discharge	-rrhea	rē-ă	16
disease	path/o	păth-ō	51
	-pathy	pă-thē	15, 52
dissimilar	anis/o	ăn-ĭ-sō	175
double	dipl-	dĭpl	33
	diplo-	dĭp-lō	33
downward displacement	-ptosis	tō-sĭs	16
dry	ichthy/o	ĭk-thē-ō	67
	xer/o	zē-rō	50, 67
duct	vas/o	văs-ō	226
dull	ambly/o	ăm-blē-ō	321
duodenum	duoden/o	dū-ŏd-ē-nō	92
dust	coni/o	kō-nē-ō	119
ear	ot/o	ō-tō	322
eardrum	myring/o	mĭr-ĭn-gō	322
	tympan/o	tĭm-pă-nō	322
eating	phag/o	făg-ō	174
	-phagia	fā-jē-ă	15, 93, 277
embryonic cell	-blast	blăst	175, 201
	blast/o	blăs-tō	173
enlargement	-megaly	mĕg-ă-lē	3, 15, 93
epididymis	epididym/o	ĕp-ĭ-dĭd-ĭ-mō	226
equal	iso-	ī-sō	175
esophagus	esophag/o	ē-sŏf-ă-gō	91
eustachian tube	salping/o	săl-pĭng-gō/săl-pĭn-jō	322
examination	-scopy	skō-pē	12, 16, 201
excess	ultra-	ŭl-tră	52
excessive	hyper-	hī-pĕr	3, 33, 68, 93
	super-	soo-pĕr	34
	supra-	soo-pră	34
excision	-ectomy	ĕk-tō-mē	12, 13
expansion	-ectasis	ĕk-tă-sĭs	14
extremity	acr/o	ăk-rō	50, 277
eye	ocul/o	ŏk-ū-lō	321
	ophthalm/o	ŏf-thăl-mō	321
	opt/o	ŏp-tō	321
eyelid	blephar/o	blĕf-ă-rō	321

English Term	Medical Word Element	Pronunciation	Page Numbers
fallopian tubes	salping/o	săl-pĭng-gō/săl-pĭn-jō	249
	-salpinx	săl-pĭnks	250
false	pseudo-	soo-dō	35
far, farthest	dist/o	dĭs-tō	49
fat	adip/o	ăd-ĭ-pō	66
	lip/o	lĭ-pō	67
	steat/o	stē-ă-tō	67
fatty plaque	ather/o	ăth-ĕr-ō	145
fear	-phobia	fō-bē-ă	15
feeling	-esthesia	ĕs-thē-zē-ă	301
female	gynec/o	gĭ-nĕ-kō/jĭn-ē-ko	249
femur	femor/o	fĕm-ō-rō	199
fibula	fibul/o	fĭb-ū-lō	199
finger	dactyl/o	dăk-tĭ-lō	200
fingers, bones of	phalang/o	făl-ăn-jō	199
first	primi-	prī-mĭ	33, 250
fixation (of a bone or joint)	-desis	dē-sĭs	14, 201
fixation (of an organ)	-pexy	pĕk-sē	14
flow	-rrhea	rē-ă	16
foot	ped/i	pĕd-ē	200
	pod/o	pō-dō	200
foreign	xen/o	zĕn-ō	51
formation	-plasia	plā-zē-ă	15
	-poiesis	poy-ē-sĭs	16, 175
forming	-gen	jĕn	14
	-genesis	jĕn-ĕ-sĭs	14, 52, 226
forming an opening (mouth)	-stomy	stō-mē	13
four	quadri-	kwŏd-rĭ	33
fracture	-clasis	klă-sĭs	14, 201
from	ab-	ăb	34, 52
front	anter/o	ăn-tĕr-ō	49
fungus	myc/o	mī-kō	67
gall	chol/e	kō-lē	92
gallbladder	cholecyst/o	kō-lē-sĭs-tō	92
gland	aden/o	ăd-ēn-ō	66, 173
glans penis	balan/o	bă-lăn-ō	226
glomerulus	glomerul/o	glō-mĕr-ū-lō	225
glue	gli/o	glē-ō	301
gonads	gonad/o	gō-năd-ō	277
good	eu-	ū-	35, 120
granule	granul/o	grăn-ū-lō	174
gray	poli/o	pōl-ē-ō	51
green	chlor/o	klor-ō	50
groin	inguin/o	ĭng-gwĭ-nō	50
growth	-physis	fī-sĭs	201, 278
	-plasia	plā-zē-ă	15
gum(s)	gingiv/o	jĭn-jĭ-vō	91
hair	pil/o	pī-lō	67
	trich/o	trĭk-ō	67
half	hemi-	hĕm-ē	33
	semi-	sĕm-ē	33
hard	kerat/o	kĕr-ă-tō	67, 322
hardening	scler/o	sklĕ-rō	67, 322
head	cephal/o	sĕf-ăl-ō	199
hearing	audi/o	aw-dē-ō	322
heart	cardi/o	kăr-dē-ō	2, 145

English Term	Medical Word Element	Pronunciation	Page Numbers
heat	therm/o	thĕr-mō	3
heel bone	calcane/o	kăl-kā-nē-ō	199
hernia	-cele	sēl	14
hidden	crypt/o	krĭp-tō	67, 226
horny tissue	kerat/o	kĕr-ă-tō	67, 321
humerus	humer/o	hū-mĕr-ō	199
ileum	ile/o	ĭl-ē-ō	92
ilium	ili/o	ĭl-ē-ō	200
imperfect	atel/o	ăt-ĕ-lō	119
in	endo-	ĕn-dō	34, 146
	in-	ĭn	34
	intra-	ĭn-tră	34
in front	ante-	ăn-tē	32
	pre-	prē	32
	pro-	prō	32
incision	-tomy	tō-mē	3, 12, 13
incomplete	atel/o	ăt-ē-lō	119
increase, abnormal	-osis	ō-sĭs	3, 15, 175
inflammation	-itis	ī-tĭs	12, 13, 15
inner ear	labyrinth/o	lăb-ĭ-rĭn-thō	322
instrument to cut	-tome	tōm	13
instrument for measuring	-meter	mē-tĕr	15
instrument for recording	-graph	grăf	15, 52, 68, 145
instrument to view or examine	-scope	skōp	16
intestine (usually small intestine)	enter/o	ĕn-tĕr-ō	92
involuntary contraction	-spasm	spăzm	16
inward	eso-	ĕ-sō	322
iris	irid/o	ĭr-ĭ-dō	321
iron	sider/o	sĭd-ĕr-ō	174
irregular	poikil/o	poy-kĭ-lō	174
ischium	ischi/o	ĭs-kē-ō	200
jejunum	jejun/o	jĕ-joo-nō	92
joined	sym-	sĭm	35
	syn-	sĭn	35
joint	arthr/o	ăr-thrō	3, 12, 200
kidney	nephr/o	nĕf-rō	2, 225
	ren/o	rē-nō	225
kneecap	patell/o	pă-tĕl-ō	200
knowing	-gnosis	nō-sĭs	52
labor	-tocia	tō-sē-ă	250
labyrinth	labyrinth/o	lăb-ĭ-rĭn-thō	322
lacrimal sac	dacryocyst/o	dăk-rē-ō-sĭs-tō	321
lamina	lamin/o	lăm-ĭ-nō	200
large	macro-	măk-rō	3, 33, 175
larynx (voice box)	laryng/o	lă-rĭng-ō	118
lens	phac/o	fā-kō	322
lip	cheil/o	kī-lō	91
	labi/o	lā-bē-ō	91, 249
little	-icle	ĭk-ăl	27
	-ole	ŏl	27
	-ula	ū-lā	27
	-ule	yool	27
liver	hepat/o	hĕp-ă-tō	92

English Term	Medical Word Element	Pronunciation	Page Numbers
lobe	lob/o	lō-bō	119
loins	lumb/o	lŭm-bō	50, 200
loosening	-lysis	lī-sĭs	14
lower	infer/o	ĭn-fĕr-ō	49
lung	pneumon/o	nū-mŏn-o	119
	pulmon/o	pŭl-mŏn-ō	119
lymph	lymph/o	lĭm-fō	174
male	andr/o	ăn-drō	225, 277
many	multi-	mŭl-tē	33, 250
	poly-	pŏl-ē	33, 175
meal	-prandial	prăn-dē-ăl	93
measuring (act of)	-metry	mĕt-rē	15
medical profession	-iatrics	ī-ăt-rĭks	26
medicine	-iatr/o	ī-ăt-rō	26
	-iatry	ī-ă-trē	26
meninges	mening/o	mĕ-nĭng-gō	301
menses	men/o	mĕn-ō	249
menstruation	men/o	mĕn-ō	249
mesh	reticul/o	rē-tĭk-ū-lō	174
metacarpus (bones of the hand)	metacarp/o	mĕt-ă-kăr-pō	199
middle	medi-	mē-dē	33, 49
	mes/o-	mĕs-ō	33
milk	galact/o	gă-lăk-tō	249
	lact/o	lăk-tō	67, 249
mind	phren/o	frĕn-ō	119
minute	-icle	ĭk-ăl	27
	-ole	ŏl	27
	-ula	ū-lă	27
	-ule	yool	27
mouth	or/o	or-ō	91
	stomat/o	stō-mă-tō	91
movement	kinesi/o	kĭ-nē-sē-ō	301
much	multi-	mŭl-tē	33
	poly-	pŏl-ē	33, 175
muscle	my/o	mī-ō	201
nail	onych/o	ŏn-ĭ-kō	67
	ungu/o	ŭng-gwō	67
narrowing	-stenosis	stĕ-nō-sĭs	16
navel (umbilicus)	omphal/o	ŏm-fă-lō	50
near	para-	păr-ă	34
	proxim/o	prŏk-sĭm-ō	49
nearest	proxim/o	prŏk-sĭm-ō	49
neck	cervic/o	sĕr-vĭ-kō	199, 249
nerve	neur/o	nū-rō	301
nervous system	neur/o	nū-rō	301
net	reticul/o	rē-tĭk-ū-lō	174
neuroglia	gli/o	glē-ō	301
night	noct/o	nŏk-tō	226
nipple	thel/o	thē-lō	67
normal	eu-	ū	35, 120
nose	nas/o	nā-zō	118
	rhin/o	rī-nō	118
not	a-	ă	34, 175, 301
	an-	ăn	34, 301
	im-	ĭm	34
	in-	ĭn	34

English Term	Medical Word Element	Pronunciation	Page Numbers
nourishment	-trophy	trō-fē	16, 277
nucleus	kary/o	kăr-ē-ō	174
	nucle/o	nū-klē-ō	49, 174
numbing	narc/o	năr-kō	301
old age	presby/o	prĕz-bē-ō	322
one	mono-	mŏn-ō	33, 175
	uni-	yoo-nē	33
one half	hemi-	hĕm-ē	33
	semi-	sĕm-ē	33
one who specializes	-ist	ĭst	26
organ (internal)	viscer/o	vĭs-ĕr-ō	51
origin	-gen	jĕn	14
	-genesis	gĕn-ĕ-sĭs	14, 52, 226
other	all-	ăl	52
out	ec-	ĕk	34
	ex-	ĕks	34
out from	ec-	ĕk	34
	ex-	ĕks	34
outside, outward	ecto-	ĕk-tō	34
	exo-	ĕks-ō	34, 322
	extra-	ĕks-tră	34, 146
ovary	oophor/o	ō-ŏf-ō-rō	249
	ovari/o	ō-văr-ē-ō	249
oviduct(s)	salping/o	săl-pĭng-gō/săl-pĭn-jō	249, 322
	-salpinx	săl-pĭnks	250
oxygen (O$_2$)	ox/o	ŏks-ō	119
pain	-algesia	ăl-gē-zē-ă	301
	-algia	ăl-jē-ă	12, 14, 301
	-dynia	dĭn-ē-ă	14
painful	dys-	dĭs	35, 93, 250
pancreas	pancreat/o	păn-krē-ă-tō	93, 277
paralysis	-plegia	plē-jē-ă	15
parathyroid glands	parathyroid/o	păr-ă-thī-roy-dō	277
partial paralysis	-paresis	pă-rē-sĭs	15
patella	patell/o	pă-tĕl-ō	200
peculiar	idi/o	ĭd-ē-ō	51
pelvis	pelv/i	pĕl-vē	50, 200
	pelv/o	pĕl-vō	50
perineum	perine/o	pĕr-ĭ-nē-ō	249
pertaining to	-ac	ăk	26
	-al	ăl	26
	-ar	ĕr	26
	-ary	ĕr-ē	26
	-eal	ē-ăl	26
	-ic	ĭk	26
	-ical	ĭk-ăl	26
	-ory	or-ē	26
	-ous	ŭs	26
	-tic	tĭk	26
phalanges (bones of fingers and toes)	phalang/o	făl-ăn-jō	199
pharynx	pharyng/o	fă-rĭng-gō	91, 118
physicians	-iatrics	ī-ăt-rĭks	26
pleura	pleur/o	ploo-rō	119
poison	-toxic	tŏks-ĭk	16, 278
porous	-porosis	pō-rō-sĭs	201

English Term	Medical Word Element	Pronunciation	Page Numbers
posterior	poster/o	pŏs-tĕr-ō	49
pregnancy	-cyesis	sī-ē-sĭs	250
	-gravida	grăv-ĭ-dă	250
pressure	ton/o	tŏn-ō	301
process	-ia	ē-ă	26
	-y	ē	26
producing	-gen	jĕn	14
	-genesis	jĕn-ĕ-sĭs	14, 52, 226
production	-poiesis	poy-ē-sĭs	16, 175
prolapse	-ptosis	tō-sĭs	16
prostate	prostat/o	prŏs-tă-tō	226
protein	-globin	glō-bĭn	175
pubis (part of hip bone)	pub/o	pū-bō	200
pulse	sphygm/o	sfĭg-mō	145
puncture	-centesis	sĕn-tē-sĭs	3, 12, 13
pupil	core/o	kō-rē-ō	322
	pupill/o	pū-pĭ-lō	322
pus	py/o	pī-ō	226
pylorus	pylor/o	pī-lō-rō	91
radiation	radi/o	rā-dē-ō	51
rapid	tachy-	tăk-ē	35, 120
record	-gram	grăm	14, 52, 68, 145
recording (instrument used for)	-graph	grăf	14, 52, 68, 145
recording (process of)	-graphy	gră-fē	14, 52, 68
rectum	proct/o	prŏk-tō	92
	rect/o	rĕk-tō	92
red	erythem/o	ĕr-ĭ-thē-mō	51
	erythr/o	ē-rĭth-rō	51, 174
	rube/o	roo-bē-ō	51
refracture	-clasis	klăh-sĭs	201
relating to	-ac	ăk	26
	-al	ăl	26
	-ar	ĕr	26
	-ary	ĕr-ē	26
	-eal	ē-ăl	26
	-ic	ĭk	26
	-ical	ĭk-ăl	26
	-ory	ŏr-ē	26
	-ous	ŭs	26
	-tic	tĭk	26
removal	-ectomy	ĕk-tō-mē	12, 13
resembling	-oid	oyd	15
retina	retin/o	rĕt-ĭ-nō	322
ribs	cost/o	kŏs-tō	199
rod-shaped (striated)	rhabd/o	răb-dō	201
rod-shaped (striated) muscle	rhabdomy/o	răb-dō-mī-ō	201
rose colored	eosin/o	ē-ō-sĭn-ō	174
rupture	-rrhexis	rĕk-sĭs	16
safe	immun/o	ĭm-ū-nō	174
saliva	sial/o	sī-ă-lō	93
salivary gland	sial/o	sī-ă-lō	93
same	home/o	hō-mē-ō	51, 277
	hom/o	hō-mō	35, 175
	is/o	ī-sō	175

English Term	Medical Word Element	Pronunciation	Page Numbers
scaly	squam/o	skwā-mō	67
	ichthy/o	ĭk-thē-ō	67
scanty	olig/o	ō-lĭg-ō	226
sclera	scler/o	sklĕ-rō	67, 322
secrete	-crine	krĭn/krīn	277
seizure	-lepsy	lĕp-sē	301
seminal vesicle	vesicul/o	vĕ-sĭk-ū-lō	226
sensation	-esthesia	ĕs-thē-zē-ă	301
separation	-lysis	lī-sĭs	14
sex glands	gonad/o	gō-năd-ō	277
shape	morph/o	mor-fō	174
side	later/o	lăt-ĕr-ō	49
sigmoid colon	sigmoid/o	sĭg-moi-dō	92
skin	cutane/o	kū-tā-nē-ō	67
	-derma	dĕr-mă	68
	derm/o	dĕr-mō	67
	dermat/o	dĕr-mă-tō	67
skull	crani/o	krā-nē-ō	199, 301
slow	brady-	brăd-ē	35, 120, 301
small	-icle	ĭk-ăl	27
	-ole	ōl	27
	micro-	mī-krō	3, 33, 175
	-ula	ū-lă	27
	-ule	yool	27
smell	-osmia	ŏz-mē-ă	120
smooth muscle	leiomy/o	lī-ō-mī-ō	201
softening	-malacia	mă-lā-shē-ă	15, 201
specialist in the study of	-logist	lō-jĭst	15, 68
speech	-phasia	fā-zē-ă	301
sperm	spermat/o	spĕr-mă-tō	226
spinal cord	myel/o	mī-ĕ-lō	174, 200, 301
spine	rachi/o	răk-ē-ō	199
spitting	-ptysis	tĭ-sĭs	120
spleen	splen/o	splē-nō	174
splitting	-schisis	skĭ-sĭs	201
standing still	-stasis	stā-sĭs	16, 175
stapes	staped/o	stā-pē-dō	322
sternum (breastbone)	stern/o	stĕr-nō	199
stiffness	ankyl/o	ăng-kĭ-lō	200
stimulate	-tropin	trō-pĭn	278
stomach	gastr/o	găs-trō	2, 3, 13, 91
stone	-lith	lĭth	15, 93
straight	orth/o	or-thō	119, 200
striated (rod-shaped) muscle	rhabdomy/o	răb-dō-mī-ō	201
stricture	-stenosis	stĕ-nō-sĭs	16
stroke	-plegia	plē-jē-ă	15
study of	-logy	lō-jē	15, 68
stupor	narc/o	năr-kō	301
sugar	gluc/o	gloo-kō	277
	glyc/o	glī-kō	277
surgical repair	-plasty	plăs-tē	14, 93, 201
suspension	-pexy	pĕk-sē	14
suture	-rrhaphy	răf-ē	14
swallowing	phag/o	făg-ō	174
	-phagia	fā-jē-ă	15, 93, 277
sweat	hidr/o	hī-drō	67
sweetness	gluc/o	gloo-kō	277
	glyc/o	glī-kō	277

English Term	Medical Word Element	Pronunciation	Page Numbers
swelling	-cele	sēl	14
tail	caud/o	kaw-dō	49
tear	dacry/o	dăk-rē-ō	321
teeth	dent/o	dĕn-tō	91
	odont/o	ŏ-dŏn-tō	91
tendon	ten/o	tĕn-ō	201
	tend/o	tĕnd-ō	201
	tendin/o	tĕn-dĭn-ō	201
tension	ton/o	tŏn-ō	301
testes	orch/i	or-kē	226
	orchi/o	or-kē-ō	226
	orchid/o	or-kĭ-dō	226
thalamus	thalam/o	thăl-ă-mō	301
thigh bone	femor/o	fĕm-ō-rō	199
thirst	-dipsia	dĭp-sē-ă	277
three	tri-	trī	33
throat	pharyng/o	fă-rĭng-gō	91, 118
through	-dia	dī-ă	34, 93
	trans-	trănz	34, 52, 146
thymus	thym/o	thī-mō	174, 277
thyroid	thyr/o	thī-rō	277
	thyroid/o	thī-roy-dō	277
tibia	tibi/o	tĭb-ē-ō	200
tissue	hist/o	hĭs-tō	49
to bear (offspring)	-para	păr-ă	15, 250
toe	dactyl/o	dăk-tĭ-lō	200
toes, bones of	phalang/o	făl-ăn-jō	199
together	sym-	sĭm	35
	syn-	sĭn	35
tone	ton/o	tŏn-ō	301
tongue	gloss/o	glŏs-ō	91
	lingu/o	lĭng-gwō	91
tonsils	tonsill/o	tŏn-sĭ-lō	118
tooth	dent/o	dĕnt-ō	91
	odont/o	ō-dŏn-tō	91
toward	ad-	ăd	34, 52
trachea	trache/o	trā-kē-ō	119
treatment	-iatry	ī-ă-trē	26
	-therapy	thĕr-ă-pē	68
tumor	-oma	ō-mă	15
turning	-tropia	trō-pē-ă	322
twitching	-spasm	spăzm	16
two	bi-	bī	33
twofold	diplo-, dipl-	dĭp-lō	33
tympanic membrane	myring/o	mĭr-ĭn-gō	322
	tympan/o	tĭm-pă-nō	322
under	hypo-	hī-pō	32, 68
	infra-	ĭn-fră	32, 52
	sub-	sŭb	32, 68, 93
unequal	aniso-	ăn-ī-sō	175
union	sym-	sĭm	35
	syn-	sĭn	35
unknown	idi/o	ĭd-ē-ō	51
upon	epi-	ĕp-ĭ	32, 68
ureter	ureter/o	ū-rē-tĕr-ō	225
urethra	urethr/o	ū-rē-thrō	225

English Term	Medical Word Element	Pronunciation	Page Numbers
urine	ur/o	ū-rō	225
	-uria	ū-rē-ă	226, 278
uterine tubes	salping/o	săl-pǐng-gō/săl-pǐn-jō	249, 322
	-salpinx	săl-pǐnks	250
uterus	hyster/o	hǐs-těr-ō	249
	metr/o	mě-trō	249
	uter/o	ū-těr-ō	249
vagina	colp/o	kǒl-pō	249
	vagin/o	vă-jǐn-ō	249
varied	poikil/o	poy-kǐ-lō	174
vas deferens	vas/o	văs-ō	226
vein	phleb/o	flěb-ō	12, 145
	ven/o	vē-nō	145
ventricle (of heart or brain)	ventricul/o	věn-trǐk-ū-lō	301
vertebrae	spondyl/o	spǒn-dǐ-lō	199
	vertebr/o	věr-tē-brō	199
vesicle, seminal	vesicul/o	vě-sǐk-ū-lō	226
vessel	angi/o	ăn-jē-ō	145
	vas/o	văs-ō	145, 226
vision	-opia	ō-pē-ă	322
	opt/o	ǒp-tō	321
visual examination	-scopy	skō-pē	12, 16, 201
voice	-phonia	fō-nē-ă	120
vomiting	-emesis	ěm-ě-sǐs	14, 93
vulva	episi/o	ē-pǐz-ē-ō	249
	vulv/o	vŭl-vō	249
water	aque/o	ā-kwē-ō	321
white	albin/o	ăl-bǐn-ō	50
	leuc/o	loo-kō	50
	leuk/o	loo-kō	50, 174
within	endo-	ěn-dō	34, 146, 250
	intra-	ǐn-tră	34
without	a-	ă	34, 175, 301
	an-	ăn	34, 301
woman	gynec/o	gǐ-ně-kō/jǐn-ē-kō	249
womb	hyster/o	hǐs-těr-ō	249
	metr/o	mě-trō	249
	uter/o	ū-těr-ō	249
wrist bones	carp/o	kăr-pō	199
record, a writing	-gram	grăm	14, 52, 68, 145
x-ray	radi/o	rā-dē-ō	51
yellow	cirrh/o	sǐr-rō	50
	jaund/o	jawn-dō	50
	xanth/o	zăn-thō	50

Appendix D

INDEX OF GENETIC DISORDERS

cretinism, Chapter 14, Endocrine System, p. 278

cystic fibrosis, Chapter 8, Respiratory System, p. 123

diabetes mellitus, Chapter 14, Endocrine System, p. 280

Down syndrome, Chapter 13, Female Reproductive System, p. 255

hemophilia, Chapter 10, Blood, Lymph, and Immune Systems, p. 177

Huntington's chorea, Chapter 15, Nervous System, p. 305

muscular dystrophy, Chapter 11, Musculoskeletal System, p. 205

retinoblastoma, Chapter 16, Special Senses, p. 326

rheumatoid arthritis, Chapter 11, Musculoskeletal System, p. 204

sickle cell anemia, Chapter 10, Blood, Lymph, and Immune Systems, Table 10–3, p. 176

spina bifida, Chapter 11, Musculoskeletal System, p. 204

spina bifida cystica, Chapter 11, Musculoskeletal System, p. 204

spina bifida occulta, Chapter 11, Musculoskeletal System, p. 204

trisomy 21, Chapter 13, Female Reproductive System, p. 255

Appendix E

INDEX OF DIAGNOSTIC IMAGING PROCEDURES

abdominal sonogram, Chapter 7, Gastrointestinal System, p. 101

aortography, Chapter 9, Cardiovascular System, p. 151

arthrography, Chapter 11, Musculoskeletal System, p. 206

barium enema, lower GI, Chapter 7, Gastrointestinal System, p. 100

bronchography, percutaneous transtracheal, Chapter 8, Respiratory System, p. 126

cardiac catheterization, Chapter 9, Cardiovascular System, p. 151

cerebral angiography, Chapter 15, Nervous System, p. 307

cerebral arteriography, Chapter 15, Nervous System, p. 307

chest radiographs (gallbladder series), Chapter 8, Respiratory System, p. 126

cholecystography, Chapter 7, Gastrointestinal System, p. 100

computed tomography (CT) scan, Chapter 5, Body Structure, p. 47

coronary angiography, Chapter 9, Cardiovascular System, p. 151

CT scan (bone), Chapter 11, Musculoskeletal System, p. 206

CT scan (joint), Chapter 11, Musculoskeletal System, p. 206

CT scan (kidney), nephrotomography, Chapter 12, Genitourinary System, p. 230

CT scan (liver, spleen), Chapter 7, Gastrointestinal System, p. 100

CT scan (pancreas, thyroid, adrenal glands), Chapter 14, Endocrine System, p. 283

CT scan (thoracic), Chapter 8, Respiratory System, p. 126

cystography, Chapter 12, Genitourinary System, p. 230

cystometrogram, cystometrography, Chapter 12, Genitourinary System, p. 230

cystourethrogram, cystourethrography, Chapter 12, Genitourinary System, p. 230

dacryocystography, Chapter 16, Special Senses, p. 328

digital radiography, Chapter 5, Body Structure, p. 53

diskography, Chapter 11, Musculoskeletal System, p. 206

echocardiography, Chapter 9, Cardiovascular System, p. 151

echocardiography, Doppler, Chapter 9, Cardiovascular System, p. 151

echoencephalography, Chapter 15, Nervous System, p. 307

electromyogram, electromyography, Chapter 12, Genitourinary System, p. 230

endoscopic retrograde cholangiopancreatography (ERCP), Chapter 7, Gastrointestinal System, p. 101

endovaginal ultrasound, Chapter 13, Female Reproductive System, p. 256

esophagram, Chapter 7, Gastrointestinal System, p. 100

eustachianography, Chapter 16, Special Senses, p. 328

excretory urography, Chapter 12, Genitourinary System, p. 230

fluorescein angiography, Chapter 16, Special Senses, p. 328

fluoroscopy, Chapter 5, Body Structure, p. 53

hysterosalpingography, hysterosalpingogram, Chapter 13, Female Reproductive System, p. 256

liver scan, Chapter 7, Gastrointestinal System, p. 101

lumbosacral spinal radiography (LS spine), Chapter 11, Musculoskeletal System, p. 206

lung perfusion studies, Chapter 8, Respiratory System, p. 126

lymphadenography, Chapter 10, Blood, Lymph, and Immune Systems, p. 180

lymphangiogram, Chapter 10, Blood, Lymph, and Immune Systems, p. 180

magnetic resonance angiography, Chapter 5, Body Structure, p. 53

magnetic resonance imaging (MRI), Chapter 5, Body Structure, p. 53

mammogram, mammography, Chapter 6, Integumentary System, p. 75

myelogram, myelography, Chapter 15, Nervous System, p. 307; Chapter 11, Musculoskeletal System, p. 206

percutaneous transtracheal bronchography, Chapter 8, Respiratory System, p. 126

phonocardiography, Chapter 9, Cardiovascular System, p. 151

positron emission tomography (PET) scan, Chapter 5, Body Structure, p. 53

positron emission tomography (PET) scan, cranial, Chapter 15, Nervous System, p. 307

radioactive iodine uptake (RAIU), Chapter 14, Endocrine System, p. 283

radiography, roentgenography, Chapter 5, Body Structure, pp. 47, 53

sialography, Chapter 7, Gastrointestinal System, p. 101

sonography, Chapter 5, Body Structure, p. 53; Chapter 7, Gastrointestinal System, p. 101

sphincter electromyography, Chapter 12, Genitourinary System, p. 230

splenography, Chapter 10, Blood, Lymph, and Immune Systems, p. 180

stereoradiography, Chapter 5, Body Structure, p. 53

subtraction angiography, Chapter 9, Cardiovascular System, p. 151

thyroid echogram (ultrasound examination of thyroid), Chapter 14, Endocrine System, p. 283

tomography (cranial), Chapter 15, Nervous System, p. 307

tomography (cranial) computed (CT scan), Chapter 15, Nervous System, p. 307

tympanography, Chapter 16, Special Senses, p. 328

ultrasonogram, ultrasonography, Chapter 5, Body Structure, p. 48; Chapter 7, Gastrointestinal System, p. 101; Chapter 13, Female Reproductive System, p. 256

ultrasound, Chapter 12, Genitourinary System, p. 230

ultrasound scrotal, Chapter 12, Genitourinary System, p. 230

upper GI, Chapter 7, Gastrointestinal System, p. 101

urography, Chapter 12, Genitourinary System, p. 230

urography, excretory, Chapter 12, Genitourinary System, p. 230

venography, Chapter 9, Cardiovascular System, p. 151

xeromammography, xeromammogram, Chapter 6, Integumentary System, p. 75

xeroradiography, Chapter 6, Integumentary System, p. 75

x-ray examination, Chapter 5, Body Structure, p. 47

INDEX OF PHARMACOLOGY

anabolic agent, Chapter 14, Endocrine System, p. 284

analgesics, Chapter 15, Nervous System, p. 308

antacids, Chapter 7, Gastrointestinal System, p. 102

antianginals, Chapter 9, Cardiovascular System, p. 154

antibacterials, Chapter 6, Integumentary System, p. 76

anticoagulants, Chapter 10, Blood, Lymph, and Immune Systems, p. 182

anticonvulsants, Chapter 15, Nervous System, p. 308

antidepressants, Chapter 15, Nervous System, p. 308

antidiarrheals, Chapter 7, Gastrointestinal System, p. 102

antiemetics, Chapter 7, Gastrointestinal System, p. 102

antiflatulents, Chapter 7, Gastrointestinal System, p. 102

antifungals, Chapter 6, Integumentary System, p. 76

antihistamines, Chapter 8, Respiratory System, p. 128

antihyperlipidemics, Chapter 14, Endocrine System, p. 284

antihypertensives, Chapter 9, Cardiovascular System, p. 154

anti-infectives, Chapter 6, Integumentary System, p. 76

anti-inflammatory drugs, Chapter 6, Integumentary System, p. 76; Chapter 11, Musculoskeletal System, p. 207

antinauseants, Chapter 7, Gastrointestinal System, p. 102

antipruritics, Chapter 6, Integumentary System, p. 76

antipyretics, Chapter 11, Musculoskeletal System, p. 207

antiseptics, Chapter 6, Integumentary System, p. 76

antispasmodics, Chapter 7, Gastrointestinal System, p. 102

antitussives, Chapter 8, Respiratory System, p. 128

aurotherapy, Chapter 11, Musculoskeletal System, p. 207

beta-adrenergic blocking agents, beta blockers, Chapter 9, Cardiovascular System, p. 154

beta-adrenergics, Chapter 16, Special Senses, p. 329

bronchodilators, Chapter 8, Respiratory System, p. 128

calcium channel blockers, Chapter 9, Cardiovascular System, p. 154

cathartics, laxatives, purgatives, Chapter 7, Gastrointestinal System, p. 103

chrysotherapy, Chapter 11, Musculoskeletal System, p. 207

contraceptives, Chapter 13, Female Reproductive System, p. 258

corticosteroids, Chapter 11, Musculoskeletal System, p. 207; Chapter 14, Endocrine System, p. 285

corticosteroids, topical, Chapter 6, Integumentary System, p. 76

cycloplegics, Chapter 16, Special Senses, p. 329

decongestants, Chapter 8, Respiratory System, p. 128

diuretics, Chapter 9, Cardiovascular System, p. 154; Chapter 12, Genitourinary System, p. 232

emetics, Chapter 7, Gastrointestinal System, p. 103

estrogen hormones, Chapter 12, Genitourinary System, p. 232; Chapter 13, Female Reproductive System, p. 258

expectorants, Chapter 8, Respiratory System, p. 128

fibrinolytics, Chapter 10, Blood, Lymph, and Immune Systems, p. 182

gold therapy, aurotherapy, chrysotherapy, Chapter 11, Musculoskeletal System, p. 207

gonadotropin, Chapter 12, Genitourinary System, p. 232

hemostatics, Chapter 10, Blood, Lymph, and Immune Systems, p. 182

heparin, Chapter 9, Cardiovascular System, p. 167

hypnotics, Chapter 15, Nervous System, p. 308

immunosuppressive agents, Chapter 10, Blood, Lymph, and Immune Systems, p. 182

inotropics, cardiotonics, Chapter 9, Cardiovascular System, p. 154

insulin, Chapter 14, Endocrine System, p. 285

keratolytics, Chapter 6, Integumentary System, p. 76

miotics, Chapter 16, Special Senses, p. 324

mucolytics, Chapter 8, Respiratory System, p. 128

mydriatics, Chapter 16, Special Senses, p. 329

opiates, Chapter 15, Nervous System, p. 308

oral contraceptives, Chapter 13, Female Reproductive System, p. 257

oral hypoglycemics, Chapter 14, Endocrine System, p. 285

oxytocins, Chapter 13, Female Reproductive System, p. 258

parasiticides, Chapter 6, Integumentary System, p. 76

peripheral vasodilators, Chapter 9, Cardiovascular System, p. 154

protectives, Chapter 6, Integumentary System, p. 76

psychotropic drugs, Chapter 15, Nervous System, p. 308

relaxants, Chapter 11, Musculoskeletal System, p. 207

sedatives, Chapter 15, Nervous System, p. 308

spermicidals, Chapter 12, Genitourinary System, p. 232; Chapter 13, Female Reproductive System, p. 258

tissue plasminogen activators, Chapter 9, Cardiovascular System, p. 154

topical anesthetics, Chapter 6, Integumentary System, p. 76

topical corticosteroids, Chapter 6, Integumentary System, p. 76

tranquilizers, Chapter 15, Nervous System, p. 308

uricosurics, Chapter 12, Genitourinary System, p. 232

vaccines, Chapter 10, Blood, Lymph, and Immune Systems, p. 182

vasodilators, Chapter 9, Cardiovascular System, p. 154

vasopressin, Chapter 14, Endocrine System, p. 285

Appendix G

INDEX OF ONCOLOGICAL TERMS

acute lymphocytic leukemia (ALL), Chapter 10, Blood, Lymph, and Immune Systems, p. 179

acute myelogenous leukemia (AML), Chapter 10, Blood, Lymph, and Immune Systems, p. 179

adenocarcinomas, Chapter 14, Endocrine System, p. 281

basal cell carcinoma, Chapter 6, Integumentary System, p. 71

breast cancer, Chapter 6, Integumentary System, p. 72

bronchogenic carcinoma, Chapter 8, Respiratory System, p. 123

carcinoma of the breast, Chapter 6, Integumentary System, p. 274

carcinoma of the prostate, Chapter 12, Genitourinary System, p. 228

cervical cancer, Chapter 13, Female Reproductive System, p. 253

chondrosarcoma, Chapter 11, Musculoskeletal System, p. 205

chronic lymphocytic leukemia (CLL), Chapter 10, Blood, Lymph, and Immune Systems, p. 179

chronic myelogenous leukemia (CML), Chapter 10, Blood, Lymph, and Immune Systems, p. 179

esophageal carcinomas, Chapter 7, Gastrointestinal System, p. 96

Ewing's sarcoma, Chapter 11, Musculoskeletal System, p. 205

fibrosarcoma, Chapter 11, Musculoskeletal System, p. 205

hepatocellular carcinomas, Chapter 7, Gastrointestinal System, p. 96

Hodgkin's disease, Chapter 10, Blood, Lymph, and Immune Systems, p. 179

intracranial neoplasms, Chapter 15, Nervous System, p. 304

intracranial tumors, Chapter 15, Nervous System, p. 303

intraorbital melanoma, Chapter 16, Special Senses, p. 326

Kaposi's sarcoma, Chapter 10, Blood, Lymph, and Immune Systems, p. 179

leukemias, Chapter 10, Blood, Lymph, and Immune Systems, p. 179

lymphosarcoma, Chapter 10, Blood, Lymph, and Immune Systems, p. 180

malignant tumors of the heart, Chapter 9, Cardiovascular System, p. 149

malignant melanoma, Chapter 6, Integumentary System, p. 72; Chapter 9, Cardiovascular System, p. 149

melanoma, Chapter 16, Special Senses, p. 326

melanoma of the choroid, Chapter 16, Special Senses, p. 326

metastatic tumors of the cranial cavity, Chapter 15, Nervous System, p. 303

myxoma, Chapter 9, Cardiovascular System, p. 149

neoplasms, Chapter 6, Integumentary System, p. 71

pancreatic cancer, Chapter 7, Gastrointestinal System, p. 281

pituitary tumors, Chapter 14, Endocrine System, p. 281

primary intracranial tumors, Chapter 15, Nervous System, p. 303

primary pulmonary cancer, Chapter 8, Respiratory System, p. 123

prostatic cancers, Chapter 12, Genitourinary System, p. 228

retinoblastoma, Chapter 16, Special Senses, p. 326

squamous cell carcinoma, Chapter 6, Integumentary System, p. 72

stomach cancer, Chapter 7, Gastrointestinal System, p. 96

thyroid cancer, Chapter 14, Endocrine System, p. 281

TNM system of staging, Chapter 6, Integumentary System, p. 72

tumor grading, Chapter 6, Integumentary System, p. 71

INDEX

Page numbers followed by "f" indicate figures; page numbers followed by "t" indicate tables.

Abbreviations, 351–359
Abdominal sonogram, 101
Abdominopelvic region, 46–47, 46f
Ablation, 53
Abortion, 255
Abruptio placentae, 255
Abscess, 72
Accommodation, 318
Achromatopsia, 326
Acidosis, 125
Acne, 72
Acquired immune system, 170
Acquired immunodeficiency syndrome
    (AIDS), 176–177
Acromegaly, 282, 283f
Activated partial thromboplastin time
    (APTT), 180
Acute lymphocytic leukemia, 179
Acute myelogenous leukemia, 179
Acute myocardial infarction, medical record
    related to, 155
Acute tubular necrosis, 228
Adams-Stokes syndrome, 149
Addison's disease, 279
Adenocarcinomas, 281
Adenohypophyseal (anterior lobe)
    hormones, functions of, 273t
Adenoids, 116, 117f
Adenomas, 279
Adhesion, 53
Adipose tissue, 65, 66f
Adnexa, 254, 326
Adrenal cortex, 275
    disorders of, 279–280
Adrenal cortical hormones, functions of, 276t
Adrenal glands
    anatomy and physiology of, 274–275
    disorders of, 279–280
    hormones of, 276t
Adrenal medulla, 275
    disorders of, 279
Adrenal medullary hormones, functions of,
    276t
Adrenalectomy, 280
Adrenocorticotropic hormone (ACTH),
    functions of, 273t
Adult respiratory distress syndrome (ARDS),
    123
Aerophagia, 98
Afferent arteriole, 223f, 224
Afferent nerves, 294

Age-related macular degeneration (ARMD),
    325
Agglutinin, 173, 173t
Agglutinogens, 173, 173t
Agnosia, 304
Agranulocytes, 167
AIDS (acquired immunodeficiency
    syndrome), 176–177
Aldosterone, 275
Alkaline phosphatase, 101
Allergy(ies), 178f, 179
Allograft, 75
Alopecia, 65, 71
Alveolus(i), 117, 117f
Alzheimer's disease, 303
Amblyopia, 325
Amenorrhea, 248
Ametropia, 323–324, 323f
Amniocentesis, 257
Amnion, 255
Amphiarthroses, 195
Amputation, 207
Anabolic agents, actions of, 284
Anacusis, 327
Analgesics, actions of, 308
Anastomosis, 54, 102, 147, 153
Anatomical directions, combining forms
    denoting, 49
Anatomical position, 43–44, 44f
Anemia(s), 176, 176t
    aplastic, 176t
    causes of, 176
    described, 176
    folic acid deficiency, 176t
    hemolytic, 176t
    iron-deficiency, 176t
    pernicious, 176t
    sickle cell, 176t
    types of, 176
Anesthetics, topical, actions of, 76
Aneurysm, 146, 149
    aortic, 150f
Angina, 147
Angina pectoris, 147
Angiography
    cerebral, 307
    coronary, 151
    fluorescein, 328
    subtraction, 151
Angioplasty, 153
    arterial balloon, 147, 147f

Anisocytosis, 180
Ankylosis, 202, 325
Anorchism, 229
Anorexia, 98, 178
Anorexia nervosa, 98
Anosmia, 125
Anoxemia, 125
Anoxia, 125
Antacids, actions of, 102
Anterior cavity, 318–319, 318f
Antianginals, actions of, 154
Antibacterials, actions of, 76
Antibody(ies), 171–172, 180
Anticoagulants, actions of, 182
Anticonvulsants, actions of, 308
Antidepressants, actions of, 308
Antidiarrheals, actions of, 102
Antiemetics, actions of, 102
Antiflatulents, actions of, 102
Antifungals, actions of, 76
Antigens, 170–171, 180
Antihemophilic factor (AHF), 178
Antihistamines, actions of, 128
Antihyperlipidemics, actions of, 284
Antihypertensives, actions of, 154
Anti-infectives, actions of, 76
Anti-inflammatory drugs, actions of, 76, 207
Antinauseants, actions of, 102
Antipruritics, actions of, 76
Antipyretics, actions of, 207
Antiseptics, actions of, 76
Antispasmodics, actions of, 102
Antitussives, actions of, 128
Antral irrigation, 128
Anuria, 228
Aorta, 140
Aortic aneurysms, 150f
Aortic semilunar valve, 140
Aortography, 151
Aphasia, 302
Aplastic anemia, 176t
Aponeurosis, 198
Apoplexy, 302
Appendicitis, 98
Appendicular skeleton, 193
Aqueous humor, 318
Arachnoid space, 300
Areola, 66, 66f
Arrest
    cardiac, 149
    circulatory, 149

Arrhythmias, 149, 302–303
Arterial balloon angioplasty, 147, 147f
Arterial blood gases (ABGs), 127
Arteriography, cerebral, 307
Arteriole(s), 138, 139f
    afferent, 223f, 224
    efferent, 223f, 224
Arteriosclerosis, 302
Artery(ies), 138, 139f
    anterior descending, left, 142
    circumflex, 142
    coronary
        left, 142
        right, 142
    pulmonary
        left, 140
        right, 140
    renal, 222, 223f
Arthralgia, 94, 149
Arthritis, 252
    gouty, 204
    rheumatoid, 204
Arthrocentesis, 207
Arthroclasia, 207
Arthrography, 206
Arthroscopy, 207
Articulate, 195
Articulations, 195
Ascending tracts, 300
Ascites, 98, 121, 177, 180
Aspartate transaminase (AST), 147
Aspermia, 229
Asphyxia, 125
Aspiration, 181
Aspiration biopsy cytology (ABC), 101
Asthenia, 302, 304
Astigmatism, 323f, 324
Astrocytes, 296
Ataxia, 302, 304
Atelectasis, 125
Atherectomy, 153
Atheromas, 146
Atherosclerosis, 146–147, 146f
Atlas, 193
Atresia, 254
Atrium
    left, 140
    right, 140, 141f, 144, 144f
Attachments, anatomy and physiology of,
    196, 197f–198f, 198
Audiometry, 328
Aura, 304
Auricle, 320, 320f
Aurotherapy, actions of, 207
Auscultation, 122
Autism, 304
Autoimmune disease, 177
Autonomic nervous system (ANS),
    298–299
Axial skeleton, 192
Axis, 193
Axon, 294, 295f
Azotemia, 228

B lymphocytes, 171
Bacteriuria, 227
Balanitis, 229
Baldness, 65
Barium enema, 100
Barrier contraceptive condom, 257
Bartholin's glands, 245, 245f, 246, 246f
Basal cell carcinoma, 71
Bell's palsy, 302
Benign prostatic hyperplasia, 227–228
Benign prostatic hypertrophy, 227–228

Beta-adrenergic blocking agents, actions of,
    154, 329
Bicuspid (mitral) valve, 140
Bilateral pneumonia, 123
Biliary lithotripsy, 102
Biliary system, combining forms related to,
    92–93
Biopsy, 54, 75, 153
    needle, 54
    punch, 54
Bladder neck obstruction, 227
Blepharectomy, 328
Blepharoplasty, 328
Blind spot, 319
Blood, 163–187
    abbreviations related to, 182
    anatomy and physiology of, 164–168,
        165f, 166f, 167t, 168t
    combining forms related to, 173–174
    diagnostic, symptomatic, and therapeutic
        terms related to, 180
    diagnostic procedures related to,
        180–181
    medical record related to, 183
    oncology of, 179
    pathology of, 176–179
    pharmacology related to, 182
    prefixes related to, 175
    suffixes related to, 175
    surgical and therapeutic procedures
        related to, 181
    worksheets for, 184–187
Blood culture, 180
Blood groups, 173, 173t
Blood pressure, anatomy and physiology of,
    142–143
Blood urea nitrogen (BUN), 231
Blood-brain barrier, 296
Body cavities, 45, 45f, 46t
Body planes, 44, 44f, 45t
Body structure, 41–61
    abbreviations related to, 54–55
    abdominopelvic region, 46–47, 46f
    anatomical position of, 43–44, 44f
    body cavities, 45, 45f, 46t
    combining forms denoting, 51
    combining forms related to, 49–51
    diagnostic, symptomatic, and therapeutic
        terms related to, 53
    diagnostic imaging of, 47–48
    diagnostic procedures related to, 53
    directional terms related to, 48–49
    disease process in, 43
    levels of organization, 42–43
    medical record related to, 55
    planes of body, 44, 44f, 45t
    prefixes related to, 52
    spine, 48
    suffixes related to, 52
    surgical and therapeutic procedures
        related to, 54
    worksheets for, 56–61
Bolus, 87
Bone(s)
    depressions in, 195, 195t
    flat, 191
    irregular, 191
    long, 190–191, 191f
    pathology of, 202–204, 203f
    projections of, 195, 195t
    short, 191
    types of, 190–195, 191f–194f
Bone grafting, 207
Bone marrow, 181
Bone marrow transplantation, 181
Borborygmus, 98

Bowel obstruction, 95–96
Bowman's capsule, 223f, 224
Bradycardia, 147
Bradykinesia, 303
Brain, anatomy and physiology of, 299–300,
    299f
Breast(s), 65–66, 66f
Breast cancer, 72
Breech presentation, 255
Bronchiole(s), 117, 117f
Bronchodilators
    actions of, 128
    for COPD, 120
Bronchography, 126
Bronchopneumonia, 122–123, 122f
Bronchoscopy, 127
Bronchus(i), 117, 117f
Bruit, 149
Buccal cavity, anatomy and physiology of,
    86
Bulbourethral (Cowper's) gland, 224f, 225
Bulimia, 98
Bulla(ae), 71
Burns, 70–71, 70f
Bursectomy, 207

Cachexia, 98
Calcitonin, functions of, 274t
Calcium channel blockers, actions of, 154
Canal of Schlemm, 318f, 319
Cancer
    cervical, 253–254
    colon, 96–97, 97f
    lung, 123–125
    pancreatic, 281
    prostate, 228
    stomach, 96–97, 97f
    thyroid, 281
Candidiasis, 251
Canthus(i), 319
Capillary(ies), 138–139, 139f
    peritubular, 223f, 224
    pulmonary, 117, 117f
Carbuncle, 72
Cardiac catheterization, 151
Cardiac enzyme studies, 153
Cardiomyopathy, 149
Cardiotonics, actions of, 154
Cardiovascular system, 137–162
    abbreviations related to, 154–155
    anatomy and physiology of, 138–144
    combining forms related to, 145
    diagnostic, symptomatic, and therapeutic
        terms related to, 149–151, 150f
    diagnostic procedures related to,
        151–153, 152f
    medical record related to, 155
    oncology related to, 149
    pathology of, 146–149
    pharmacology related to, 154
    prefixes related to, 146
    suffixes related to, 145
    surgical and therapeutic procedures
        related to, 153
    worksheets for, 156–162
Carpal tunnel syndrome (CPT), 205
Cast(s), 227
Casting, 207
Cataracts, 324
Cathartics, actions of, 103
Catheterization, cardiac, 151
Cauterize, 54
Cell(s), 42
Cell body, 294, 295f
Cellular immunity, 171

Cellular respiration, anatomy and physiology of, 116
Cellular structure, combining forms denoting, 49
Cellulitis, 72
Central nervous system (CNS), 296–299, 296f–298f
Central venous catheter, 152f
Cerclage, 257
Cerebellum, 299f, 300
Cerebral angiography, 307
Cerebral arteriography, 307
Cerebral cortex, 299f, 300
Cerebral palsy, 304
Cerebrospinal fluid (CSF) analysis, 308
Cerebrovascular accident, 302
Cerebrovascular disease, 302
Cerebrum, 299–300, 299f
Cerumen, 320
Cervical cancer, 253–254
Cervical cap, 257
Cervicitis, 251, 253
Cervix, 246, 246f
Cervix uteri, 246, 246f
Cesarean birth, 257
Chalazion, 326
Chancre, 252
Change of life, 248
Chest radiographs, 126
Cheyne-Stokes respiration, 125
Chlamydia, 252–253
Chloasma, 73
Choked disc, 326
Cholecystography, 100
Cholelithiasis, 98
Chondrosarcoma, 205
Chorea, Huntington's, 305
Choriocarcinoma, 254
Chorionic villus sampling (CVS), 256
Choroid, 318, 318f
Chronic lymphocytic leukemia, 179
Chronic myelogenous leukemia, 179
Chronic obstructive pulmonary disease (COPD), 120–121
Chronic renal failure, 229
Chrysotherapy, actions of, 207
Chyme, 88
Cicatrix, 70
Ciliary body, 318, 318f
Circulation, fetal, anatomy and physiology of, 144, 144f
Circumcision, 231
Circumflex artery, 142
Cirrhosis, 99
Claudication, 205
Cleft palate, 99
Climacteric, 248
Clitoris, 245, 245f
Clonic spasm, 304
Closed head trauma, 304
Closed reduction of fractures, 207
Coarctation, 149
Coccyx, 193, 194f, 195
Cochlea, 320, 320f
Colic, 99
Colitis
  granulomatous, 99
  ulcerative, 94
Collecting tubule, 223f, 224
Colon
  anatomy and physiology of, 88f, 89
  combining forms related to, 92
Colon cancer, 96–97, 97f
Colonoscopy, 101
Color(s), combining forms denoting, 50–51
Colostomy, 102

Colpectomy, 257
Colpocleisis, 257
Colpoperineoplasty, 257
Colpoperineorrhaphy, 257
Colposcopy, 256
Coma, 304
Combining forms, 2, 49–51
  blood-related, 173–174
  body structure–related, 51
  cardiovascular system–related, 145
  defined, 2
  denoting anatomical directions, 49
  denoting cellular structure, 49
  denoting colors, 50–51
  denoting regions of body, 50
  endocrine system–related, 277
  examples of, 2
  female reproductive system–related, 249
  genitourinary system–related, 225–226
  immune system–related, 173–174
  integumentary system–related, 66–67
  lymph system–related, 173–174
  musculoskeletal system–related, 199–201
  nervous system–related, 301
  respiratory system–related, 118–119
  special senses–related, 321–322
Comedo, 73
Commissurotomy, 148
  mitral, 153
Common bile duct, 90, 90f
Compact bone, 190, 191f
Complete blood cell (CBC) count, 180
Compliance, 125
Computed tomography (CT), 47, 100, 126, 206, 283, 307
Concussion, 304
Conduction impairment, 327
Conductive tissue, 142
Cones, 318f, 319
Congestive heart failure (CHF), 121, 149
Conization, 257
Conjunctiva, 318, 318f, 319, 319f
Conjunctivitis, 326
Contraception, 257
Contraceptive(s), actions of, 258
Contraceptive implant, 257
Contracture, 205
Contusion, 69
Convergence, 326
Convulsions, 302–303
COPD. See Chronic obstructive pulmonary disease
Cordocentesis, 257
Coredialysis, 324
Corium, 64f, 65
Cornea, 318, 318f
Coronary angiography, 151
Coronary artery
  left, 142
  right, 142
Coronary artery disease, 147, 147f, 148f
  causes of, 147
Corpus callosum, 299f, 300
Corpus luteum, 254
Corpuscles, renal, 223–224, 223f
Cortex
  cerebral, 299f, 300
  renal, 222, 223f
Corticosteroids, actions of, 76, 207, 285
Coryza, 125
Costal cartilage, 194
Cough, productive, 120
Cowper's gland, 224f, 225
Crackle, 126
Cranial nerves, 296–299, 296f–298f
Creatine kinase (CK), 147

Creatine phosphokinase (CPK), 147
Crepitation, 205
Crest, 195
Cretinism, 278
Crohn's disease, 99
Croup, 125
Crushing, suffixes denoting, 14
Crustations, 68
Cryocautery, 257
Cryoprobe, 324
Cryosurgery, 257, 308
Cryptorchidism, 228
C-section, 257
Curettage, 54
Cushing's syndrome, 279
Cyanosis, 123
Cyclodialysis, 328
Cycloplegics, actions of, 329
Cyst(s), ganglion, 205
Cystic duct, 90, 90f
Cystic fibrosis, 123, 124f
Cystitis, 227, 252
Cystography, 230
Cystometrography, 230
Cystoscopy, 230
Cystourethrography, 230
Cytology, 42
  exfoliative, 256

Dacryocystography, 328
Debridement, 75
Decongestants, actions of, 128
Decortication, 128
Decubitus ulcer, 73
Degenerative joint disease, 204
Deglutition, 99
Dehiscence, 53
Dementia, 304
Demyelination, 303
Dendrites, 294, 295f
Dentin, 86f, 87
Dermabrasion, 75
Dermatomycosis, 73
Dermatoplasty, 71
Dermis, 64f, 65
Descending tracts, 300
Desquamation, 73
Diabetes, gestational, 281
Diabetes mellitus
  hyperparathyroidism and, medical record related to, 286
  insulin-dependent, 280, 280t
  non–insulin-dependent, 280, 281t
Diabetic retinopathy, 327
Diagnostic imaging procedures, index of, 383–384
Dialysis, 231
Diaphoresis, 147
Diaphragm, 45, 45f, 46t, 117f, 118, 118f, 257
Diaphragmatic hernia, 95
Diaphysis, 190, 191f
Diarrhea, 94
Diarthroses, 195
Diastole, 142
Diencephalon (interbrain), 299f, 300
Differential count, 181
Digestion, accessory organs of, 89–90, 90f
  combining forms related to, 92–93
Digital radiography, 53
Dilatation and curettage (D&C), 257
Directional terms, 48–49
Disc(s)
  choked, 326
  intervertebral, 193

Disease, process of, 43
Diskography, 206
Distal tubule, 223f, 224
Diuresis, 280, 282
Diuretics, actions of, 154, 232
Diverticula, 96
Diverticulectomy, 96
Diverticulitis
Diverticulosis, 96, 97f
Doppler echocardiography, 151
Dorsal cavity, 45, 45f, 46t
Dorsal vertebrae, 193
"Double" pneumonia, 123
Down syndrome, 255
Drusen, 325
Ductus arteriosus, 144, 144f
Ductus deferens, 224f, 225
Ductus venosus, 144, 144f
Duodenum, 87, 87f
Dura mater, 300
Dyscrasia, 180
Dysentery, 99
Dysmenorrhea, 250
Dyspareunia, 254
Dyspepsia, 99
Dysphagia, 99, 179, 205
Dysphasia, 302
Dyspnea, 32, 147, 149, 179
Dysrhythmias, 149, 302–303
Dystocia, 255
Dysuria, 229, 252

Ear(s), anatomy and physiology of,
        320–321, 320f
Ecchymosis, 73, 73f
Echocardiography, 151
Echoencephalography, 307
Echogram, thyroid, 283
Eclampsia, 255
Ectopic pregnancy, 255
Ectropion, 326
Eczema, 73
Edema, 177
    localized, 177
    pulmonary, 126, 149
Efferent arteriole, 223f, 224
Efferent nerves, 294
Effusion(s), pleural, 121
Ejaculatory duct, 224f, 225
Electrocardiography (ECG), 142, 152
Electroencephalography (EEG), 307
Electromyography (EMG), 205, 230, 307
Electronystagmography, 328
Embolectomy, 149
Embolus(i), 149
    pulmonary, 126
Emetics, actions of, 103
Empyema, 122
Encephalocele, 95
Endarterectomy, 147
Endocarditis, infective, 148
Endocervicitis, 254
Endocrine system, 269–291
    abbreviations related to, 285
    anatomy and physiology of, 270–276,
        270t, 271f, 272f, 273t–276t
    combining forms related to, 277
    diagnostic, symptomatic, and therapeutic
        terms related to, 282, 283f
    diagnostic procedures related to,
        283–284
    medical record related to, 286
    oncology of, 281
    pathology of, 278

    pharmacology related to, 284–285
    suffixes related to, 277–278
    surgical and therapeutic procedures
        related to, 284
    worksheets for, 287–291
Endometrial biopsy, 256
Endometrial smear, 256
Endometriosis, 251
Endometritis, 251
Endomysium, 198
Endoscopic retrograde
        cholangiopancreatography (ERCP),
        101
Endovaginal ultrasound, 256
Enteritis, regional, 99
Entropion, 326
Enucleation, 326, 328
Enuresis, 229
Ependyma, 296
Epidermis, 64, 64f
Epididymis, 224f, 225
Epiglottis, 86f, 87, 117, 117f
Epiglottitis, 125
Epilepsy, 302–303
    petit mal, 302
Epimysium, 198
Epinephrine, functions of, 276t
Epiphora, 326
Epiphysis, 190, 191f
Episiorrhaphy, 257
Episiotomy, 257
Epispadias, 229
Epistaxis, 125
Equilibrium, 321
Errors of refraction, 323–324, 323f
Eructation, 99
Erythema, 70, 73
Erythrocyte(s), 164–166
Erythrocyte sedimentation rate (ESR), 181
Erythropenia, 176
Erythropoiesis, 164, 191
Eschar, 73
Esophagogastroduodenoscopy, 101
Esophagoscopy, 101
Esophagram, 100
Esophagus, 86f, 87, 87f
    combining forms related to, 91
Esotropia, 325
Estrogen hormones, actions of, 232, 258
Estrogen replacement therapy (ERT), 248
Eupnea, 32
Eustachian tube, 320f, 321
Eustachianography, 328
Evisceration, 328
Ewing's sarcoma, 205
Exacerbation, 205
Excoriation, 68–69
Exfoliative cytology, 256
Exophthalmos, 278, 326
Exotropia, 324–325, 324f
Expectorants
    actions of, 128
    for COPD, 121
External auditory meatus, 320, 320f
External ear, 320
External respiration, anatomy and
        physiology of, 116
Extracapsular extraction, 324
Eye(s), anatomy and physiology of, 318–319

Fallopian tubes, 244–246, 245f
False ribs, 194
Fasting blood sugar (FBS), 101, 284
Fecalith, 96, 99

Fetal circulation, anatomy and physiology of,
        144, 144f
Fibrillation, 150
Fibrinolytics, actions of, 182
Fibroids, 254
Fibromyoma uteri, 254
Fibrosarcoma, 205
Fibrous attachments, 196, 197f–198f, 198
Filtrate, 224
Fimbriae, 246–247, 246f
Fistula, 229
Flatus, 99
Fleshy attachments, 196, 197f–198f, 198
Floating ribs, 194
Fluorescein angiography, 328
Fluoroscopy, 53
Folic acid deficiency anemia, 176t
Follicle-stimulating hormone (FSH),
        functions of, 273t
Foramen ovale, 144, 144f
Foreskin, 224f, 225
Fovea, 318f, 319
Fractures
    closed reduction of, 207
    open reduction of, 207
    types of, 202, 203f
Frequency, 229
Frontal lobe, 299f, 300
Frostbite, 71
Frozen section, 54
Fulguration, 75
Fundus, 87f, 88, 246, 246f

Gallbladder, 90, 90f
Gallbladder series, 100
Ganglion cyst, 205
Gastroesophageal hernia, 95
Gastroesophageal reflux disease, 100
Gastrointestinal system, 85–113
    abbreviations related to, 103–104
    accessory organs of, 89–90, 90f
    anatomy and physiology of, 86–89, 86f
    combining forms related to, 91–93
    diagnostic, symptomatic, and therapeutic
        terms related to, 98–100
    diagnostic procedures related to, 100–102
    medical record related to, 104
    oncology of, 96–97, 97f
    pathology of, 94–97
    pharmacology related to, 102–103
    prefixes related to, 93
    suffixes related to, 93
    surgical and therapeutic procedures
        related to, 102
    worksheets for, 105–113
Gastroscopy, 101
Genetic disorders, index of, 381
Genital herpes, 252, 253f
Genitourinary system, 219–241
    abbreviations related to, 232–233
    anatomy and physiology of, 220–225,
        220f–224f
    combining forms related to, 225–226
    diagnostic, symptomatic, and therapeutic
        terms related to, 228–229
    diagnostic procedures related to, 230–231
    macroscopic structures of, 220f, 221–222,
        221f, 222f
    medical record related to, 233
    microscopic structures of, 222–224, 223f
    oncology of, 228
    pathology of, 227–228
    pharmacology related to, 232
    suffixes related to, 226

surgical and therapeutic procedures related to, 231, 232f
worksheets for, 234–241
Gestation, 247, 255
Gestational diabetes, 281
Gingiva, 87
Gingivitis, 178
Gland(s). *See also specific type, e.g.,* Pituitary gland
sebaceous, 64f, 65
sudoriferous, 64f, 65
Glandular tissue, 65–66, 66f
Glans penis, 224f, 225
Glaucoma, 324
Glomerulonephritis, 227
Glomerulus, 223–224, 223f
Glucagon, 282
functions of, 276t
Glucocorticoids, 275
functions of, 276t
Glucose, 282
Glucose tolerance test (GTT), 101, 284
Glucosuria, 282
Glutamic oxaloacetic transaminase (GOT), 147
Glycosuria, 280, 282
Goiter, toxic, 278
Gold therapy, actions of, 207
Gonadotropin, actions of, 232
Gonioscopy, 327
Gonorrhea, 252
Gout, 204
Gouty arthritis, 204
Graft *versus* host reaction (GVHR), 180
Grand mal seizures, 303
Granulocytes, 167, 167t
Granulomatous colitis, 99
Graves' disease, 278
Gravida, 255
Growth hormone (GH), functions of, 273t
Guillain-Barré syndrome, 304
Gynecology, 254
Gyrus(i), 299f, 300

Hair, 65
Hair follicle, 64f, 65
Hair root, 64f, 65
Hair shaft, 64f, 65
Hairs of Corti, 321
Halitosis, 100
Hard palate, 86f, 87
Head trauma, closed, 304
Hearing, 320–321, 320f
Heart
anatomy and physiology of, 140–142, 141f
conduction system of, anatomy and physiology of, 142, 143f
Heberden's nodes, 204
Hemarthrosis, 178, 205
Hematemesis, 100
Hematocrit, 176, 181
Hematomas, 178, 202
Hematopoiesis, 164, 190
Hematuria, 227
Hemiparesis, 302
Hemiplegia, 302
Hemocytoblast, 164, 165f
Hemodialysis, 231
Hemoglobin, 164–165, 181
Hemolysis, 180
Hemolytic anemia, 176t
Hemophilia, 177–178
Hemopoiesis, 164, 165f
Hemoptysis, 123

Hemorrhage, 176t
subarachnoid, medical record related to, 309
Hemorrhoids, 96
Hemosiderin, 164–165
Hemostasis, 150, 180
Hemostatics, actions of, 182
Hemothorax, 122
Heparin, 167
actions of, 154
Hepatic duct, 90, 90f
Hepatitis, viral, 96
Hepatitis panel, 102
Hepatomegaly, 178
Hernia(s), 94–95, 95f
diaphragmatic, 95
gastroesophageal, 95
hiatal, 95
inguinal, 95
umbilical, 95
Herniated nucleus pulposus (HNP), 194
Hernioplasty, 95
Herniorrhaphy, 95, 228
Herpes
genital, 252, 253f
medical record related to, 260
Herpes zoster, 304, 305f
Hesitancy, 229
Hiatal hernia, 95
Hilum, 221f, 222
Hip girdle, 194–195, 194f
Hirsutism, 73, 280, 282
Histamines, 167
Hives, 178f, 179
Hodgkin's disease, 179
Holter monitor test, 152
Homeostasis, 43, 270, 282
Hordeolum, 326
Hormonal contraception, 257
Hormone(s). *See also specific types, e.g.,* Adrenal cortical hormones
definition and characteristics of, 270, 270t
estrogen, actions of, 232, 258
Humoral immunity, 171
Huntington's chorea, 305
Hyaline membrane, 123
Hyaline membrane disease (HMD), 123
Hydrocele, 229
Hydrocephalus, 301, 305
Hydronephrosis, 227
Hydrothorax, 122
Hymenotomy, 258
Hypercalcemia, 228, 282
Hypercholesterolemia, 146
Hyperesthesia, 70
Hyperglycemia, 280
Hyperkalemia, 279, 282
Hyperlipidemia, 150
Hypermenorrhea, 251
Hypermetropia, 323–324, 323f
Hyperopia, 323–324, 323f
Hyperparathyroidism, 279
and diabetes mellitus, medical record related to, 286
Hyperplasia
nodular, 227–228
prostatic, benign, 227–228
Hypertension, 143, 150
Hypertrophy, prostatic, 227
benign, 227–228
Hypervolemia, 282
Hypnotics, actions of, 308
Hypocalcemia, 279
Hypochromasia, 176
Hypochromic, 176

Hypodermis, 64f, 65
Hypoglycemia, 280
Hypoglycemics, oral, actions of, 285
Hypokinesia, 303
Hyponatremia, 279, 282
Hypoparathyroidism, 279
Hypophysis, 270, 273t–274t
Hypoplastic anemia, 176t
Hypoproteinemia, 177
Hypospadias, 229
Hypotension, 143
Hypothalamus, 299f, 300
Hypotonia, 205
Hypoxemia, 125
Hypoxia, 125
Hysterectomy, 253, 258
Hysterosalpingography, 256

Icterus, 96
Ilium, 194, 194f
Imaging procedures, diagnostic, index of, 383–384
Immune system, 163–187
abbreviations related to, 182
anatomy and physiology of, 170–173
combining forms related to, 173–174
diagnostic, symptomatic, and therapeutic terms related to, 180
diagnostic procedures related to, 180–181
medical record related to, 183
oncology of, 179
pathology of, 176–179
pharmacology related to, 182
prefixes related to, 175
suffixes related to, 175
surgical and therapeutic procedures related to, 181
Immunity
cellular, 171
humoral, 171
Immunosuppressive agents, actions of, 182
Impetigo, 73
Impotence, 229
Incision(s), suffixes denoting, 13
Incision and drainage (I&D), 54
Incontinence, 229
Incus, 320, 320f
Infant respiratory distress syndrome (IRDS), 123
Infarct, 150
Infectious mononucleosis, 178
Infective endocarditis, 148
Inferior vena cava, 140, 144, 144f
Infertility, 254
Influenza, 121
Infusion, 153
Inguinal hernia, 95
Inotropics, actions of, 154
Insufflation, 258
Insula, 299f, 300
Insulin
actions of, 285
functions of, 276t
Insulin tolerance test, 284
Insulinoma, 282
Integumentary system, 63–84
abbreviations related to, 76
anatomy and physiology of, 64–68
diagnostic, symptomatic, and therapeutic terms related to, 72–75, 73f, 74f
diagnostic procedures related to, 75
medical record related to, 77
pathology of, 68–72
pharmacology related to, 76

Integumentary system—Continued
    prefixes related to, 68
    suffixes related to, 68
    surgical and therapeutic procedures
        related to, 75
    worksheets for, 78–84
Interbrain, 299f, 300
Internal respiration, anatomy and physiology
    of, 116
Interstitial cell–stimulating hormone (ICSH),
    functions of, 273t
Intervertebral discs, 193
Intracapsular extraction, 324
Intraocular pressure, 324
Intrauterine devices (IUDs), 258
Intussusception, 95
Iridectomy, partial, 324
Iridodialysis, 324
Iris, 318f, 319
Iron-deficiency anemia, 176t
Irritable bowel syndrome, 100
Ischemia, 146, 150, 302
Ischium, 194, 194f
Islets of Langerhans, anatomy and
    physiology of, 275–276
Isthmus, 271

Jaundice, 96
Joint capsule, 195
Joints, 195
    pathology of, 204

Kaposi's sarcoma, 179
Keloids, 70
Keratitis, 302
Keratocentesis, 328
Keratolytics, actions of, 76
Keratosis, 73
Keratotomy, 328
Ketoacidosis, 280
Kyphosis, 203

Labia majora, 245, 245f
Labia minora, 245, 245f
Labor and childbirth, stages of, 247, 248f
Labyrinth, 320
Labyrinthitis, 327
Lacerations, 69
Lacrimal canals, 319, 319f
Lacrimal glands, 319, 319f
Lactate dehydrogenase (LD), 147
Lactiferous duct, 66, 66f
Laminectomy, 207
Laparoscopy, 256
Large bowel, anatomy and physiology of,
    88f, 89
Large intestine
    anatomy and physiology of, 88f, 89
    combining forms related to, 92
Laryngopharynx, 116, 117f
Laryngoscopy, 127
Larynx, 116–117, 117f
Laser surgery, 54
Lavage, 128
Laxatives, actions of, 103
Left anterior descending artery, 142
Left atrium, 140
Left coronary artery, 142
Left pulmonary artery, 140
Left pulmonary veins, 140
Left ventricle, 140
Leiomyomas, 253
Lens, 318, 318f

Lentigo, 73
Leptomeninges, 303–304
Lesions, skin. See Skin lesions
Lethargy, 305
Leukemia, 179
Leukocytes, 164, 166–167, 167t, 168f
    mononuclear, 167, 167t
Leukoplakia, 100
Leukopoiesis, 164, 165f, 191
Leukorrhea, 251
Ligaments, suspensory, 318, 318f
Ligation, 54
Ligation and stripping, 153
Lipid profile, 153
Lithotripsy, biliary, 102
Liver, 89–90, 90f
    combining forms related to, 92–93
    disorders of, 96
Liver biopsy, 102
Liver scan, 101
Lobar pneumonia, 123
Loop of Henle, 223f, 224
Loosening, suffixes denoting, 14
Lordosis, 204
Lower esophageal (gastroesophageal)
    sphincter, 88
Lumbar vertebrae, 193
Lumbosacral spinal radiography (LS spine),
    206
Lumpectomy, 75
Lung(s)
    left, 117, 117f
    postural drainage of, positions for, 123, 124f
    right, 117, 117f
Lung cancer, 123–125
Lung perfusion studies, 126
Lunula, 65
Luteinizing hormone (LH), functions of,
    273t
Lymph nodes, major groups of, 172f
Lymph system, 163–187
    abbreviations related to, 182
    anatomy and physiology of, 168–170,
        169f–172f
    combining forms related to, 173–174
    diagnostic, symptomatic, and therapeutic
        terms related to, 180
    diagnostic procedures related to, 180–181
    medical record related to, 183
    oncology of, 179
    pathology of, 176–179
    pharmacology related to, 182
    prefixes related to, 175
    suffixes related to, 175
    surgical and therapeutic procedures
        related to, 181
Lymph vessels, system of, 172f
Lymphadenography, 180
Lymphadenopathy, 177, 179, 180
Lymphangiectomy, 181
Lymphangiogram, 180
Lymphocyte(s)
    B, 171
    T, 171
Lymphosarcoma, 180, 205

Macrocytic, 176
Macrophages, 170–171
Macular degeneration, 325
Magnetic resonance angiography (MRA), 53
Magnetic resonance imaging (MRI), 47, 53
Malabsorption syndrome
Malaise, 149
Malignant melanoma, 72, 149
Malleus, 320, 320f

Mammography, 75
Mammoplasty, 75
Mantoux, 127
Mastectomy, 75
Mastication, 87
Mastoid antrotomy, 329
Mastoiditis, 325
Meatus, 224f, 225
Mediastinoscopy, 127
Mediastinum, 117, 117f
Medical word(s)
    building of, rules for, 3–4
    defining of, rules for, 4
    elements of, 1–9, 361–380
        combining forms, 2
        prefixes, 3
        suffixes, 2–3
        word roots, 2
        worksheets for, 7–9
    pronunciation guidelines for, 5–6
Medulla, 299f, 300
    adrenal, 275
        disorders of, 279
    renal, 222, 223f
Medullary cavity, 190–191, 191f
Melanocytes, 72
Melanoma, 326
    malignant, 149
Melena
Menarche, 254
Ménière's disease, 327
Meninges, 300
    anatomy and physiology of, 300–301
Meningocele, 204
Meningomyelocele, 204
Menopause, 248
Menorrhagia, 251
Menstrual cycle, 247
    phases of, 247
Menstrual disturbances, 250–251
Metamorphopsia, 326
Metrorrhagia, 250
Microcytic, 176
Microglia, 296
Microneurosurgery of pituitary gland, 284
Midbrain, 299f, 300
Mineralocorticoids, 275
    functions of, 276t
Miotics, 324
    actions of, 329
Mitral commissurotomy, 153
Mitral valve prolapse (MVP), 151
Mixed nerves, 297–298
Mononuclear leukocytes, 167, 167t
Mononucleosis, infectious, 178
Monospot, 181
Motor neurons, 294
Mouth
    anatomy and physiology of, 86–87, 86f
    combining forms related to, 91
Mucolytics
    actions of, 128
    for COPD, 120
Mucus, 125
Multigravida, 255
Multipara, 255
Multiple myeloma, 205
Multiple sclerosis, 303
Murmur, 149
Muscle(s)
    actions of, 196, 196f, 197t
    anatomy and physiology of, 195–196,
        196f, 197t
    cardiac, 196
    pathology of, 204–205
    skeletal, 196

smooth, 196
striated, 196
voluntary, 196
Muscular dystrophy, 205
Musculoskeletal system, 189–217
    abbreviations related to, 208
    anatomy and physiology of, 190–198
    combining forms related to, 199–201
    diagnostic, symptomatic, and therapeutic
        terms related to, 205–206
    diagnostic procedures related to, 206
    medical record related to, 208–209
    oncology of, 205
    pathology of, 202–205
    pharmacology related to, 207
    suffixes related to, 201
    surgical and therapeutic procedures
        related to, 207
    worksheets for, 210–217
Myasthenia gravis, 177, 204
Mydriatics, actions of, 329
Myelin sheath, 294, 295f
Myelocele, 204
Myelography, 206, 307
Myeloma, multiple, 205
Myocardial infarction, 147, 148f
    acute, medical record related to, 155
Myomectomy, 258
Myopia, 323–324, 323f
    unilateral, 325
Myringoplasty, 329
Myringorrhexis, 325
Myringotomy, 325
Myxedema, 278
Myxoma, 149

Nails, 65
Nares, 123
Nasal cavity, 116, 117f, 319, 319f
Nasopharynx, 116, 117f
Neoplasms. See Tumor(s)
Nephrolithiasis, 227, 279
Nephrolithotomy, 231
Nephropexy, 231
Nephroscopy, 230
Nephrotic syndrome, 229
Nephrotomography, 230
Nervous system, 293–315
    abbreviations related to, 308–309
    anatomy and physiology of, 294–301,
        295f–298f
    combining forms related to, 301
    diagnostic, symptomatic, and therapeutic
        terms related to, 304–306, 306f
    diagnostic procedures related to, 307
    medical record related to, 309
    oncology of, 303–304
    pathology of, 302–304
    pharmacology related to, 308
    prefixes related to, 302
    subdivisions of, 296–299, 296f–298f
    suffixes related to, 301
    surgical and therapeutic procedures
        related to, 308
    worksheets for, 310–315
Nervous tissue, anatomy and physiology of,
    294–296, 295f
Neural tube, 305
Neuroglia, 294, 296
Neurohypophyseal (posterior lobe)
    hormones, functions of, 274t
Neurolemma, 294, 295f
Neurolemmal sheath, 294, 295f
Neuron(s), 294–296, 295f
    motor, 294

olfactory, 116
sensory, 294
structures of, 294, 295f
Neurotransmitter, 294–295
Nipple, 66, 66f
Nocturia, 229
Node of Ranvier, 294, 295f
Nodular hyperplasia, 227–228
Norepinephrine, functions of, 276t
Normochromic, 176
Nuclear medicine, 53
Nucleus, 294, 295f
Nyctalopia, 326
Nycturia, 229
Nystagmus, 326

Obesity, 282
Obstetrician, 255
Obstetrics, 255
    female, 255
Obstipation, 96
Occipital lobe, 299f, 300
Occlusion, 146
Occult blood, 102
Olfactory neurons, 116
Oligodendrocytes, 296
Oligomenorrhea, 254
Oliguria, 228, 229
Oncology
    blood-related, 179
    cardiovascular system–related, 149
    endocrine system–related, 281
    female reproductive system–related, 253–
        254
    gastrointestinal system–related, 96–97, 97f
    genitourinary system–related, 228
    immune system–related, 179
    integumentary system–related, 71–72, 71t
    lymph system–related, 179
    musculoskeletal system–related, 205
    nervous system–related, 303–304
    respiratory system–related, 123–125
    special senses–related, 326
    terms related to, index of, 387–388
Oophoritis, 251, 252
Open reduction of fractures, 207
Ophthalmoscopy, 327
Opiates, actions of, 308
Optic disc, 319
Optic nerve, 319
Oral cavity, anatomy and physiology of, 86
Oral contraceptive pills (OCP), 257
Oral hypoglycemics, actions of, 285
Orchiectomy, 231
Orchiopexy, 228
Organisms, 43
Organs, 42–43
Oropharynx, 116, 117f
Orthopnea, 121
Orthoptic training, 325
Osteitis deformans, 202
Osteitis fibrosa cystica, 279
Osteoarthritis, 204
Osteoblasts, 191
Osteomas, 205
Osteomyelitis, 202
Osteophyte, 205
Osteoporosis, 202–203, 248, 279
Otitis externa, 327
Otitis media, 325
Otoencephalitis, 325
Otoplasty, 329
Otopyorrhea, 325
Otosclerosis, 325
Otoscopy, 327

Oval window, 321
Ovaries, 244–245, 245, 245f, 246f
Oxytocins
    actions of, 258
    functions of, 274t

Paget's disease, 202
Palatine tonsils, 116, 117f
Pallor, 73, 147
Pancreas, 90, 90f
    anatomy and physiology of, 275–276
    combining forms related to, 92–93
    disorders of, 280–281, 280t, 281t
    hormones of, 276t
Pancreatic cancer, 281
Panhypopituitarism, 282
Papanicolaou (Pap) test, 256
Papilla(ae), 64f, 65, 86f, 87
Papilledema, 304, 326
Para, 255
Paracentesis, 324
Parametritis, 251
Paraplegia, 305
Parasiticides, actions of, 76
Parasympathetic nervous system, 299
Parathyroid disorders, 279
Parathyroid glands
    anatomy and physiology of, 274
    hormones of, 275t
Parathyroid hormone (PTH), functions of,
    275t
Parathyroidectomy, 284
Paresis, 305
Paresthesia, 306
Parietal lobe, 299f, 300
Parietal pleura, 117, 117f
Parkinson's disease, 303
Partial iridectomy, 324
Partial thyroidectomy, 284
Parturition, 247, 255
Patent, 151
Patent ductus arteriosus, 151
Pathogenesis, 43
Pathology, 43
Pediculosis, 73
Pelvic (hip) girdle, 194–195, 194f
Pelvic infections, 251
Pelvimetry, 255
Pemphigus, 74
Penis, 224f, 225
Peptic ulcer, 94
Percussion, 122
Percutaneous transluminal coronary
    angioplasty, 153
Perforated ulcer, 94
Perforation, 94
Pericardiocentesis, 153
Pericardium, 140
Perimysium, 198
Perineal prostatectomy, 228
Perineum, 254
Periosteum, 191, 191f
Peripheral nervous system (PNS), 296–299,
    296f–298f
Peritoneal dialysis, 231
Peritoneoscopy, 256
Peritonitis, 95
Peritubular capillaries, 223f, 224
Pernicious anemia, 176t
Pertussis, 125
Petechia(ae), 74
Petit mal epilepsy, 302
Phacoemulsification, 324, 328
Phantom limb, 206
Pharmacology, index of, 385–386

Pharyngeal tonsils, 116, 117f
Pharynx, 86f, 87
    combining forms related to, 91
Pheochromocytoma, 279, 282
Phimosis, 229
Phlebitis, 148–149
Phlebotomy, 153
Phlegm, 125
Phonocardiography, 151
Photocoagulation, 325
Photophobia, 326
Photopigments, 319
Pia mater, 300
Pineal gland, anatomy and physiology of, 276
Pinealectomy, 284
Pinna, 320, 320f
Pituitary disorders, 278
Pituitary gland
    anatomy and physiology of, 270, 273t–274t
    hormones of, functions of, 273t–274t
    microneurosurgery of, 284
Pituitary tumors, 281
Placenta, 144, 144f
Placenta previa, 255
Plaques, 303
Plasma, 168
Plasma cells, 171
Plasmapheresis, therapeutic, medical record related to, 183
Platelet(s), 167
Pleura, 117, 117f
Pleural cavity, 117, 117f
Pleural effusions, 121
Pleurectomy, 128
Pleurisy, 126
Pleuritis, 126
Pneumoconiosis, 126
Pneumonectomy, 128
Pneumonia
    bilateral, 123
    "double," 123
    lobar, 123
Pneumothorax, 122
Poliomyelitis, 306
Polydipsia, 280
Polymorphonuclear cells, 167
Polyp, 53
Polyphagia, 280
Pons, 299f, 300
Pore(s), 65
Positron emission tomography (PET), 53, 307, 307f
Postural drainage, 126
Pott's disease, 204
Prefix(es), 3, 31–39
    blood-related, 175
    body structure–related, 52
    cardiovascular system–related, 146
    defined, 3
    of direction, 34
    examples of, 3
    female reproductive system–related, 25
    gastrointestinal system–related, 93
    immune system–related, 175
    integumentary system–related, 68
    lymph system–related, 175
    of negation, 34
    nervous system–related, 302
    of number and measurement, 33
    of position, 32–33
    respiratory system–related, 120
    special senses–related, 322
    worksheets for, 36–39

Pregnancy, 247
    ectopic, 255
Premenstrual syndrome, 251
Prepuce, 224f, 225
Presbyacusia, 327
Presbycusis, 327
Presbyopia, 323–324
Pressure-equalizing tubes, 327
Primigravida, 255
Primipara, 255
Process, 195
Proctosigmoidoscopy, 101
Productive cough, 120
Pronunciation guidelines, 5–6
Prostate cancer, 228
Prostate gland, 224f, 225
Prostatectomy
    perineal, 228
    suprapubic, 228
Prostatic hyperplasia, benign, 227–228
Prostatic hypertrophy, 227
    benign, 227–228
Prosthesis, 206
Protective(s), actions of, 76
Protein-bound iodine (PBI), 284
Proteinuria, 227
Prothrombin time (PT), 181
Proximal convoluted tubule, 223f, 224
Pruritus, 74, 179, 251
Psoriasis, 74
Psychotropic drugs, actions of, 308
Puberty, 254
Pubis, 194, 194f
Puerperium, 255
Pulmonary artery
    left, 140
    right, 140
Pulmonary capillaries, 117, 117f
Pulmonary edema, 126, 149
Pulmonary embolus, 126
Pulmonary function studies, 127
Pulmonary semilunar valve, 140
Pulmonary veins
    left, 140
    right, 140
Pulp, 87
Pupil(s), 318f, 319
Purgatives, actions of, 103
Purpura, 74
Pyelogram, 230
Pyelonephritis, 227
Pyloric sphincter, 87f, 89
Pyloric stenosis
Pyloromyotomy, 102
Pylorus, 87f, 88
Pyogenesis, 94
Pyopneumothorax, 122
Pyosalpinx, 254
Pyuria, 227

Quadriplegia, 306

Rachitis, 206
Radical dissection, 54
Radioactive iodine uptake (RAIU), 283
Radiofrequency (RF) waves, 47
Radiography, 47
    chest, 126
    digital, 53
Radiopaque materials, 47
Radiopharmaceutical, 53
Rale, 126
RBC indices, 181

Reconstructive surgeries, suffixes denoting, 14
Red blood cells (erythrocytes), 164–166
Refracturing, suffixes denoting, 14
Regional enteritis, 99
Regions of body, combining forms denoting, 50
Regurgitation, 148
Relaxants, actions of, 207
Renal artery, 221f, 222
Renal corpuscle, 223–224, 223f
Renal cortex, 222, 223f
Renal dialysis, 231
Renal failure, chronic, 229
Renal medulla, 222, 223f
Renal tubule, 223–224, 223f
Renal vein, 221f, 222
Reproductive system
    abbreviations related to, 259–260
    combining forms related to, 249
    diagnostic procedures related to, 256
    female, 243–268
        anatomy and physiology of, 244–248, 244f–246f, 248f
        anterior view of, 244f
        diagnostic and symptomatic terms related to, 254–255
        internal organs, 245–246, 246f
    male
        anatomy and physiology of, 224–225, 224f
        diagnostic, symptomatic, and therapeutic terms related to, 229
    medical record related to, 260
    oncology of, 253–254
    pathology of, 250–254, 252f, 253f
    pharmacology related to, 258
    prefixes related to, 250
    structures of, 244–245, 245f
    suffixes related to, 25
    surgical and therapeutic procedures related to, 257–258
    worksheets for, 261–268
Resection, 54, 128, 231
Respiration
    cellular, anatomy and physiology of, 116
    Cheyne-Stokes, 125
    external, anatomy and physiology of, 116
    internal, anatomy and physiology of, 116
Respiratory distress syndrome (RDS), 123
Respiratory system, 115–135
    abbreviations related to, 128–129
    anatomy and physiology of, 116–118, 117f
    combining forms related to, 118–119
    diagnostic, symptomatic, and therapeutic terms related to, 125–126
    diagnostic procedures related to, 126–127
    medical record related to, 129
    oncology of, 123–125
    pathology of, 120–125
    pharmacology related to, 128
    prefixes related to, 120
    suffixes related to, 120
    surgical and therapeutic procedures related to, 128
    worksheets for, 130–135
Reticulocyte(s), 164–165
Retina, 318, 318f
Retinoblastoma, 326
Retinopathy, 327
    diabetic, 327
Retinoscopy, 327
Retroversion, 254
Reye's syndrome, 306
RF detector coil, 47

Rheumatoid arthritis, 204
Rhinoplasty, 128
Rhonchus(i), 126
Rickets, 206
Right atrium, 140, 141f, 144, 144f
Right coronary artery, 142
Right pulmonary artery, 140
Right pulmonary veins, 140
Right ventricle, 140, 141f, 144, 144f
Rods, 318f, 319
Roentgenography, 47
Rubin's test, 258
Rugae, 87f, 88, 222, 222f

Sacrum, 193, 194f, 195
Salpingitis, 251, 252
Salpingo-oophorectomy, 258
Saphenous vein, 147
Sarcoma, 205
Scabies, 74
Schilling test, 181
Schwann cell, 294, 295f
Sciatica, 306
Sclera, 318, 318f
Sclerostomy, 329
Scoliosis, 203
Scrotum, 224f, 225
Sebum, 64f, 65
Sedatives, actions of, 308
Seizure(s), grand mal, 303
Seizure disorders, 302–303
Semen analysis, 231
Semicircular canals, 320f, 321
Seminal duct, 224f, 225
Seminal vesicle, 224f, 225
Seminiferous tubules, 224f, 225
Senile cataract, 324
Senses, special, 317–337
    abbreviations related to, 329–330
    anatomy and physiology of, 318–321
    combining forms related to, 321–322
    diagnostic, symptomatic, and therapeutic
        terms related to, 326–327
    diagnostic procedures related to, 327–328
    medical record related to, 330
    oncology of, 326
    pathology of, 323–326
    pharmacology related to, 329
    prefixes related to, 322
    suffixes related to, 322
    surgical and therapeutic procedures
        related to, 328–329
    worksheets for, 331–337
Sensory neurons, 294
Sepsis, 53
Septicemia, 180
Septum, 116, 117f
Sequestrectomy, 207
Sequestrum, 206
Seroconversion, 177
Serology, 180
Sexually transmitted diseases (STDs),
    251–253, 252f, 253f
Shingles, 304, 305f
Sialography, 101
Sickle cell anemia, 176t
Sigmoidoscopy, 101
Skeletal system
    anatomy and physiology of, 190–195,
        191f–194f, 195t
    bone of, 190–195, 191f–194f
    functions of, 190
    structure of, 190–195, 191f–194f
Skeleton, anterior view of, 192–193, 192f

Skin
    anatomy and physiology of, 64–68
    appendages of, 65–66, 66f
    combining forms related to, 66–67
    ecchymosis on, 73f
    functions of, 64–65, 64f
    structure of, 64, 64f
Skin graft, 75
Skin lesions
    primary, 68, 69f, 69t
    secondary, 68–70
    types of, 69t
Small bowel, anatomy and physiology of,
    88f, 89
Small intestine
    anatomy and physiology of, 88f, 89
    combining forms related to, 92
Soft palate, 87
Somatic nervous system (SNS), 298–299
Sonography, 53, 101
Spasm, clonic, 304
Specific immune system, 170
Spermicidals, actions of, 232
Spina bifida, 204
Spina bifida cystica, 204
Spina bifida occulta, 204
Spinal cord, 298f
    anatomy and physiology of, 300
Spinal disorders, 203–204
Spinal nerves, 296–299, 296f–298f, 298f
Spinal puncture, 308
Spinal tap, 308
Spine
    cervical and lumbar, radiology report of,
        medical record related to, 55
    curvature of, 203
    section of, 48
Spirometry, 127
Splenography, 180
Splenolaparotomy, 181
Splenomegaly, 178
Splenorrhexis, 178
Splinting, 207
Spondylitis, 204
Spondylolisthesis, 206
Spondylosis, 206
Spongy bones, 191, 191f
Sprain, 206
Sputum, 126
Sputum culture, 127
Squamous cell carcinoma, 72
Stapedectomy, 325
Stapes, 320, 320f
Steatorrhea
Stereoradiography, 53
Stereotaxy, 308
Sterility, 229, 254
Sternum, 194
Stoma, 94
Stomach
    anatomy and physiology of, 87–89, 87f,
        88f
    cancer of, 96–97, 97f
    combining forms related to, 91
Stool culture, 102
Storm, thyroid, 282
Strabismus, 324–325, 324f
Strabotomy, 325
Strain, 206
Strata, 64, 64f
Stratified squamous epithelium, 64, 64f
Stratum corneum, 64, 64f
Stratum germinativum, 64, 64f
Stress test, 152
Stridor, 126

Sty, 326
Subarachnoid hemorrhage, medical record
    related to, 309
Subarachnoid space, 300
Subcutaneous tissue, structure of, 64, 64f
Subdural space, 300
Subluxation, 206
Subtotal thyroidectomy, 284
Subtraction angiography, 151
Sudden infant death syndrome (SIDS), 126
Suffix(es), 2–3, 11–23, 25–30
    adjective, 26
    blood-related, 175
    body structure–related, 52
    cardiovascular system–related, 145
    defined, 2–3
    described, 12
    diagnostic, 14–16
    diminutive, 26–27
    endocrine system–related, 277–278
    examples of, 3
    female reproductive system–related, 25
    gastrointestinal system–related, 93
    genitourinary system–related, 226
    immune system–related, 175
    integumentary system–related, 68
    lymph system–related, 175
    musculoskeletal system–related, 201
    nervous system–related, 301
    noun, 26
    plural, 27
    related, 14–16
    respiratory system–related, 120
    special senses–related, 322
    surgical, 13–14
        denoting incisions, 13
        denoting reconstructive surgeries, 14
        denoting refracturing, loosening, or
            crushing, 14
    symptomatic, 14–16
    uses of, 12–13
    worksheets for, 17–23, 28–30
Sulcus(i), 299f, 300
Superior vena cava, 140
Suppurative, 53
Suprapubic prostatectomy, 228
Suprarenal glands, 274–275
Suspensory ligaments, 318, 318f
Sweat test, 127
Sympathetic nervous system, 299
Symphysis pubis, 194f, 195
Synapse, 294, 295f
Synaptic knob, 294–295
Synarthroses, 195
Syncope, 306
Synovectomy, 207
Synovial fluid, 195
Synovial membrane, 195
Syphilis, 252
System(s), 43
Systole, 142

T lymphocytes, 171
Tachycardia, 147
Tachypnea, 123
Talipes, 206
Target organs, 270, 271f
Target tissues, 270, 271f
Teeth, 86f, 87
Temporal lobe, 299f, 300
Tendons, 198
Testis(es), 224f, 225
Tetany, 279
Tetralogy of Fallot, 151

Thalamotomy, 308
Thalamus, 299f, 300
Thoracentesis, 128
Thoracic vertebrae, 193
Thoracocentesis, 128
Thorax, 194, 194f
Throat culture, 127
Thrombocyte(s), 164
Thrombolysis, 149, 153
Thrombophlebitis, 148–149
Thrombopoiesis, 164
Thrombosis, 146
Thrombus(i), 148, 151
Thymectomy, 284
Thyroid cancer, 281
Thyroid disorders, 278–279
Thyroid echogram, 283
Thyroid function test, 284
Thyroid gland
    anatomy and physiology of, 271, 274t
    hormones of, 274t
Thyroid storm, 282
Thyroidectomy
    partial, 284
    subtotal, 284
Thyroid-stimulation hormone (TSH),
        functions of, 273t
Thyrotropin, functions of, 273t
Thyroxine (T_4), functions of, 274t
Tinea, 74
Tinnitus, 325, 327
Tissue(s), 42
    types of, 42
Tissue plasminogen activators (TPAs),
        actions of, 154
TNM system of staging, 72t
Tomography, 307
Tongue, functions of, 86
Tonometer, 324
Tonometry, 328
Tonsils
    palatine, 116, 117f
    pharyngeal, 116, 117f
Total calcium, 284
Toxic goiter, 278
Trachea, 86f, 87, 117, 117f
Trachoma, 327
Traction, 207
Tractotomy, 308
Tranquilizers, actions of, 308
Transfusion, 181
    autologous, 181
    homologous, 181
Transient ischemic attack (TIA), 302, 306
Transplantation, 181
    bone marrow, 181
Trauma, head, closed, 304
Trephination, 308
Trichomoniasis, 253
Tricuspid valve, 140
Trigone, 222, 222f
Triiodothyronine (T_3), functions of, 274t
Trisomy 21, 255
True ribs, 194
Tubal ligation, 258

Tuberculin test, 127
Tuberculosis, 122
Tubule(s)
    collecting, 223f, 224
    distal, 223f, 224
    proximal convoluted, 223f, 224
    renal, 223–224, 223f
    seminiferous, 224f, 225
Tumor(s), 71
    pituitary, 281
    uterine, 253
    Wilms', 229
Tumor grading, 71t
Tumor staging, TNM, 72t
Tunica intima, 146, 146f
Tympanic cavity, 320
Tympanic membrane, 320
Tympanography, 328
Tympanoplasty, 329
Tympanorrhexis, 325
Tympanotomy, 325
Tympanum, 320

Ulcer(s), 70, 94
    decubitus, 73
    peptic, 94
    perforated, 94
Ulcerative colitis, 94
Ultrasonography, 48, 101, 230, 256
    endovaginal, 256
Umbilical cord, 144, 144f
Umbilical hernia, 95
Umbilical vein, 144, 144f
Unilateral myopia, 325
Uremia, 228
Ureter, 221f, 222, 222f
Ureteral opening, 222, 222f
Urethra, 222, 222f, 224f, 225
Urethral orifice (meatus), 224f, 225
Urethritis, 252
Urethrorrhaphy, 231
Urethroscopy, 230
Urethrotomy, 231
Urgency, 229
Uricosurics, actions of, 232
Urinalysis, 231
Urinary system
    anatomy and physiology of, 220–224,
        220f–223f
    diagnostic, symptomatic, and therapeutic
        terms related to, 228–229
Urine culture and sensitivity (C&S), 231
Urography, 230
Urolithiasis, 229
Urticaria, 75, 178f, 179
Uterine tumors, 253
Uterus, 245, 245f, 246, 246f
Uvula, 87

Vaccines, actions of, 182
Vagina, 245, 245f, 246, 246f
Vaginal atrophy, 248
Vaginal infections, 251

Vaginectomy, 257
Vaginismus, 254
Vaginitis, 251
Vagotomy, 308
Valvotomy, 148, 153
Varicocele, 229
Varicose veins, 148–149
Vas deferens, 224f, 225
Vascular system, anatomy and physiology of,
        138–140, 139f
Vasectomy, 231, 232f
    reversal of, 232f
Vasodilators, actions of, 154
Vasopressin, actions of, 285
Vegetations, 148
Vein(s), 139–140, 139f
    pulmonary
        left, 140
        right, 140
    saphenous, 147
    umbilical, 144, 144f
    varicose, 148–149
Vena cava
    inferior, 140, 144, 144f
    superior, 140
Venipuncture, 153
Venography, 151
Ventral cavity, 45, 45f, 46t
Ventricles, 300–301
    left, 140
    right, 140, 141f, 144, 144f
Verruca, 75
Vertebra(ae), cervical, 193
Vertebral column, 193–194, 193f
Vertigo, 327
Vesicles, 71
Vestibule, 320f, 321
Viable, 255
Viral hepatitis, 96
Virile, 282
Virilism, 282
Visceral pleura, 117, 117f
Viscus, 95
Visual acuity test, 328
Visual field, 327
Vitiligo, 75
Vitreous chamber, 318f, 319
Vitreous humor, 318f, 319
Volvulus, 95
von Recklinghausen's disease, 279

Wheeze, 126
White blood cells (leukocytes), 166–167,
        167t, 168f
Wilms' tumor, 229
Word roots, 2
    defined, 2
    examples of, 2

Xenograft, 75
Xeromammography, 75
Xeroradiography, 75
X-ray examination, 47